PET/CT and PET/MR in Melanoma and Sarcoma

Amir H. Khandani

Editor

PET/CT and PET/MR in Melanoma and Sarcoma

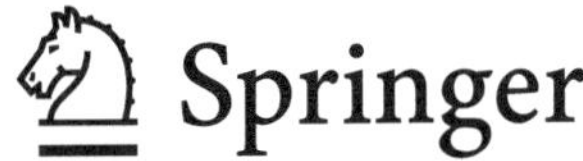

Editor
Amir H. Khandani
Department of Radiology, UNC School of Medicine
Division of Molecular Imaging and Therapeutics (Mit)
Chapel Hill, NC
USA

ISBN 978-3-030-60431-8   ISBN 978-3-030-60429-5   (eBook)
https://doi.org/10.1007/978-3-030-60429-5

This Springer imprint is published by the registered company Springer Nature Switzerland AG
The registered company address is: Gewerbestrasse 11, 6330 Cham, Switzerland

To my beautiful, talented and accomplished wife, Romina, for all her love and support. For taking a journey across continents to allow me to pursue my career.

To our daughters, Hannah and Sienna. Thank you for the endless joy and the love you bring to my life every day.

To my mother, Parvin, for enduring separation after I left home at a young age in search of a new life and a new future.

To my late father, Abbas, for his dedication to the education of his children.

To my uncle Mahmoud and my aunt Cornelia for giving me the opportunity for new possibilities.

To many mentors throughout my career for teaching me nuclear medicine and caring for the sick.

Preface

The purpose of this book is:

1. To serve as a comprehensive guide for imaging specialists for patient preparation as well as image acquisition and image interpretation in PET/CT and PET/MR in general and specifically as they relate to melanoma and sarcoma.
2. To illustrate for referring physicians the role of PET/CT and PET/MR in patient management in melanoma and sarcoma from the surgeon's and oncologist's point of view.
3. To cover biological and physical underpinning of PET with FDG and other novel radiotracer with reference to melanoma and sarcoma and in general.
4. For a large portion of the target audience in countries where PET is an emerging technology, this book should serve as a primer for PET/CT and PET/MR in general beyond melanoma and sarcomas.

Chapel Hill, NC, USA   Amir H. Khandani

Contents

Contributors

Adeet Amin, MD UTHealth Department of Orthopaedics, McGovern School of Medicine, Houston, TX, USA

Ea-sle Chang, MD Department of Surgery, St. Louis University, St. Louis, MO, USA

Ernest U. Conrad III, MD FACS UTHealth Department of Orthopaedics, McGovern School of Medicine, Houston, TX, USA

Ian J. Davis, MD, PhD Department of Pediatrics, University of North Carolina School of Medicine, Chapel Hill, NC, USA

Lineberger Comprehensive Cancer Center, University of North Carolina School of Medicine, Chapel Hill, NC, USA

Farrokh Dehdashti, MD Edward Mallinckrodt Institute of Radiology, Washington University in St. Louis, St. Louis, MO, USA

Janet F. Eary, MD National Institutes of Health/NCI/DCTD, Bethesda, MD, USA

Stuart H. Gold, MD Department of Pediatrics, University of North Carolina School of Medicine, Chapel Hill, NC, USA

Lineberger Comprehensive Cancer Center, University of North Carolina School of Medicine, Chapel Hill, NC, USA

Brett L. Hayden, MD UTHealth Department of Orthopaedics, McGovern School of Medicine, Houston, TX, USA

Eddy C. Hsueh, MD Department of Surgery, St. Louis University, St. Louis, MO, USA

Marija Ivanovic, PhD Department of Radiology, Division of Molecular Imaging and Therapeutics, University of North Carolina, Chapel Hill School of Medicine, Chapel Hill, NC, USA

Amir H. Khandani, MD Department of Radiology, Division of Molecular Imaging and Therapeutics, University of North Carolina, Chapel Hill School of Medicine, Chapel Hill, NC, USA

Stephen M. Moerlein, PharmD, PhD Edward Mallinckrodt Institute of Radiology, Washington University in St. Louis, St. Louis, MO, USA

Mitchel Muhleman, MD Department of Radiology, Division of Molecular Imaging and Therapeutics, University of North Carolina, Chapel Hill School of Medicine, Chapel Hill, NC, USA

Jorge Daniel Oldan, MD Department of Radiology, Division of Molecular Imaging and Therapeutics, University of North Carolina, Chapel Hill School of Medicine, Chapel Hill, NC, USA

David W. Ollila, MD Department of Surgery, Division of Surgical Oncology, University of North Carolina at Chapel Hill, Chapel Hill, NC, USA

Sally W. Schwarz, RPh, MS Edward Mallinckrodt Institute of Radiology, Washington University in St. Louis, St. Louis, MO, USA

Arif Sheikh, MD Icahn School of Medicine, The Mount Sinai Hospital, New York, NY, USA

Andrew B. Smitherman, MD MSc Department of Pediatrics, University of North Carolina School of Medicine, Chapel Hill, NC, USA

Lineberger Comprehensive Cancer Center, University of North Carolina School of Medicine, Chapel Hill, NC, USA

Eric Wolsztynski, PhD Insight Centre for Data Analytics, School of Mathematical Sciences, University College Cork, Cork, Ireland

What Is Positron Emission Tomography?

Jorge Daniel Oldan, Marija Ivanovic, and Amir H. Khandani

Introduction: What Is Positron Emission Tomography?

While other modalities such as computed tomography (CT) and magnetic resonance imaging (MRI or MR) have excellent spatial resolution and soft tissue contrast, they may still fail to detect smaller metastases. In addition, response to treatment is usually assessed by observing a decrease in tumor size, which can take weeks to months to manifest.

Nuclear medicine is the only clinical discipline to use intracellular contrast agents in imaging and therefore can detect certain disease processes where other anatomic modalities may not. The best-known is radioiodine for diagnosis (and treatment) of thyroid cancer. However, problems persist with low specificity (since a variety of biological processes can produce any given change in tracer distribution) and spatial resolution of many nuclear imaging systems.

Nuclear medicine involves the use of a radiotracer, where a radioactive atom (the radionuclide) is bound to a pharmaceutical (the tracer) to produce a radiotracer. The pharmaceutical determines the biological activity, and the radionuclide allows for visualization. Two radiopharmaceuticals with the same radionuclide but different radiopharmaceuticals will behave completely differently, whereas two radiopharmaceuticals with the same pharmaceutical but different radionuclides will differ primarily in imaging and physical parameters such as tracer half-life, the number of photons emitted per second, and the energy of the photon, which can have a significant effect on the what is seen on the images. Examples are 123-MIBG and 131-MIBG [1].

Positron emission tomography (PET) is a particular modality of nuclear medicine (the others being single-photon emission tomography, or SPECT, and planar gamma imaging) where the radionuclide is a positron emitter, most commonly fluorine-18 [1]. Other commonly used radionuclides are gallium-68, nitrogen-13, and rubidium-82. PET became clinically useful in the past few decades with the advent of 18F-fluorodeoxyglucose (FDG), an analog of glucose, which has greatly improved diagnosis, staging, and restaging in oncology. Non-oncologic applications exist as well; it can also be used in neurology to find seizure foci and infectious diseases to find foci of occult infection. Rubidium-82 and nitrogen-13 ammonia have applications in myocardial perfusion imaging, and there are a variety of tracers for evaluating

J. D. Oldan (✉) · M. Ivanovic · A. H. Khandani
Department of Radiology, Division of Molecular
Imaging and Therapeutics, University of North
Carolina, Chapel Hill School of Medicine,
Chapel Hill, NC, USA
e-mail: jorge_oldan@med.unc.edu;
Marija.Ivanovic@unchealth.unc.edu;
khandani@med.unc.edu

© Springer Nature Switzerland AG 2021
A. H. Khandani (ed.), *PET/CT and PET/MR in Melanoma and Sarcoma*,
https://doi.org/10.1007/978-3-030-60429-5_1

amyloid plaques (and one recently approved tracer for tau protein) in dementia.

Recently, other tracers such as 18F-FES for estrogen-receptor positive cancers (including breast and endometrial), 18F-FACBC for prostate cancer (with other prostate cancer tracers in the pipeline), Ga68-DOTATATE and DOTATOC for neuroendocrine tumors, and 18F-sodium fluoride for bone metastases have been approved [2]. However, as of yet, there are no dedicated melanoma or sarcoma tracers, and generally FDG is the only tracer that is used for melanoma or sarcoma.

PET has four main applications in oncology: diagnosing cancer, such assessing solitary pulmonary nodule for malignancy; staging, or determining where in the body a cancer has spread; response assessment, or determining whether a tumor has responded to therapy and, if so, how much; and surveillance and restaging, or determining if a cancer has returned and, if so, and how widespread is the recurrence. Additionally, in particular in sarcoma, it may be used to assess the most malignant portion of a lesion in order to guide biopsy.

Physics of PET

When a radionuclide used in PET decays, it does so by emitting a positron, or positively charged antimatter electron (Fig. 1.1). After travelling a few millimeters in tissue, it collides with a normal electron and, being antimatter, annihilates the entire mass of both itself and the electron, which is changed into two photons with energy of 511 keV each travelling 180 degrees apart. The PET scanner is a ring or ring of detectors positioned around the patient which can detect these photons and verify that they reached the detector at the same time (or times within a specified timing window in the case of time-of-flight scanners); this is known as coincidence detection (Fig. 1.2), which allows the placement of the originating photon along a line of response (Fig. 1.3). Coincidence detection allows a higher

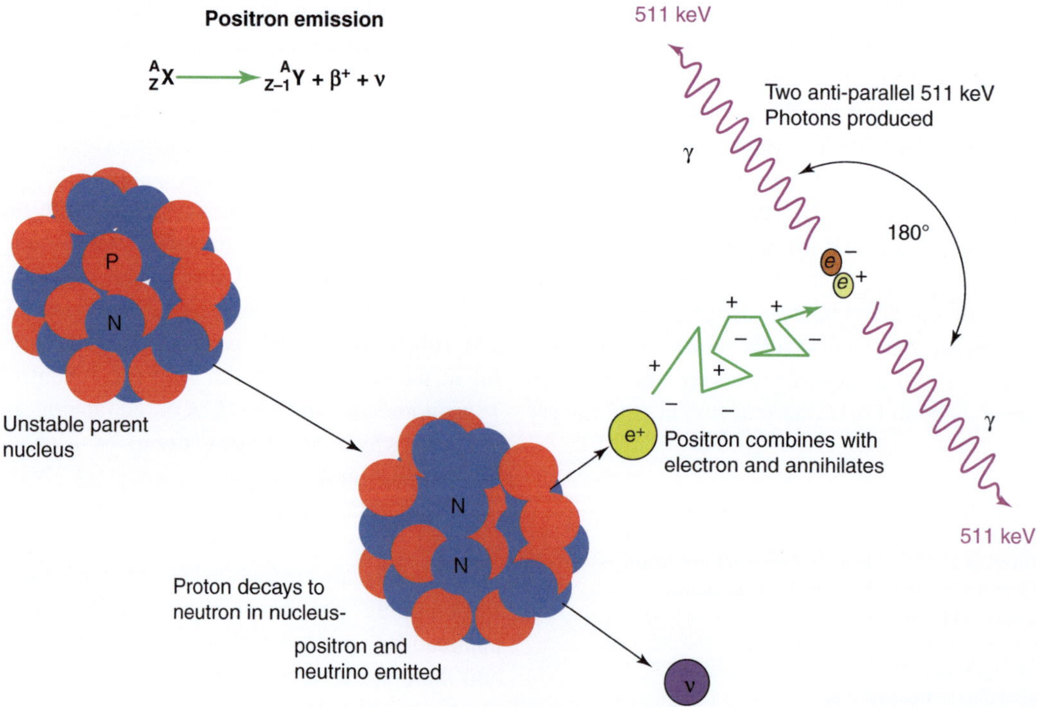

Fig. 1.1 Positron emission and annihilation

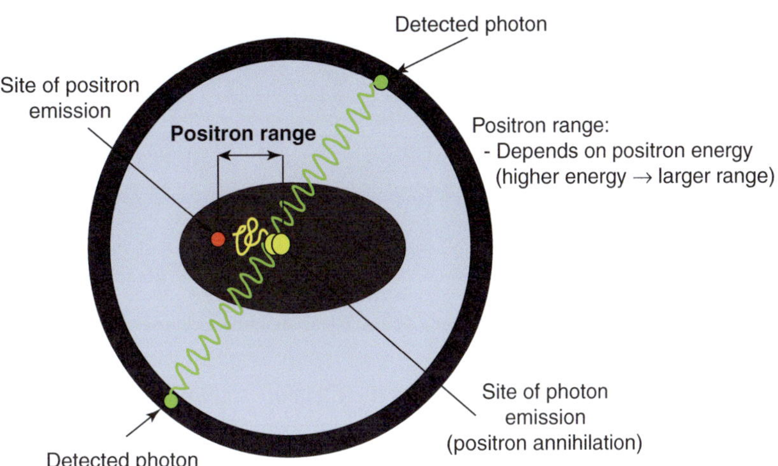

Fig. 1.2 Photon emission and detection

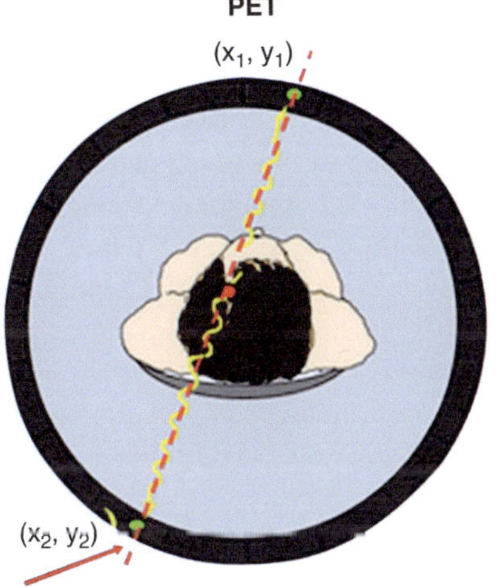

Coordinates of a two simultaneously detected photons determine the line of photon emission (line of response-LOR)

Fig. 1.3 Line of response reconstruction

resolution relative to SPECT and planar gamma imaging and, with attenuation correction as described below, allows for quantitative measurement of uptake in a given volume [3]. Some scanners (those with rapid scintillation crystals and the appropriate software) allow for time-of-flight (TOF) imaging, which uses very precise (picosecond-level) timing of the arrival of the photons to help further localize the origin of the arriving photons.

As the photons move through the body, they are absorbed, or attenuated. This causes underestimation of radioactivity in the center of the body. There is also apparent overestimation of radioactivity at the surface of the body (as well as in low-attenuation structures like the lungs). This is corrected for in the modern era using a CT scan; CT data provide the information on the tissue type and density which is needed for PET attenuation correction. In addition, of course, a CT is a diagnostic imaging scan that can also be useful, both for localizing areas of radioactivity within the body and as a diagnostic scan in its own right [3]. While the CT was initially done without contrast and used solely for anatomic localization and attenuation correction, the CT is now sometimes done as a full diagnostic scan with oral and intravenous contrast. The CT can usually be done within a few seconds, whereas PET acquisition time will usually be a few minutes per bed position for a total time of 20–25 minutes for a whole-body melanoma scan. Fused PET/CT images can be produced that show both anatomic and physiologic information, with the PET displayed as a colored "ghost" over the CT (Fig. 1.4).

Of course, if the patient moves (voluntarily or involuntarily such as breathing motion) between the PET and CT scans, lesions will be mislocalized and interpreting physicians must be careful interpreting areas of high motion such as the chest and abdomen near the diaphragm, as well as any

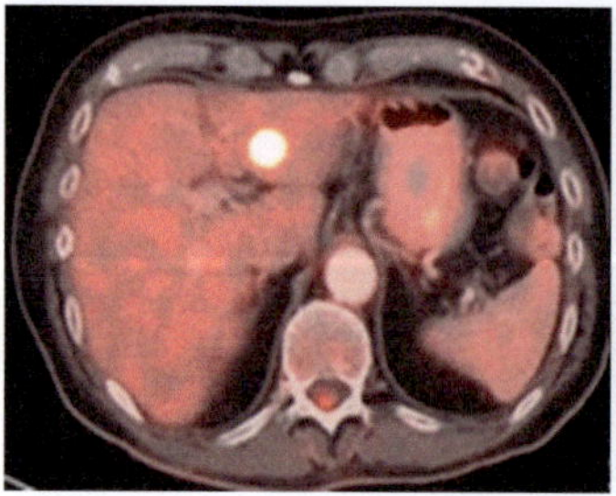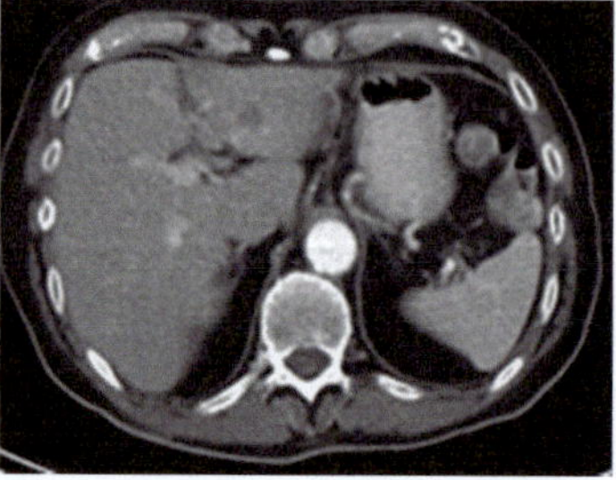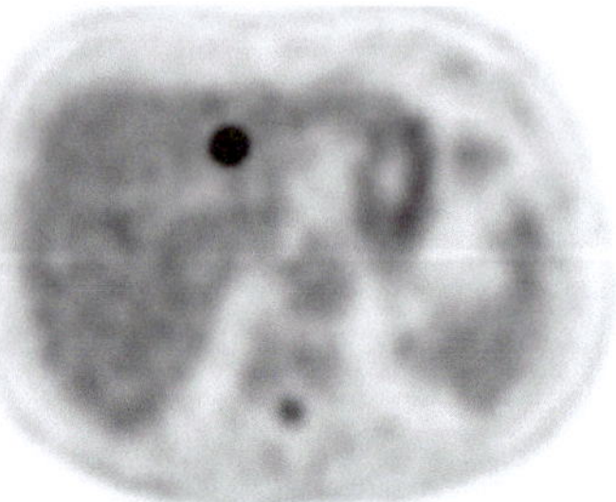

Fig. 1.4 Fused image (left), with component CT (middle) and PET (right) images

location where image fusions suggest the CT and PET do not coincide. In such cases reference to the non-attenuation-corrected images is useful. Additionally, breathing motion causes "smearing" and decrease in registered signal on PET.

Seeing Tumors on PET

As previously discussed, the most commonly used tracer in clinical PET imaging is FDG, or 2-[18f]-fluoro-2-deoxy-D-glucose. FDG is similar enough to glucose to be taken up by glucose transporters and phosphorylated to FDG-6-phosphate. However, both cancer cells and normal cells are unable to further break down FDG-6-phosphate due to the replacement of a hydroxyl group with a fluorine atom, and it is trapped there. In addition, cancers disproportionately consume glucose due to a breakdown in aerobic metabolism (known as the Warburg effect) and tend to have lower expression of an enzyme known as glucose-6-phosphatase which can dephosphorylate the molecule and allow it to leave the cell. Together, these factors increase the accumulation of FDG in cancer cells and allow us to visualize them on PET [1].

Intensity of a malignant tumor is correlated with a number of factors. The number of malignant cells in the tumor mass is the most important factor; thus sparse tumors such as invasive lobular breast carcinoma or tumors that produce a noncellular substance such as mucinous tumors will be less avid. The overall anaerobic metabolic activity (in terms of glucose consumption) is also relevant, with more aggressive tumors generally being more FDG-avid. In addition, most effective therapies will decrease the number or metabolic activity of malignant cells or both, decreasing the amount of FDG uptake. This allows monitoring of response to therapy by PET much more closely than with CT or MR as the metabolic signal decreases much faster after effective therapy than size. One cannot exclude that microscopic disease, undetectable by PET, might remain in tumor. The likelihood of this to happen depends on the type tumor (e.g., lymphoma vs lung cancer) and its overall prognosis. In such cases, a short-tem (e.g., 6 weeks) follow-up PET would be beneficial to capture any regrowth of cancer cells in an early stage.

It is worth noting that white blood cells and fibroblasts are also highly FDG-avid, causing uptake in benign processes such as infection and inflammation (Fig. 1.5). The best way to avoid false positives is to look at the pattern of uptake (focal mostly indication cancer vs diffuse or linear mostly indicating inflammation) and to obtain the medical history and determine any history of infectious or inflammatory processes. We often tell referring clinicians to defer obtaining PET scans on patients with active infection until such infection has resolved (where possible), unless the indication is to look for infection. Unfortunately, there is no consensus on how long to wait after chemotherapy, surgery, or radiation to significantly decrease the risk of a false positive [4].

A possible cause of false negatives is physiologic FDG uptake by muscle (Fig. 1.6), drawing off glucose from the tumor. The most common causes of physiologic muscle uptake are due to exercise or insulin secretion, either

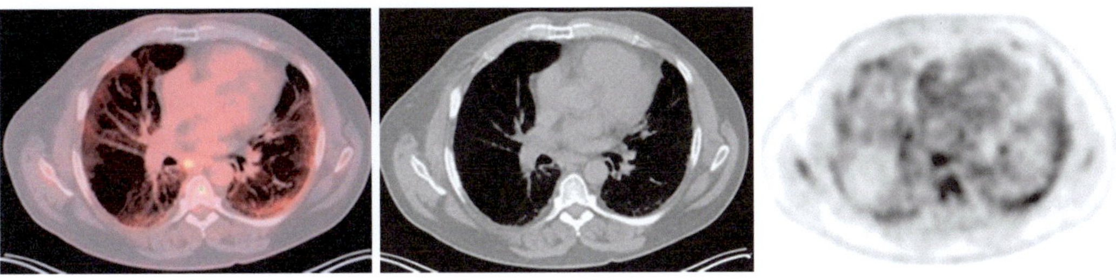

Fig. 1.5 Lung uptake on fused images (left), CT (middle), and PET (right) showing the correspondence of uptake to areas of active inflammation

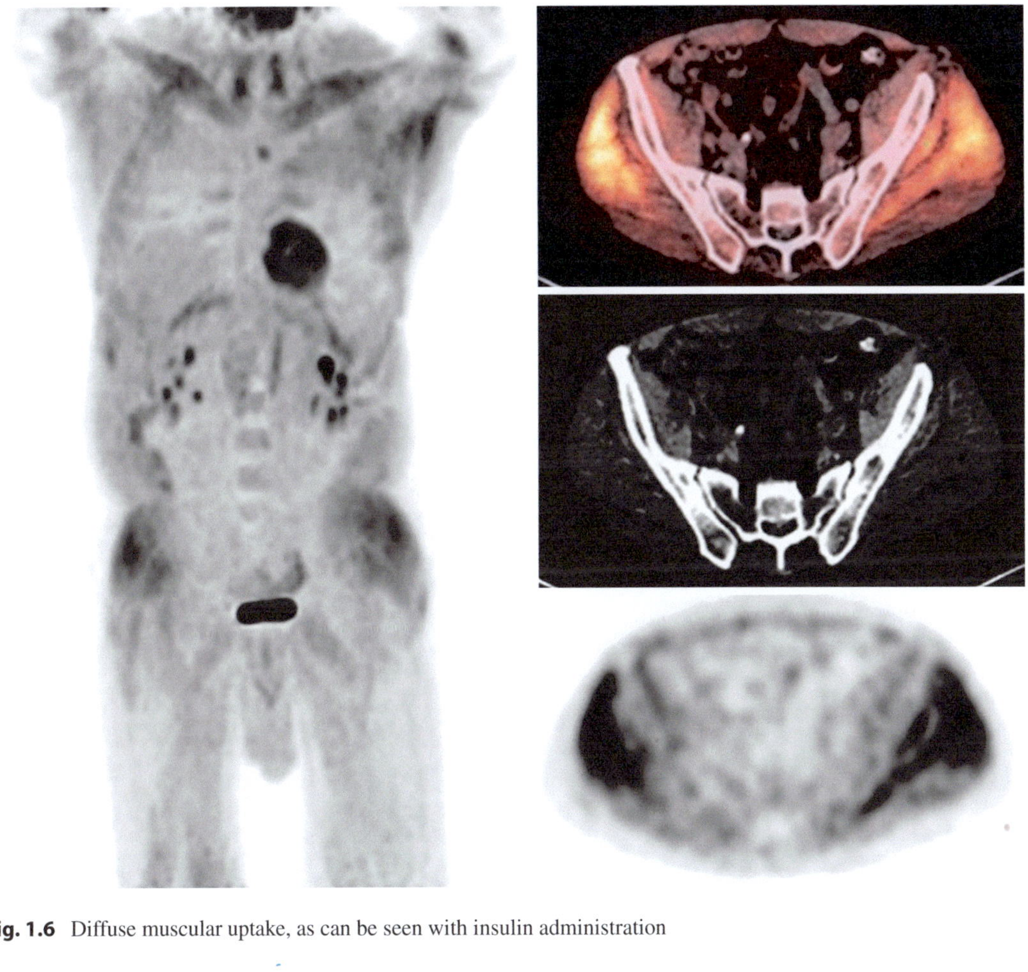

Fig. 1.6 Diffuse muscular uptake, as can be seen with insulin administration

exogenous or physiologic from food consumption. As a result, patients are instructed to avoid excessive physical activity for 24 hours before their appointment and fast (including glucose-containing drinks and intravenous glucose) for at least 4–6 hours beforehand as well. In addition, fasting lowers the serum glucose level to decrease competition for glucose uptake sites in the tumor. For similar reasons, high glucose levels in diabetics (above about 200–250 mg/dL) may decrease sensitivity, and institutions will usually try to wait to perform PET until diabetes is sufficiently controlled. Of course, this may not be possible in all cases, and in such situations image quality should be assessed and discussed in the report if necessary [2].

Brown fat may be present in the neck and supraclavicular regions (as well as in the posterior mediastinum and upper abdomen less frequently), particularly in younger patients and women and on unusually cold days (Fig. 1.7), and is often intensely avid and can obscure pathology in these areas. Use of benzodiazepines before the examination can reduce uptake, and warm blankets can be used as well. In general, it is preferable to have uptake rooms as warm as possible [2].

Finally, attempts have been made to create a quantitative analog to the Hounsfield unit for CT in the form of the SUV, or standardized uptake value. It is a unitless, semiquantitative measure of tracer uptake in a region of interest, normalized to injected dose and body weight. (Technically, it is counts × weight/dose.) As the SUV is a number with a different value at each point in space resolvable by the scan, some summary statistic is necessary. The most commonly used is the SUVmax, the *most intense* pixel in the tumor. SUVmax is less dependent on reader and region

of interest (ROI) because the most intense pixel is almost always agreed upon by different observers. On the other hand, SUVmean, the average of SUVs of pixels in a defined volume, is very much dependent on the size and contour of ROI. With other words, SUVmax is much more reproducible than SUVmean, although it tends to underestimate the signal intensity due to small size of a single pixel. Other metrics include the SUVpeak, the average of the SUVs in a sphere with a diameter of 1 cm centered around the most intense area [5].

These parameters generally cannot differentiate malignant from benign tumors and are influenced by additional factors such as uptake time, body weight, blood glucose, and technical factors affecting image quality such as scanner resolution and image reconstruction algorithm. However, they can be useful in research studies to compare subjects and in clinical settings to assess response to therapy [6, 7] (assuming factors such as scanner type and uptake time can be controlled for). An association of SUVmax with prognosis (higher SUVmax has worse prognosis, likely reflecting a more aggressive tumor) has

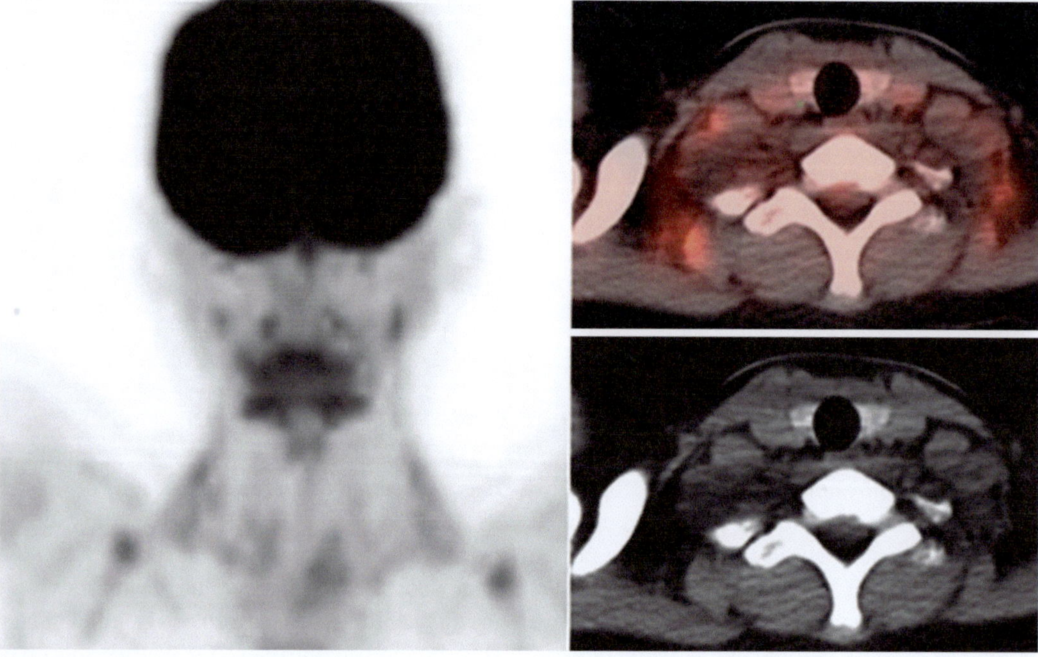

Fig. 1.7 Maximum intensity projection (left), fused (right-top), and CT (right-bottom) images of brown fat

been demonstrated across multiple tumor types and settings. In melanoma, a higher SUVmax correlates with risk of recurrence and poorer survival [8, 9], although other parameters such as MTV (metabolic tumor volume, the total amount of metabolically active tumor) and TLG (total lesion glycolysis, the SUV integrated over the MTV) may be more useful [10]. In sarcoma as well, a higher SUVmax correlates with more dedifferentiated tumors [4] and poorer survival [11, 12], although again MTV and TLG may be more useful [13].

References

1. Mettler FA, Guiberteau MJ. Radioactivity, radionuclides, and radiopharmaceuticals. In: Essentials of nuclear medicine. 7th ed. Philadelphia: Elsevier; 2019. p. 1–18.
2. Mettler FA, Guiberteau MJ. Hybrid PET/CT neoplasm imaging. In: Essentials of nuclear medicine. Philadelphia: Elsevier; 2019. p. 328–61.
3. Mettler FA, Guiberteau MJ. Instrumentation and quality control. In: Essentials of nuclear medicine. 7th ed. Philadelphia: Elsevier; 2019. p. 19–59.
4. Macpherson RE, Pratap S, Tyrrell H, Khonsari M, Wilson S, Gibbons M, et al. Retrospective audit of 957 consecutive (18)F-FDG PET-CT scans compared to CT and MRI in 493 patients with different histological subtypes of bone and soft tissue sarcoma. Clin Sarcoma Res. 2018;8:9.
5. Burger IA, Huser DM, Burger C, von Schulthess GK, Buck A. Repeatability of FDG quantification in tumor imaging: averaged SUVs are superior to SUVmax. Nucl Med Biol. 2012;39(5):666–70.
6. Schmitt RJ, Kreidler SM, Glueck DH, Amaria RN, Gonzalez R, Lewis K, et al. Correlation between early 18F-FDG PET/CT response to BRAF and MEK inhibition and survival in patients with BRAF-mutant metastatic melanoma. Nucl Med Commun. 2016;37(2):122–8.
7. Zukotynski K, Yap JT, Giobbie-Hurder A, Weber J, Gonzalez R, Gajewski TF, et al. Metabolic response by FDG-PET to imatinib correlates with exon 11 KIT mutation and predicts outcome in patients with mucosal melanoma. Cancer Imaging. 2014;14:30.
8. Malik D, Sood A, Mittal BR, Basher RK, Bhattacharya A, Singh G. Role of (18)F-fluorodeoxyglucose positron emission tomography/computed tomography in restaging and prognosis of recurrent melanoma after curative surgery. World J Nucl Med. 2019;18(2):176–82.
9. Kang S, Ahn BC, Hong CM, Song BI, Lee HJ, Jeong SY, et al. Can (18)F-FDG PET/CT predict recurrence in patients with cutaneous malignant melanoma? Nuklearmedizin. 2011;50(3):116–21.
10. Son SH, Kang SM, Jeong SY, Lee SW, Lee SJ, Lee J, et al. Prognostic value of volumetric parameters measured by pretreatment 18F FDG PET/CT in patients with cutaneous malignant melanoma. Clin Nucl Med. 2016;41(6):e266–73.
11. Hwang JP, Lim I, Kong CB, Jeon DG, Byun BH, Kim BI, et al. Prognostic value of SUVmax measured by pretreatment Fluorine-18 fluorodeoxyglucose positron emission tomography/computed tomography in patients with Ewing sarcoma. PLoS One. 2016;11(4):e0153281.
12. Kubo T, Furuta T, Johan MP, Ochi M. Prognostic significance of (18)F-FDG PET at diagnosis in patients with soft tissue sarcoma and bone sarcoma; systematic review and meta-analysis. Eur J Cancer. 2016;58:104–11.
13. Chen L, Wu X, Ma X, Guo L, Zhu C, Li Q. Prognostic value of 18F-FDG PET-CT-based functional parameters in patients with soft tissue sarcoma: a meta-analysis. Medicine (Baltimore). 2017;96(6):e5913.

Patient Preparation for FDG PET with an Emphasis on Soft Tissue Sarcoma and Melanoma: What Matters (and What Doesn't)

Mitchel Muhleman and Amir H. Khandani

Biological Background and Mechanism of F-18 FDG PET/CT

The purpose of functional imaging is to assess certain systems or functions of the body in the most unaltered state as possible. As such, in the evaluation of malignancy or potential malignancy with PET/CT, patient preparation is extremely important when assessing metabolic status with fluorine-18 fluorodeoxy-glucose (F-18 FDG or FDG). For many malignant cells, although not all and not all to the same degree, there is a higher level of metabolic activity compared to the normal surrounding tissue. This increase in metabolic activity increases the need for glucose. This was first studied by Warburg, who examined carbohydrate metabolism in rapidly growing dedifferentiated tumors and demonstrated that there was an increase in aerobic glycolysis and a decrease in cellular respiration. In his study, he used the example of normal liver cells compared to a hepatoma and proposed that a neoplastic change occurred when there was damage to the cellular respiration process, causing the cell to respond with an increase in its aerobic glycoly-

sis to maintain normal ATP production (Fig. 2.1). This concept has since been named the Warburg effect [1, 2]. With an increase in metabolic demand for rapid growth, the tumor cells adapt to increase the efficiency of the metabolic pathway. These adaptations include an increase in the number of glucose membrane transporters (GLUTs), increased activity of hexokinase II (HX II), and a decreased level of glucose-6-phosphatase (G-6-P). These adaptations facilitate tumor growth by (a) increasing the amount of glucose entering into the cell through GLUT, (b) increasing the rate of phosphorylation by HX II to have glucose in the cell available for metabolism, and (c) decreasing the rate of dephosphorylating due to very low level of G-6-P that results in a decrease in the rate, if not the cessation, of the diffusion of G-6-P out of the cell (Fig. 2.2a and b).

The ability of PET/CT to evaluate the status of the metabolic activity of a cell is due to the use of the glucose analog fluorine-18 fluorodeoxy-glucose (FDG). F-18 FDG is taken into cells and phosphorylated by the same mechanism as natural glucose. To extract glucose from the blood circulation, cells use three independent mechanisms which include (1) diffusion; (2) protein-mediated, bidirectional, facilitated diffusion; and (3) active, protein-mediated transport [3]. The cell uses predominantly two families of glucose transporters: the GLUTs, which are the major glucose facilitators, and to a lesser degree sodium-driven glucose symporters (SGLT) to

M. Muhleman (✉) · A. H. Khandani
Department of Radiology, Division of Molecular Imaging and Therapeutics, University of North Carolina, Chapel Hill School of Medicine, Chapel Hill, NC, USA
e-mail: mitchel_muhleman@med.unc.edu; khandani@med.unc.edu

© Springer Nature Switzerland AG 2021
A. H. Khandani (ed.), *PET/CT and PET/MR in Melanoma and Sarcoma*,
https://doi.org/10.1007/978-3-030-60429-5_2

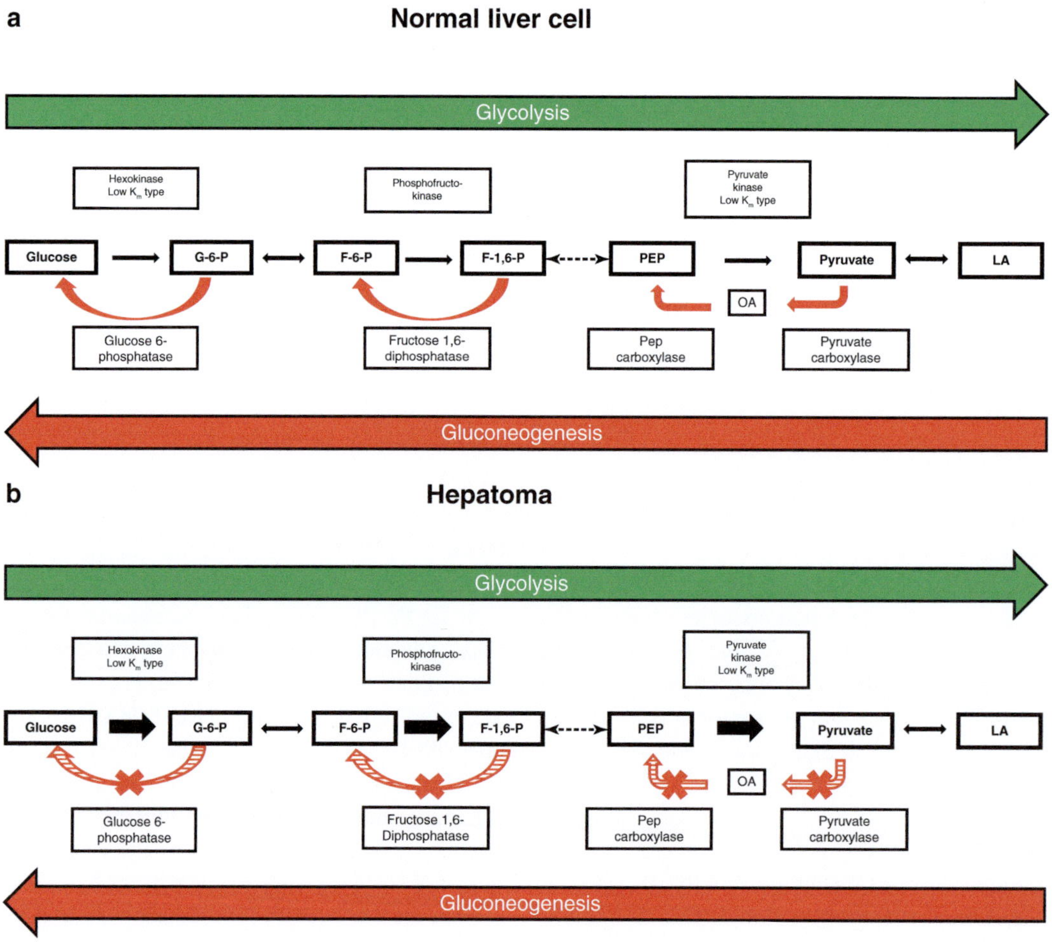

a **Normal liver cell**

b **Hepatoma**

Fig. 2.1 Illustration of carbohydrate metabolism in a normal liver cell (**a**) compared to that of a hepatoma (**b**). Abbreviations: G-6-P glucose-6-phosphate, F-6-P fructose-6-phosphate, F-1,6-P fructose-1,6-phosphate, PEP phosphoenolpyruvic acid, OA oxaloacetate, and LA lactic acid

actively transport glucose into the cells [4]. The major glucose transporter family, the GLUTs, are comprised of 14 isoforms, although GULT-1 to GLUT-7 and GLUT-10 to GLUT-12 are the major transporters responsible for the active transport of F-18 FDG into the cells [4, 5]. Once F-18 FDG enters the cell, it is immediately phosphorylated by the hexokinase isozymes (HX I to IV). The phosphorylation creates F-18 FDG-6-phosphate (F-18 FDG-6-P), which is unable to diffuse out of the cell and awaits the next step in the gly-colysis pathway. In tumor cells the GLUT-1 and HX II subtypes are the most important. However, unlike natural d-glucose, once F-18 FDG is phos-phorylated into F-18 FDG-6-P, it is unable to

continue through the pathway. F-18 FDG-6-P is not a substrate in the glycolysis pathway – this is because the next step in the pathway requires an oxygen atom at the C-2 position, which is miss-ing in F-18 FDG-6-P [5]. Inside the cell there is an alternative pathway to glycolysis where the G-6-P/F-18 FDG-6-P can diffuse out of the cell. As mentioned previously, this pathway uses the enzyme glucose-6-phosphatase (G-6-P), which causes dephosphorylation of glucose-6-phosphate/F-18 FDG-6-P, allowing diffusion of glucose/F-18 FDG out of the cell. Certain cells in the body have an increased level of this enzyme naturally (i.e., liver and bowel), and thus there can be a lower concentration of F-18 FDG in

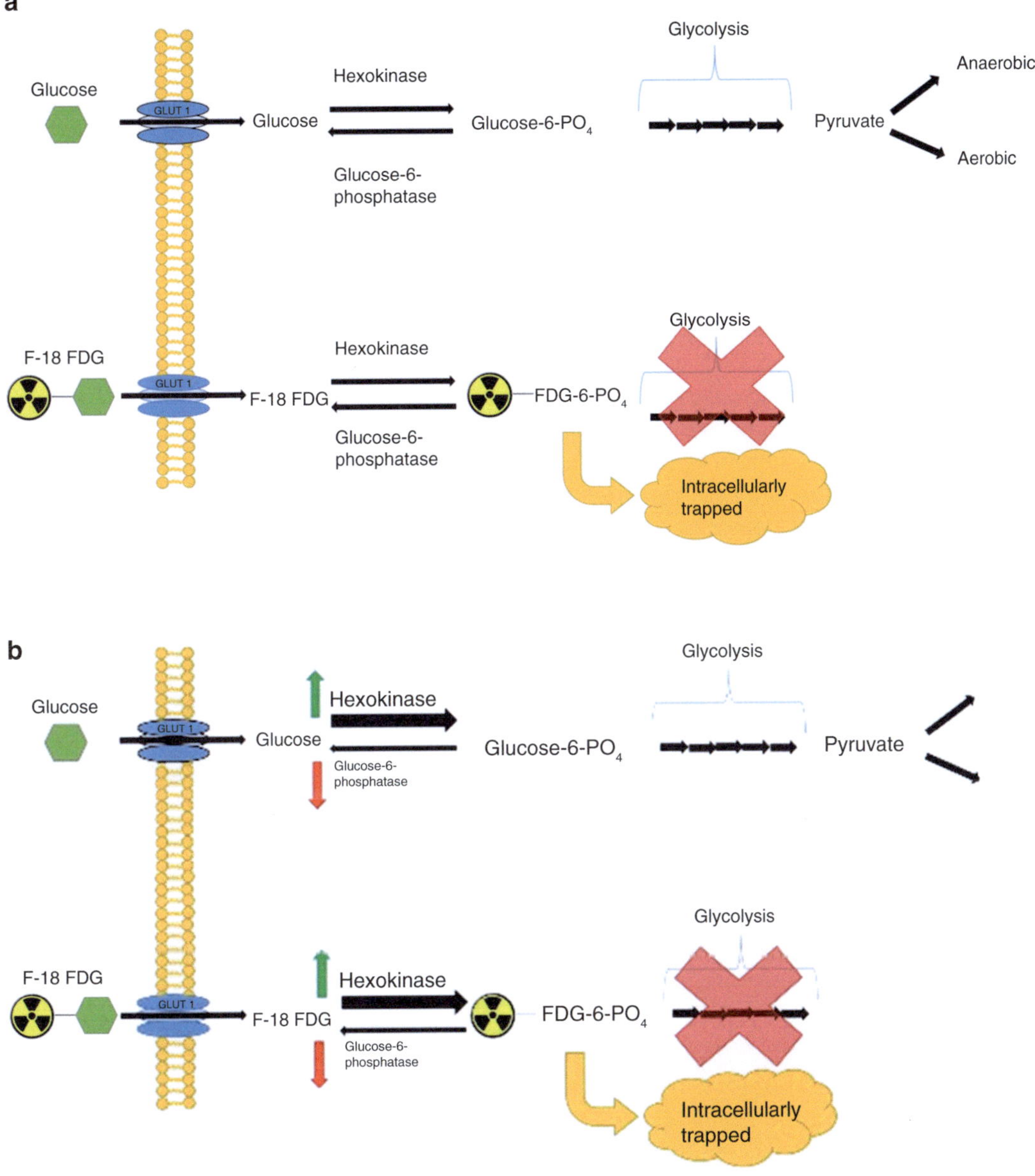

Fig. 2.2 (**a**) Normal cell and (**b**) cancer cell. Normal D-glucose and F-18 fluorodeoxy-glucose (F-18 FDG) import and trapping in normal and malignant cells

these cells. Other tissues in the body have a lower level of this enzyme (i.e., the brain and heart), and so there is higher concentration of F-18 FDG in these tissues [5]. Like the brain and heart, there are decreased levels of G-6-P in most malignant cells, which decreases the diffusion of F-18 FDG out of the cell and increases the intracellular concentration.

Following intravenous injection of F-18 FDG, the molecule is rapidly distributed throughout the body. The background activity, from circulating F-18 FDG, decreases as cellular uptake and excretion occurs. The main route of excretion of F-18 FDG is through the kidneys. Approximately 75% of the injected dose of F-18 FDG is still in circulation throughout the body 2 h after injection where it undergoes beta+ radioactive decay, with a physical half-life of almost 110 min [6]. Beta+ decay occurs in proton-rich elements that have a minimum excess energy of 1.011 MeV, which convert a proton into a neutron and a positively charged electron. The positively charged electron is ejected and collides with a negatively charged electron to produce two 511 keV gamma photons, which are emitted at an angle of approximately 180 degree and are detected by the detectors assembled in a ring in the PET scanner. This beta+ decay by the fluorine-18 element to an oxygen-18 element transforms the molecule from a fluorine-18 glucose-6-phosphate to oxygen-18 glucose-6-phosphate. This new molecule is now able to be metabolized through glycolysis like an ordinary molecule of glucose to produce non-radioactive end-products [7, 8]. The retained F-18 FDG is cleared from non-cardiac tissues within 3–24 h post injection, while clearance from cardiac tissue may take up to 96 h [9].

The main excretion pathway of F-18 FDG is through the renal system and, to a much less extent, the bowel. Within approximately 33 min after injection, 3.9% of the injected activity is cleared by the kidneys and within 2 h 20.6% is cleared [9]. These account for the biological half-life, approximately 16 min, which is much shorter than the physical half-life of 110 min. The significantly shorter biological half-life goes along with the structural difference between F-18 FDG and natural glucose. This structural difference is the reason why F-18 FDG is not reabsorbed by the proximal tubules to be retained by the kidneys, in contrast to natural glucose [10]. The retention of natural glucose by the kidneys is a normal mechanism to keep a baseline concentration of glucose in the circulating blood and low levels of glucose in the urine. There is also a small amount of F-18 in the urine that is no longer attached to the FDG [6].

The distribution of F-18 FDG is grossly reflective of the glucose distribution and metabolism in the various organs and systems of the body. One organ that normally shows a significantly high concentration of F-18 FDG is the brain, largely because it is an obligate glucose user. The urinary system is another organ system (kidneys, ureters, bladder, and sometimes the urethra) that shows increased FDG presence, primarily due to the renal system being the main route of clearance. In the liver there is moderate and occasionally heterogeneous uptake – this is due to the high level of glucose-6-phosphatase, which allows F-18 FDG to diffuse out of the tissue (Fig. 2.3). Other organ systems show variable uptake activity, such as the heart, gastrointestinal tract, salivary glands, and testes (Fig. 2.4). The uterus can show increased uptake in the endometrium, which can be normal in age-appropriate patients due to the phase of the ovulatory and menstrual cycles. Diffuse low uptake throughout the bone marrow is common and expected. Bone marrow uptake can be increased when it is in a reactive state, such as in anemia or reacting to chemotherapy treatment. The percentage of the injected dose of F-18 FDG to these organ systems is approximately as follows: urine 20–40%, brain 7%, liver 4.5%, heart 3.3%, bone marrow 1.7%, kidneys 1.3%, and lungs 0.9% [11, 12].

Patient Preparation

There are many factors that can affect F-18 FDG distribution, uptake, and clearance from the body. These factors include, but are not limited to, diet, medications, hydration, physical activity, and uptake time. When developing a protocol for conducting PET, PET/CT, or PET/MR studies with FDG, these factors, alone or in combination, will affect the performance of FDG. There are multiple societies that have developed guidelines for performing PET, PET/CT, and PET/MRIs, which include the Society of Nuclear Medicine and Molecular Imaging (SNMMI), the European Association of Nuclear Medicine (EANM), the American College of Radiology (ACR), the National Cancer Institute (NCI), and the Netherlands Society of Nuclear Medicine. The guidelines from these societies attempt to set

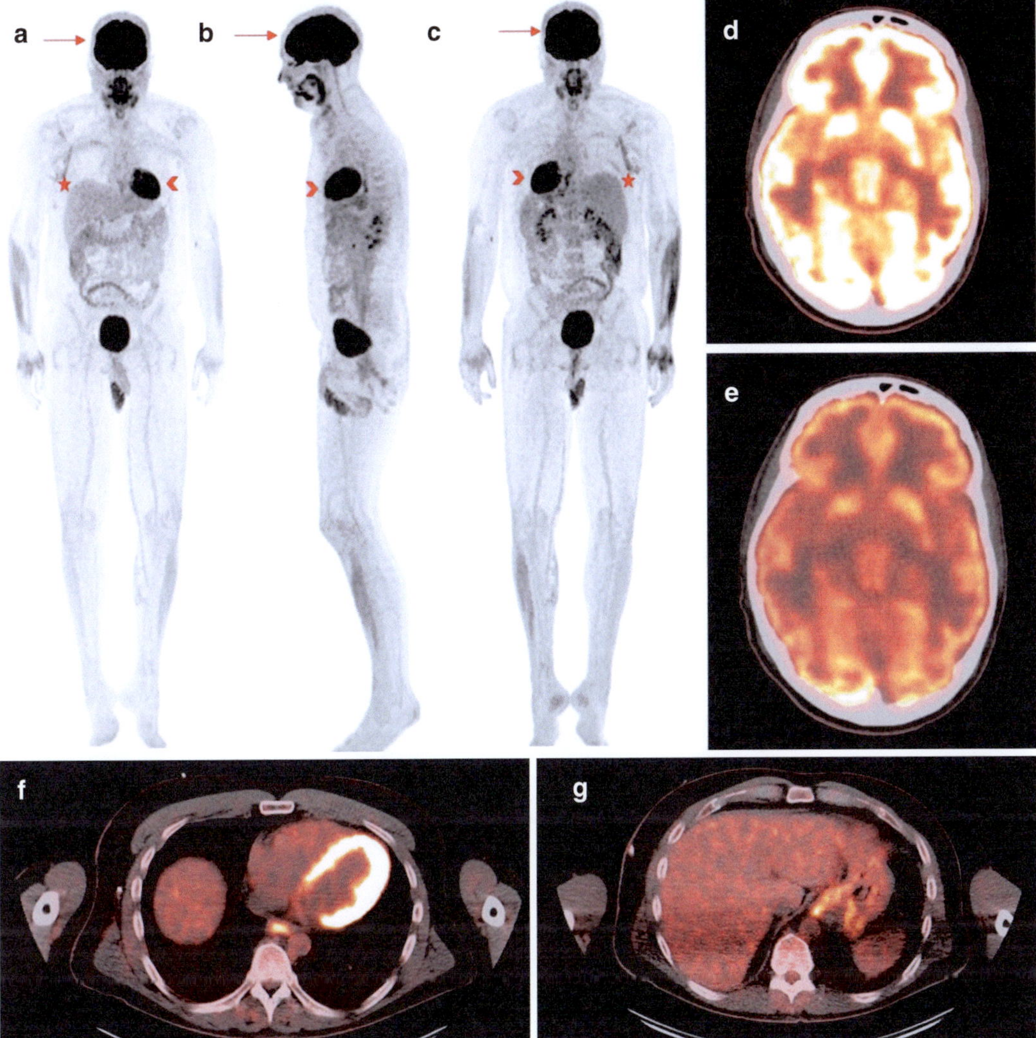

Fig. 2.3 Example of a normal F-18 FDG PET/CT showing a normal biodistribution of F-18 FDG. (**a–c**) MIP images in anterior, left lateral, and posterior views showing normal intense uptake in the brain (arrow) and heart (arrowhead). Heterogeneous FDG uptake in the liver and spleen (star). There is also normal increased activity in the kidneys and bladder due to normal excretion. (**d–e**) Intense activity in the brain at a normal intensity setting and a decrease in the intensity level showing normal increased activity in the gray matter. (**f**) Intense FDG activity in the myocardium of the right and left ventricle which can be variable. (**g**) Normal heterogeneous FDG activity in the liver and the spleen along with increased FDG uptake in the stomach possibly due to inflammation

standards for performing FDG PET studies and include patient preparation and image acquisition parameters, to produce good-quality images [13].

Dietary The use of FDG in the evaluation of metabolic activity of malignancy or suspected malignancy can be complicated by the diet of the patient. The effects of diet on the scan involve several factors: type of food ingested, timing of the meal, total glucose released (ingested along with endogenously released), and serum insulin (endogenous and administered) levels.

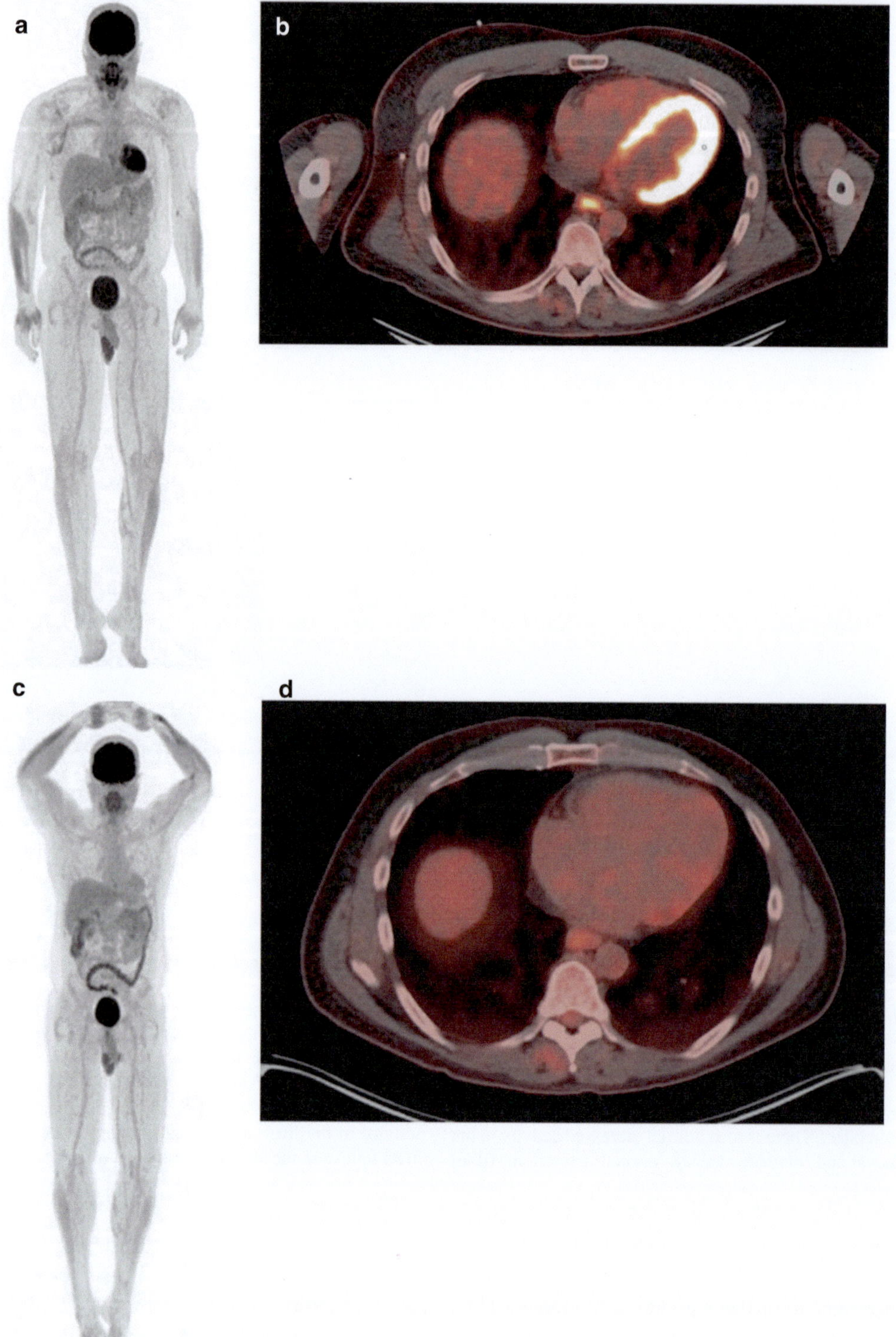

Fig. 2.4 Example of normal variable F-18 FDG uptake in the myocardium of the previous patient from two different F-18 FDG PET-CTs 1 year apart. (**a**) Anterior MIP image and (**b**) axial fused image illustrating the intense uptake in the myocardium. (**c**) Anterior MIP image and (**d**) axial fused image of the same patient 1 year later showing minimal F-18 FDG uptake in the myocardium

Fasting The ingestion of food is known to increase total blood glucose level, followed by an increase in serum insulin levels. These increases alter the distribution of normal glucose and its analog FDG by (1) causing competition between glucose and FDG for uptake by normal and malignant cells and (2) shunting delivery of FDG from malignant cells towards tissues such as fat, skeletal, and cardiac muscle by increasing the expression of insulin-dependent GLUT4 transporters in those organs. The blood glucose increases, not only from the release of glucose from the food ingested but also from the ongoing endogenous release, by gluconeogenesis and glycogenolysis via the liver and adipose tissue. The endogenous release of glucose is normally suppressed in non-diabetic patients by insulin, but in type 2 diabetic patients, this suppression can be impaired resulting in an excessive release of glucose into the circulation [14]. The first 90–120 min postprandial period shows the greatest increase in blood glucose levels, followed by a steady drop in blood glucose levels, and a subsequent increase and then drop in serum insulin over a 6 h period [14, 15] (Figs. 2.5 and 2.6).

All of the protocols from the major recognized societies require some period of fasting, ranging from 4 to 6 h prior to injection of the F-18-FDG, in order to minimize the blood levels of glucose, which competes with the injected FDG [13]. In addition to keeping the blood glucose levels at a basal state, this period of fasting will also keep the endogenous insulin levels to a basal level to prevent insulin-mediated altered biodistribution. This fasting includes tube feeding, intravenous fluids containing dextrose, and parenteral nutrients. Patients are allowed water with no added sugar or carbohydrates. The fasting recommendations also include refraining from chewing gum and ingesting candy, including breath mints [13].

Glucose When discussing preparations prior to a PET/CT, the pre-injection blood glucose level is one, if not the major, focus. This focus comes from multiple early studies like those by Wahl et al. and Lindholm et al., which showed a decrease in the FDG uptake in glucose-dependent tissues and tumor tissues with concurrent increase in the FDG uptake in skeletal muscle [13, 16–21] (Fig. 2.7). The focus of pre-injection blood glucose was so strongly accepted from these studies that the SNMMI and other societies recommend measuring blood glucose prior to FDG PET. The recommended blood glucose level cutoff for performing a scan ranges from 120 to 200 mg/dL. Some authorities, such as the NCI, separate the cutoff levels based on non-diabetic versus diabetic status – with the cutoff of 120 mg/dL (6.7 mmol/L) and 150–200 mg/dL (8.3–11.1 mmol/L), for non-diabetic and diabetic patients, respectively. In instances where blood glucose levels are greater than the cutoff for diabetic patients, some of the societies state that

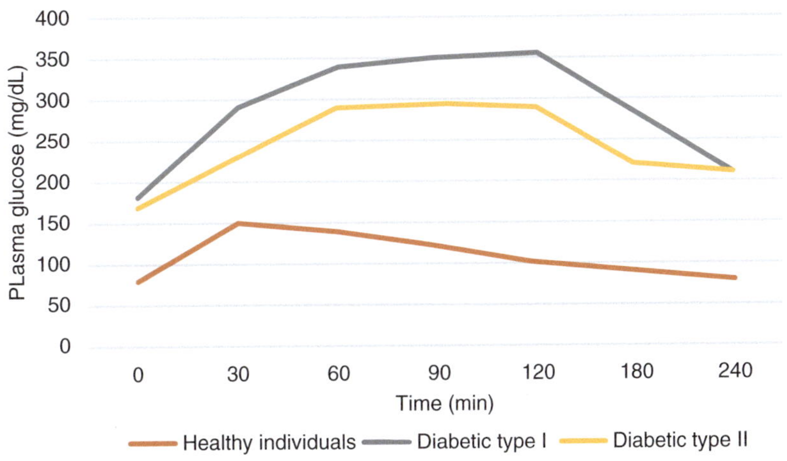

Fig. 2.5 A comparrison of the postprandial glucose response in healthy, diabetic type I, and diabetic type II individuals. Reproduced with permission from Bantle et al. [1], Copyright Massachusetts Medical Society

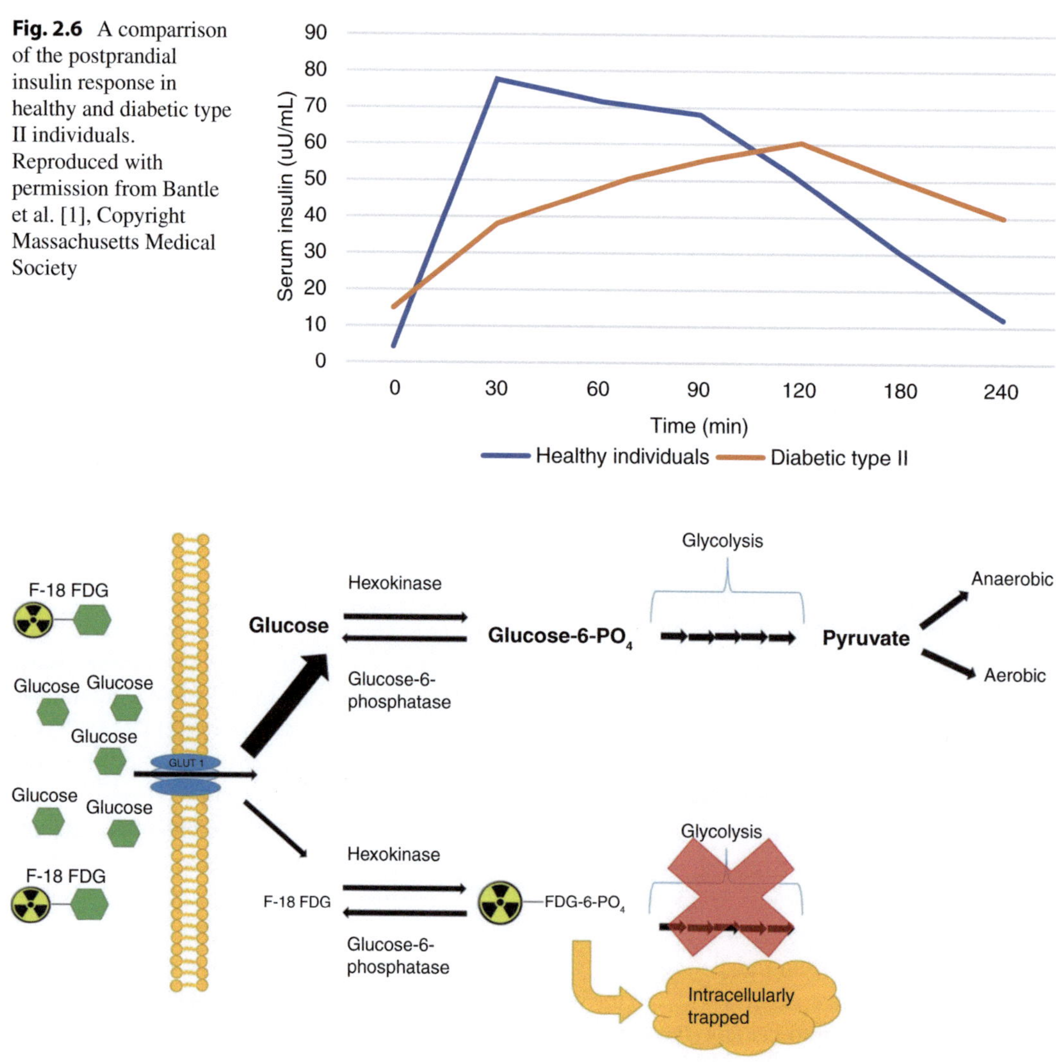

Fig. 2.6 A comparrison of the postprandial insulin response in healthy and diabetic type II individuals. Reproduced with permission from Bantle et al. [1], Copyright Massachusetts Medical Society

Fig. 2.7 Normal D-glucose and F-18 fluorodeoxy-glucose (F-18 FDG) import and trapping in a hyperglycemic state

administration of insulin can be considered. For example, the SNMMI recommends the administration of insulin but also recommends that the injection of FDG be delayed, with the duration of the delay depending on the type of insulin and the route used for administration. The EANM suggests that, if insulin is given, the delay for FDG injection should be more than 4 h, no matter the type or route of insulin given. Contrastingly, the NCI suggests that when blood glucose levels are more than 200 mg/dL (11.1 mmol/L), the study should be rescheduled, and insulin should not be given to adjust the blood glucose level [13].

Despite these recommendations, most newer studies would suggest that there is essentially no evidence that a higher glucose level, as a single factor, negatively impacts the readout of FDG PET scan. There is in fact some data indicating that this is probably not the case [22, 23]. It should be noted that the limited available original data examining the effect of glucose on tumor uptake, which are cited in the current societal recommendations mentioned above, were obtained in non-diabetic patients with normal glucose levels [18, 24]. In reality, these data indicate the effect of high insulin, and not high glucose, on FDG uptake in malignant tumors, a situation that does not apply to diabetic patients who lack insulin.

Timing is also a critical issue in the decision of whether the advantages of attempting to lower blood glucose prior to conducting a PET scan outweigh the disadvantages. In our institution, we obtain blood glucose prior to FDG injection in every patient. However, based on more recent literature and our experience of performing several thousand FDG PET annually, we usually go ahead with scanning the patient and account for the high blood glucose and the negative effect that it might have on the PET scan at the time of readout. This approach is due to the fact that the results of FDG PET are very often needed within a short time period in order to render a diagnosis or decide on treatment. This time period is usually shorter than the time that would be needed to obtain better blood glucose control. It should be kept in mind that if someone is under active medical care, as is the case in cancer patients, and still has a high blood glucose level, the attempts to gain better blood glucose control have probably been exhausted. As such, it is highly unlikely that delaying the PET scan will lead to a lower or normal glucose level within a timeframe that would allow for the PET scan to still be obtained and have an impact on patient's management. As is often the case in the practice of medicine, the correct course of action is a weighing of cost and benefit to the patient.

This is not to say that a patient's blood glucose should be completely discounted when conducting PET scans. There are factors that we are mindful of and to take into consideration when a patient presents for FDG PET:

1. The tumor type and its FDG avidity. Sarcomas are generally less and heterogeneously FDG avid, while melanomas are invariably intense on FDG PET. As such, melanomas are much less likely to be affected by high glucose level than sarcomas.
2. The expected location of potential findings. For instance, the PET signal from a tumor deep in the pelvis or retroperitoneum is much more likely to be attenuated than the signal from a tumor in the chest.

3. Body habitus. In a larger patient, PET signal is more attenuated than in a smaller patient.

We take into account the abovementioned factors when reading FDG PET in a diabetic patient with blood glucose higher than 200 mg/dL. Besides reading the scan under the abovementioned considerations, we adopted the following maneuvers for image acquisition in these patients:

1. Longer uptake time. We wait 90 or 120 min after FDG injection instead of the standard 60 min. The longer uptake time leads to increased tumor uptake and decreased background activity, allowing for better visualization of the tumor.
2. Longer acquisition time for the entire PET or certain bed positions, i.e., areas where abnormal findings are expected and/or are more prone to attenuation, such as the pelvis. Also, some institutions give patients water to drink to increase the washout of radiotracer and decrease background PET signal. With this practice of acquiring and interpreting FDG PET, if we still feel that we may be missing important findings – for instance, based on the overall poor quality of images or recent CT or MR findings that we cannot convincingly confirm as positive or negative on FDG PET – we offer the referring physician to repeat the scan at no cost after reducing the blood glucose level.

In our experience the quality of FDG PET images is sometimes actually much more severely affected in non-diabetic patients. This practically happens when they undergo PET as inpatient. This is due to the fact that they receive intravenous glucose infusion along with insulin, which leads to shifting of FDG away from tumor tissue and towards muscle and fat. The resulting decreased FDG availability for uptake in tumor and increased background signal in muscle and fat decreases the diagnostic value of the scan. Of course, these patients have a normal glucose level when arriving in PET suite. This normal glucose level is due to their non-diabetic state. This scenario, although uncommon, also indicates that measuring blood glucose prior to FDG PET has limited utility and may actually be misleading by diverting the attention away from other factors that have an influence on FDG distribution and FDG PET image quality (Fig. 2.8).

On a similar note, the value of measuring blood glucose prior to FDG PET in non-diabetic patients should be questioned. Our group studied a cohort of 117 patients with 574 scans: 91 non-diabetic patients with 429 scans and 26 diabetic patients with 145 scans. The goal was to determine the frequency of blood glucose level higher than 150 mg/dL at the time of FDG PET scan in non-diabetic patients. The cutoff of 150 mg/dL was selected based on the SNMMI guideline, recommending measuring blood glucose prior to

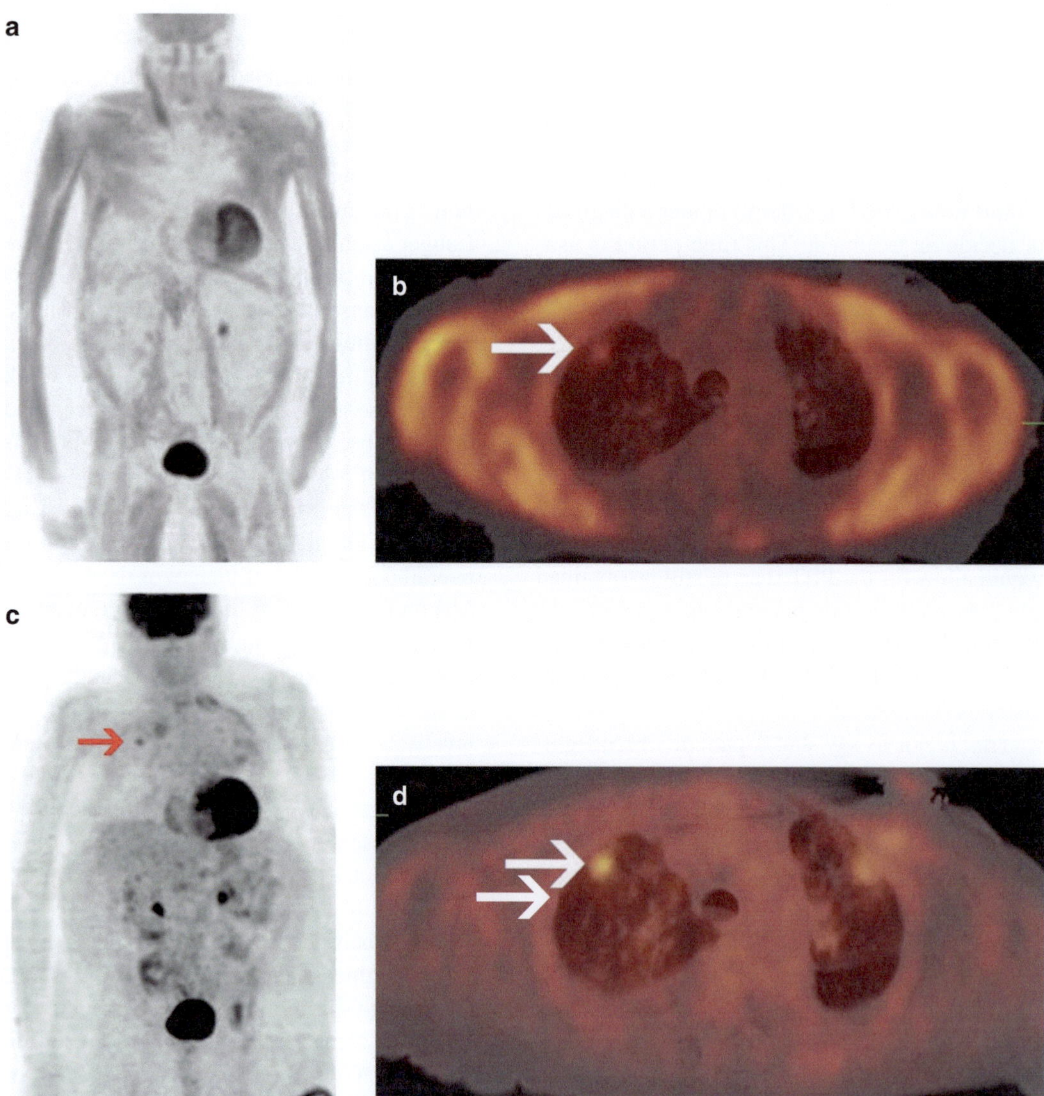

Fig. 2.8 Example of 2 FDG PET/CTs of a non-diabetic patient with normal glucose. (**a**) Anterior MIP images showing an altered biodistribution after 6 h of fasting but with IV glucose stopped shortly before imaging. Glucose was 127 mg/dL at the time. (**b**) Axial fused images showing high fat and muscle uptake with low lesion (white arrow) uptake. (**c**) Anterior MIP images of a next day repeat PET/CT after 6 h of fasting and without IV glucose, showing normal biodistribution and right lung lesion (red arrow). Glucose was 108 mg/dL at the time. (**d**) Axial fused images showing low soft tissue uptake and increased lesion (white arrow) uptake

FDG PET in every patient and not performing FDG PET if blood glucose is higher than 150–200 mg/dL. In our study, blood glucose level ranged from 44 to 259 mg/dL: 44 to 144 mg/dL in non-diabetic patients and 73 to 259 mg/dL in diabetic patients. There was no non-diabetic patient with a glucose level higher than 150 mg/dL at the time of any scan. Only one scan was performed with a blood glucose of 144 mg/dL in a non-diabetic. All other scans were performed in non-diabetic patients with a glucose level less than 140 mg/dL. Our data indicated that blood glucose level measurement prior to FDG PET could potentially be omitted in non-diabetic patients without missing any patient with blood glucose of higher than 150 mg/dL [25].

Blood Glucose Level Effects on Soft Tissue Sarcoma Evaluation Due to the generally low level and heterogeneous uptake and high recurrence and metastatic rate of the STSs, it is important to perform FDG PET with the least effect of high glucose or high insulin on FDG uptake as outlined above. Remember that the evaluation of STSs with PET/CT is twofold: (1) the identification of the most metabolically active site for biopsy and (2) the identification of local/regional or distant metastases. The presence of high blood glucose potentially decreases the FDG uptake in metabolically active regions and increases the overall background activity of the images. These alterations in the FDG distribution would potentially decrease the FDG uptake – specifically of those tumor types that are low-grade, resulting in a decrease in the sensitivity to localize the best biopsy site or identify local, regional, or distant metastases. Therefore, a "sensitive read" vs "conventional read" may be needed in order to not miss important findings – i.e., taking into account the fact that the FDG uptake in metabolically active tissue is lower even when glucose and insulin levels are normal.

Blood Glucose Level Effects on Melanoma Evaluation Melanoma is one of the most FDG-avid malignancies. The effects of a high blood glucose level would potentially have little effect on the sensitivity and accuracy of PET/CT evalu-ation due to this intense FDG avidity. Recall that the role of PET/CT in the evaluation for melanoma is reserved for those patients that have been categorized as stage III or IV, assessing for local, regional, or distant metastatic disease and disease burden. Nevertheless, a high blood glucose level would potentially decrease the sensitivity and accuracy of FDG PET in detecting smaller metastases potentially below the resolution of PET, which may be undetectable even in a low blood glucose state due to partial volume effect. There is also the potential of a decrease in sensitivity for the identification of residual disease post-resection as well as specificity for the identification of absence of residual disease and presence of post-resection change. Regardless, it is still important to minimize the alteration of biodistribution caused by a high blood glucose and continue to follow the proposed guidelines.

Insulin Although the focus of the competitive effects of serum glucose on the biodistribution of FDG is important, insulin plays just as important of a role. Glucose enters cells through three independent mechanisms, with the use of GLUTs as the major point of entry as described earlier. Insulin has the ability to alter the serum levels and biodistribution of both glucose and FDG, via a direct effect on the concentration of the insulin-dependent GLUT4 at the surface of the cell. When insulin levels are low, GLUT4 stays within the cytoplasmic vesicles where they are inactive. As the level of insulin rises and insulin binds to its receptors on the cells, the vesicles bind with the plasma membrane. Once the vesicles bind, the GLUT4 transporters are inserted into the plasma membrane, allowing for the cell to more efficiently take up glucose. As the level of insulin decreases, the GLUT4 transporters are sequestered back into the cytoplasmic vesicles. These transporters and this process occur in the skeletal and myocardial muscle, as well as adipose tissue [26]. Throughout the remaining tissues, other GLUTs are constantly present that are not insulin dependent. For example, the liver and brain use GLUT1 and GLUT3, which do not require insulin to be inserted to import glucose into the cell (Fig. 2.9). Also, GLUTs expressed

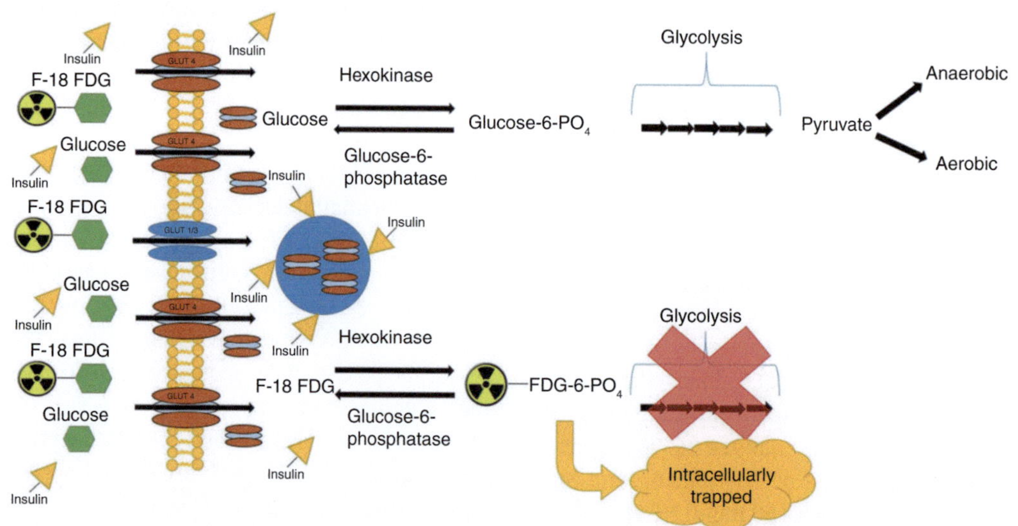

Fig. 2.9 Normal D-glucose and F-18 fluorodeoxy-glucose (F-18 FDG) import and trapping in a hyperinsulinemia

in cancer cells, mainly GLUT1 and GLUT3, are insulin independent.

An additional mechanism of insulin that alters the serum glucose level and biodistribution is its effect on the liver and its production of glycogen. Of the absorbed glucose, a large portion is quickly taken up by the hepatocytes and converted to glycogen. Insulin stimulates the production of glycogen in multiple steps. First, insulin activates hexokinase, which phosphorylates and traps glucose into the cell. With the activation of hexokinase, there is inhibition of glucose-6-phosphatase – this decreases the amount of glucose that diffuses from the cell. It has been shown by Iozzo et al. that in a hyperinsulincmic state, there is enhanced hepatic glucose influx and phosphorylation of FDG. This effect by insulin is similar in insulin-sensitive and insulin-resistant individuals. This same study also showed that even though there was an overall enhancement of phosphorylation, there was a lower ratio of phosphorylation to dephosphorylation in the low insulin-sensitive group compared to the normal insulin- and high insulin-sensitive group. This resulted in a decrease in the trapping of FDG in individuals resistant to insulin [27]. Further into the production of glycogen, which FDG does not

enter, insulin activates multiple enzymes such as phosphofructokinase and glycogen synthase to produce glycogen (Fig. 2.10).

When imaging diabetic patients who use insulin, consideration needs to be given to when the patient normally takes his or her medication in the context of determining the timing of the FDG injection and imaging. At our institution, we typically coordinate the scheduling of the diabetic patients to minimize any possible interference with blood glucose and insulin level and quality of PET images. Diabetic patients are either (1) scheduled for early morning, around 8 am, and instructed to eat and take their insulin and other diabetic medications the evening before, around 10 pm, or (2) scheduled for an early afternoon slot, around 1 pm, with food and insulin and medication taken early in the morning, around 6 am. In any case, we are watchful of the blood glucose level of the diabetic patients not only to obtain high-quality PET images but also out of concern for the safety of the patient. The instruction to take diabetic medications and food at certain times and arrive on time for PET has to be communicated to the patient very clearly and may necessitate the help of the referring physician or physician familiar with patient's diabetes treatment. We also instruct the diabetes patients to bring food and their medications with them to the PET appointment. They very often eat and take their medication before leaving our PET facility.

Increased Serum Insulin Levels with Soft Tissue Sarcoma Evaluation More pronounced compared to the effects of a high blood glucose state, an increase in serum insulin levels could potentially decrease FDG uptake in STSs. The altered biodistribution in a high insulin state results from the shunting of glucose and FDG to insulin-dependent GLUT4s. The shunting of glucose and FDG is directed towards tissues like skeletal muscle, myocardial muscle, and adipose tissue and could potentially decrease the sensitivity in identification of the most metabolically active region of the primary tumor and/or local, regional, or distant metastatic disease. In a group of tumors that already have a mild and heterogeneous uptake pattern, it is important to minimize the potential impact of postprandial high insulin levels on biodistribution by adhering to the proposed fasting time.

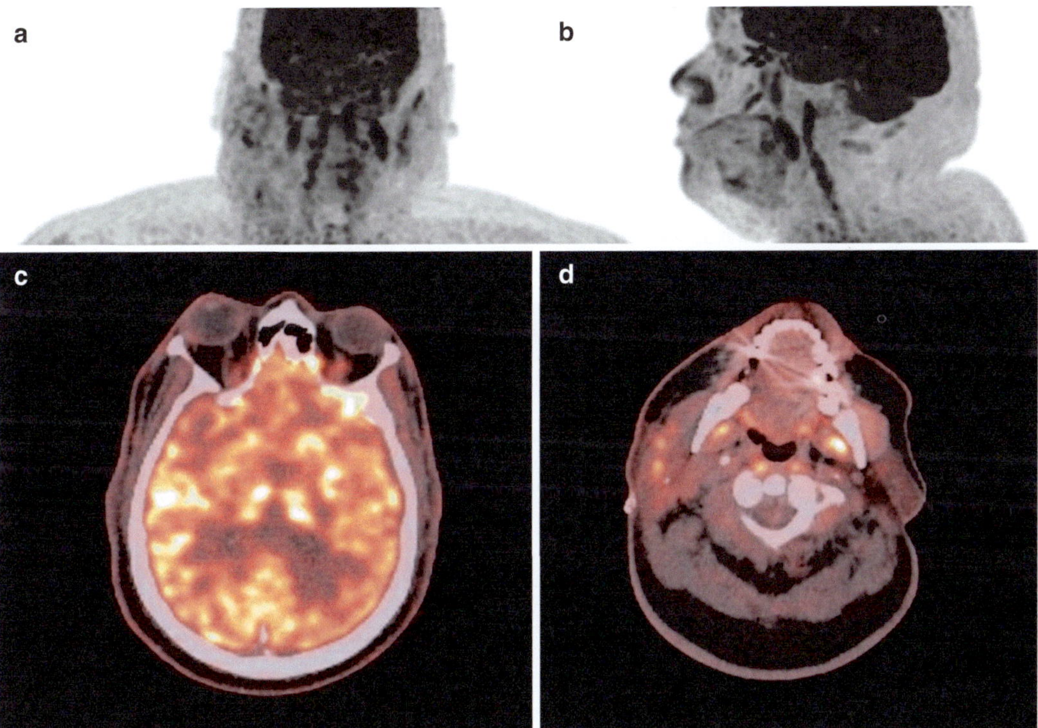

Fig. 2.10 A 69-year-old diabetic male with a right-sided parotid tumor and F-18 FDG PET/CT with altered biodistribution due to administered insulin prior to imaging. (**a, b**) Anterior and left lateral MIP images of the head and neck and whole body illustrating decreased uptake in the brain. (**c**) Axial fused PET/CT image illustrating overall decreased FDG uptake throughout the brain. (**d**) Axial fused PET/CT image showing mild increase in F-18 FDG uptake in the right parotid gland relative to the surrounding tissue most consistent with residual tumor. (**e, f**) Anterior and left lateral MIP images of the body showing increased shunting of F-18 FDG to the soft tissue and myocardium along with decreased FDG uptake in the liver and spleen. (**g**) Axial fused PET/CT image showing increased shunting of F-18 FDG to the myocardium. (**h**) Axial fused PET/CT image showing overall decrease in F-18 FDG uptake in the liver and spleen but with increased uptake in the crural muscles. (**i**) Axial fused PET/CT image showing increased uptake in the gluteal muscles bilaterally illustrating shunting of FDG to insulin-dependent tissue

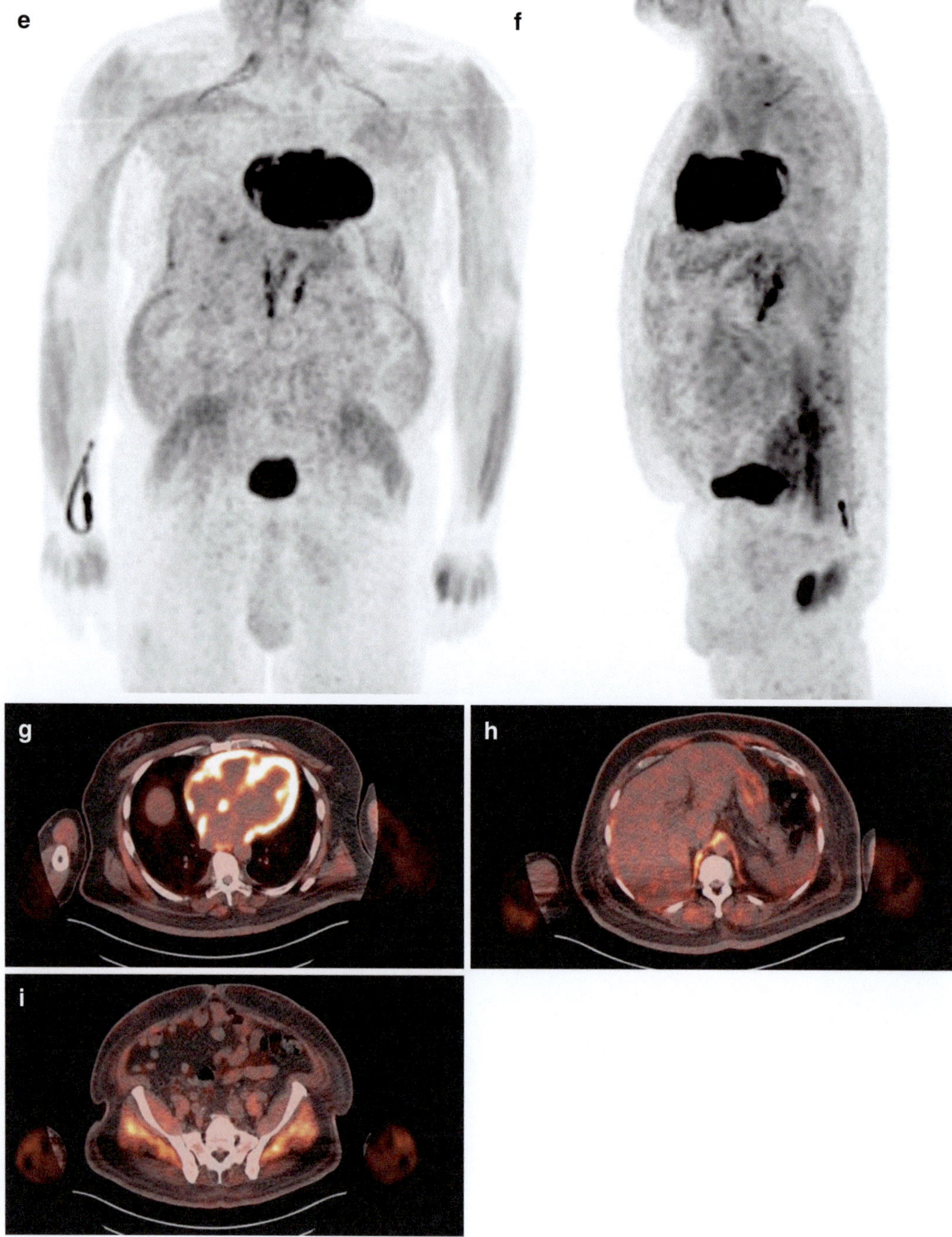

Fig. 2.10 (continued)

Increased Serum Insulin Levels with Melanoma Evaluation Although more pronounced compared to the effect of high blood glucose levels, the effects of a high insulin state on the sensitivity for the detection of metastatic melanoma may still be minimal. The high metabolic rate of melanoma would potentially still create a high target-to-background ratio, allowing for acceptable sensitivity rates. There is however a chance that there would be a decrease in sensitivity of metastatic disease potentially below the resolution threshold of PET and/or recurrent/residual disease due to the shunting of FDG into non-glucose-dependent tissue. These smaller metastases and/or recurrent/residual disease may not be detectable even under normal insulin levels, but efforts to keep insulin levels acceptable should be made to produce the best-quality images possible (Fig. 2.11).

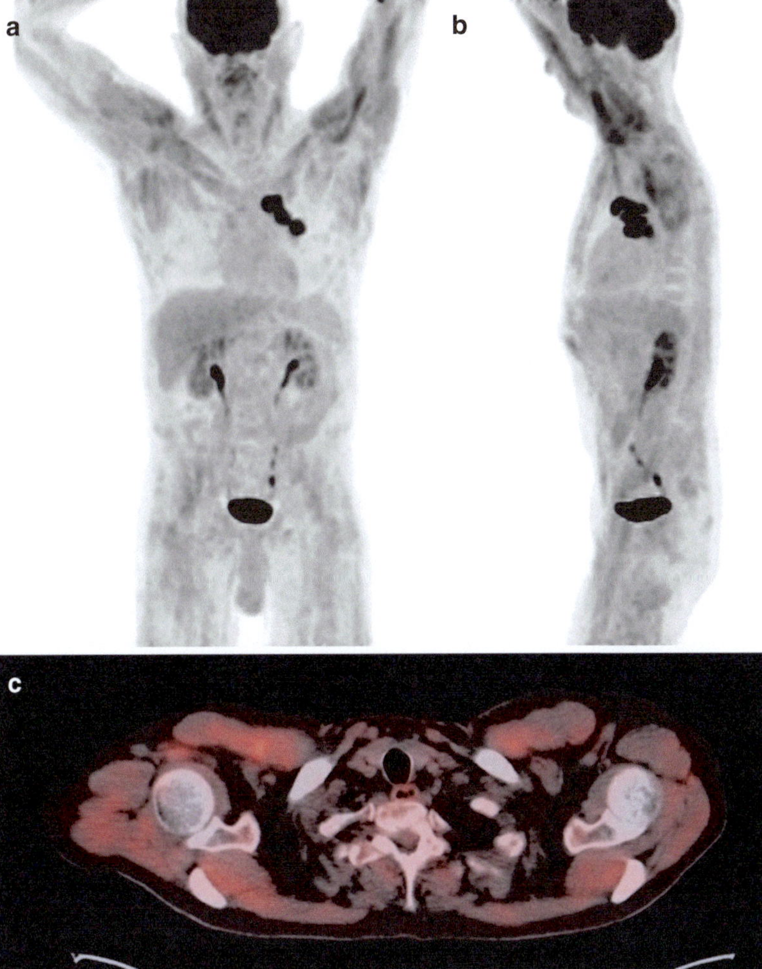

Fig. 2.11 PET image illustrating postprandial imaging. (**a**, **b**) Anterior and left lateral MIP images showing diffuse increase in F-18 FDG throughout the soft tissue and musculature. (**c**) Axial fused image of the upper thorax/upper extremities showing the increased F-18 FDG uptake in the musculature without anatomical abnormalities. (**d**) Axial fused image of the abdomen illustrating F-18 FDG uptake in the paraspinal muscle equal to that in the liver and spleen

Fig. 2.11 (continued)

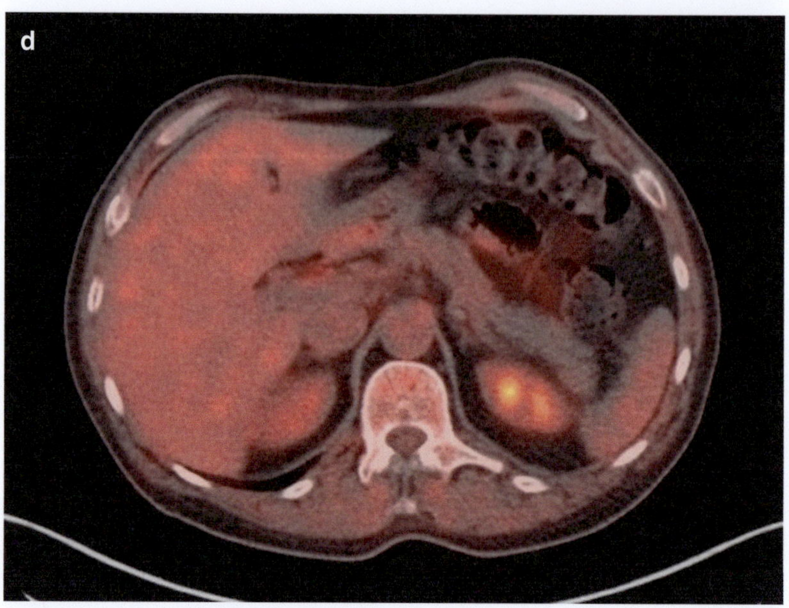

Other factors that indirectly through an increase in insulin can influence the distribution of FDG away from tumor and to the muscles and fat include long-standing eating habits and physical activity.

Additional Dietary Recommendations Many groups, societies, and institutions recommend an altered diet prior to FDG PET. The recommended altered diet consists of a high-protein, low-carbohydrate diet for 24 h prior to scanning. The reduction in carbohydrates is intended to decrease the blood glucose, and resulting insulin levels, which may still exist after normalization of blood glucose levels. Another dietary recommended protocol is a high-fat, high-protein, and low-carbohydrate diet. This diet is routinely used when assessing the FDG uptake in the heart for a myocardial sarcoidosis patient being evaluated for inflammation and active sarcoidosis of the myocardium. In this setting, the assumption is that the resulting low insulin decreases the FDG uptake in normal myocardium; hence, inflamed myocardium can be better visualized. A high-fat, high-protein, and low-carbohydrate diet for 72 h has been shown to successfully suppress the normal physiologic uptake of FDG in the heart [28]. It has been proposed that this same diet could be used for oncological studies in lieu of fasting only. However, one mouse model study showed that there was no difference in tumor FDG uptake with a 72 h high-fat diet compared to overnight fasting alone [29]. We do not restrict the diet of our patients for oncology FDG PET since we overall have not observed any notable interference. Restricting diet is also a matter of practicability and patient compliance. Our overarching approach has been to limit the patients' instructions to a necessary minimum in order to achieve a good image quality across the board in a busy academic PET facility.

An alteration in the types of foods consumed is not the only dietary recommendation. It is also recommended that the patient abstain from the ingestion of caffeine and nicotine for at least 12 h prior to the study. It has been shown that caffeine is an alkaloid that increases the activity of the sympathetic nervous system, which results in an increase in thermogenesis. Nicotine is another alkaloid that increases norepinephrine turnover and thermogenesis. The effects of both caffeine and nicotine are more prominent in the brown adipose tissue. Consequently, the use of nicotine has shown a decrease in the FDG uptake in the stomach and muscle [30]. But again, also here we do not put any restriction on the patients prior to their FDG PET scan.

When evaluating such malignancies such as STSs or malignant melanoma with FDG PET/CT, an altered diet, such as the high-protein, low-carbohydrate or high-fat, high-protein, low-carbohydrate diet used in cardiac imaging, is not needed. The potential added control from the implementation of these diets is not as beneficial as the patient adhering to fasting overnight or at least for 4–6 h prior to imaging. The abstinence from caffeine and nicotine is another suggestion that could be beneficial but is not required. In the time prior to injection, keeping the patient warm will help to decrease the physiologic uptake of FDG by the brown fat more significantly than the abstinence of caffeine and nicotine.

Physical Activity An increase in activity prior to the injection and during the uptake time can cause an increase in the uptake of FDG into the musculature (Fig. 2.12). The avoidance of a wide range of strenuous activities is recommended for a period of at least 6 h (more commonly 24 h) prior to the study, including but not limited to exercising (running, biking, weightlifting, etc.), house/yard work, and sexual activity. Some societies also recommend the avoidance of chewing gum, not only during the uptake period but also 24 h prior to injection. The abstinence from chewing gum decreases uptake in the masseter muscles, which is particularly helpful when evaluating patients with head and neck cancer [13]. But again, also here, as a matter of practicability, we do not put any restriction on the patients prior to their FDG PET scan.

The increased uptake in the skeletal muscle has the potential to decrease the available circulating FDG; mask smaller, more discreet lesions; and

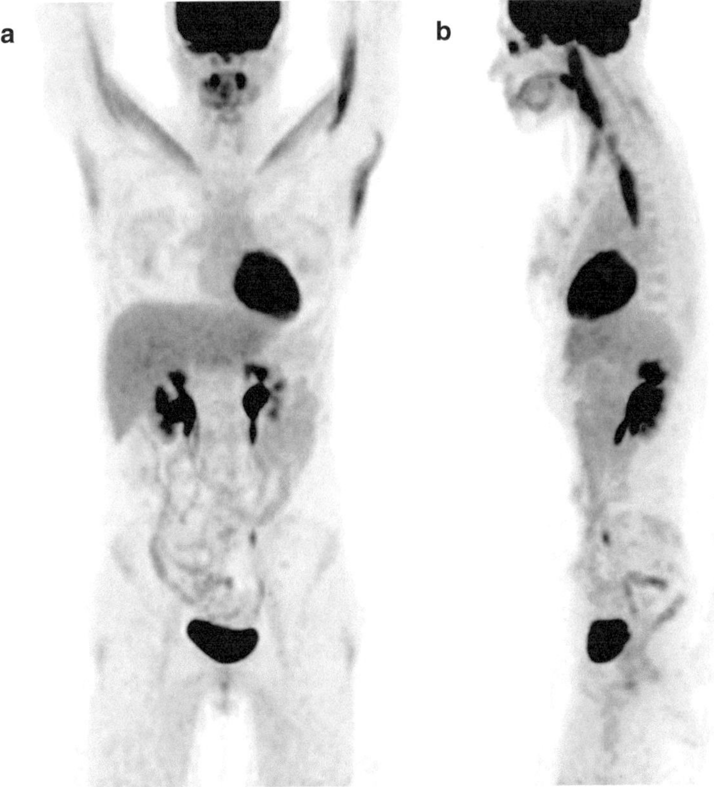

Fig. 2.12 An example of a PET image illustrating muscular uptake post-exercise. (**a**, **b**) Anterior and left lateral MIP images showing increased F-18 FDG in the bilateral upper extremities and central and lateral chest areas. (**c**, **d**) Axial fused image showing increased F-18 FDG in the bilateral biceps, pectoralis, and latissimus muscles

Fig. 2.12 (continued)

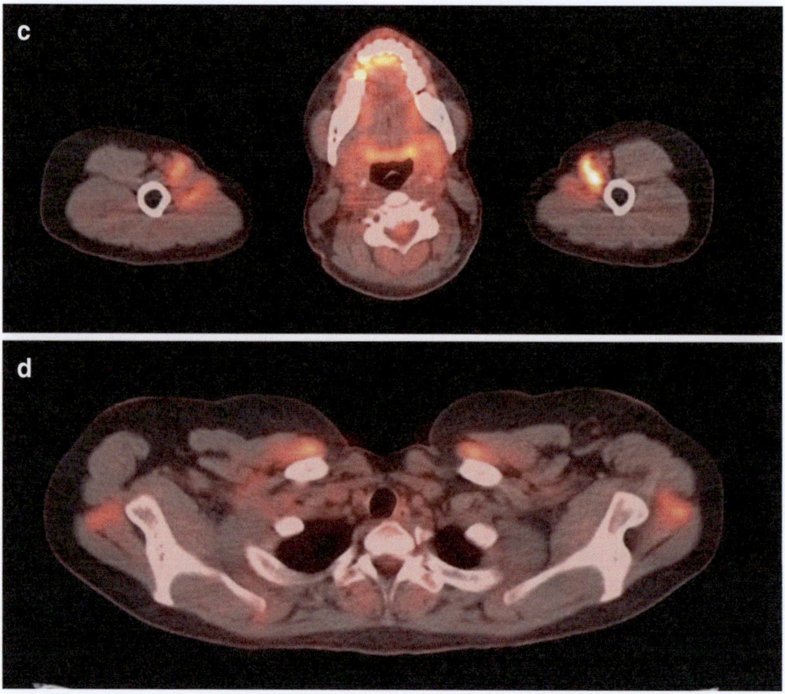

decrease the target-to-background ratio. These potential alterations are less likely to negatively affect the identification of sites of metastatic melanoma due to the high target-to-background ratio uptake. In the case of STSs, however, these alterations in distribution may decrease any subtle focal increases in low-grade tumors, thus decreasing the sensitivity required to successfully locate the most aggressive site for biopsy. There also may be blurring of the tumor edge if there is surrounding skeletal muscle with increased uptake.

Uptake Time When using FDG PET/CT, there are recommended preprocedural processes to attempt to capture the body in a basal metabolic state. Prior to the FDG injection, optimally, particularly pediatric patients should be kept in a warm room for approximately 30–60 min [31]. The patient is kept warm to try and minimize normal brown fat uptake (Fig. 2.13). After FDG injection, the patient is kept in a quiet and warm room and asked not to talk excessively, in order to try to minimize resulting increased uptake in the tongue and vocal cords (Fig. 2.14). Reading or watching TV should not create any significant muscle uptake and is permissible at our institution. In some patients, when claustrophobia is a concern, sedatives can be administered during this time. The administration of beta-blockers or benzodiazepines can also be used for prevention of normal brown fat uptake, though effectiveness varies and is mostly not needed in the area of PET/CT, since the fused images are helpful in distinguishing brown fat uptake from pathology [31].

Once the dose is injected, there is a period of time that is needed for circulation, uptake, and clearance of the tracer. Multiple studies have been conducted to evaluate for the optimal time for scanning post radiotracer administration, which is important not only for the visual quality but even more for the quantitative measurements such as SUVs. The original studies, investigating the optimal uptake time, were performed using homogenous brain tissue in order to calculate the time of the plateau phase of uptake, which was found to be 45–60 min.

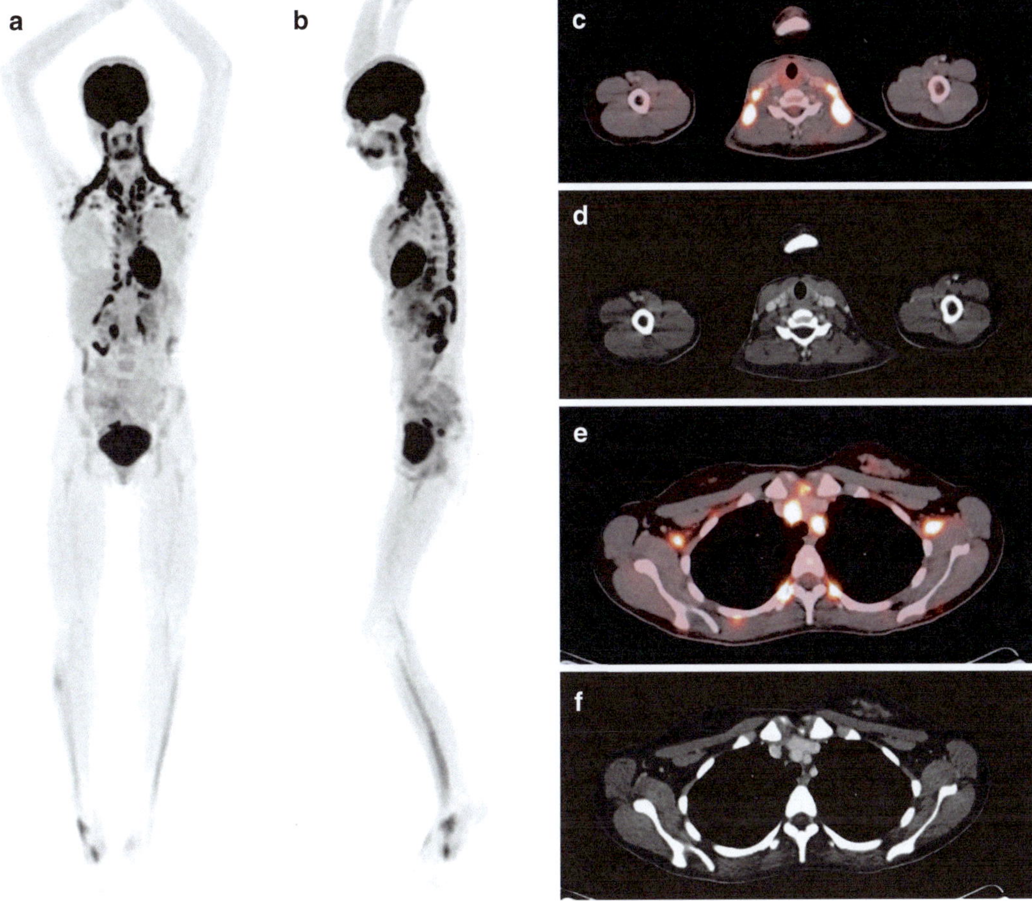

Fig. 2.13 Example of a F-18 FDG PET/CT illustrating physiologic increase in uptake in brown fat. (**a, b**) Anterior and left lateral MIP image showing symmetrical increased uptake in the bilateral cervical and paraspinal regions. (**c, d**) Axial fused and low-dose non-contrast CT showing increased F-FDG uptake in the bilateral cervical fat planes. (**e, f**) Axial fused and low-dose non-contrast CT showing increased F-18 FDG in the mediastinum, bilateral axial, and paraspinal fat spaces

Multiple studies since have looked at the many factors affecting the uptake of FDG including multi-compartment/rate constant equations, heterogeneous tissues, tumor/normal tissue uptake ratios, biological constructs of specific tumors, and multiple biological rates. The biological rates included uptake, phosphorylation, dephosphorylation, and clearance rates. These later studies concluded that the uptake time of 45–60 min underestimates the calculated SUVmax values and showed that, for many tumors, the FDG uptake did not plateau until several hours after injection. Additional studies investigated other factors such as treatment changes and specific tumor types. An example of such a study that investigated the plateau time of malignant tissue was by Hamberg et al.; this study showed that with stage III lung cancer, the average time to plateau was 298 min (before treatment) and 154 min (posttreatment) [17, 18]. A study conducted by Lodge et al. looked at the uptake peak time in malignant soft tissue masses versus benign lesions, specifically high-grade sarcomas. In this study, 29 patients with soft tissue masses (12 malignant and 8 benign) were evaluated. It was found that peak FDG uptake was at approximately 4 h post-injection in malignant tumors, whereas benign tumors peaked around 30 min.

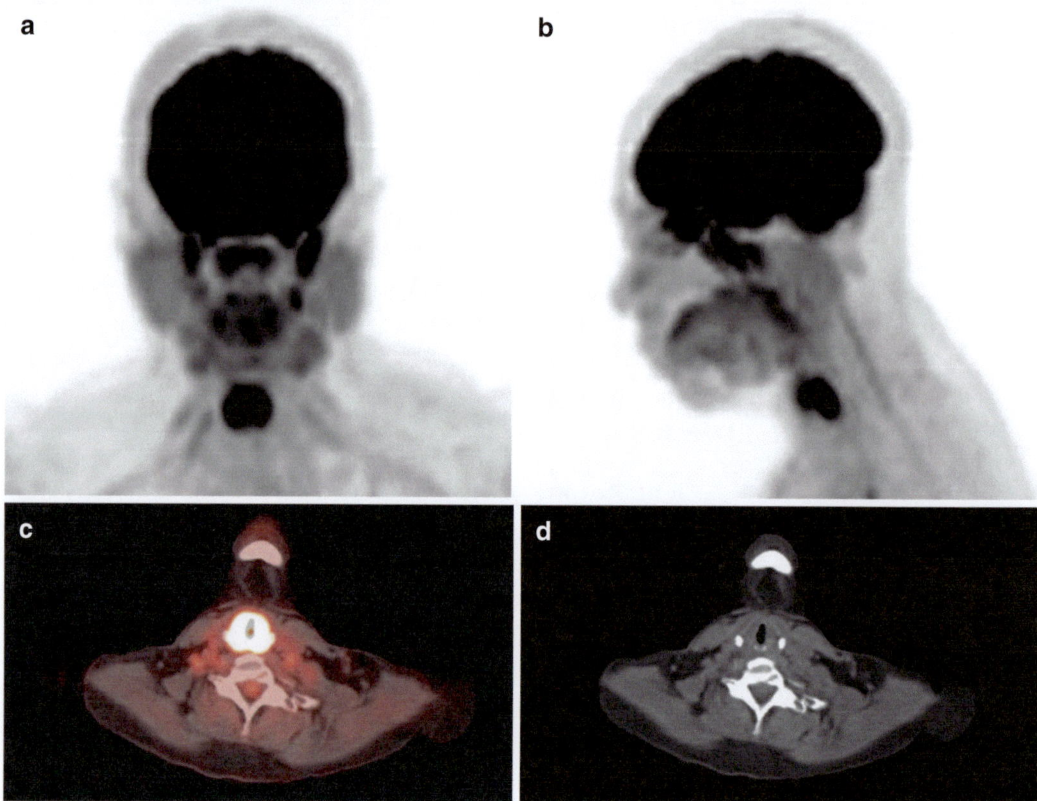

Fig. 2.14 Example of normal physiologic uptake in the vocal cords due to patient talking during the uptake time. (**a, b**) MIP images showing the intense uptake in the ante-rior lower neck. (**c, d**) Axial fused F-18 FDG PET/CT and low-dose non-contrast CT localizing the increased uptake in the vocal cord without anatomical abnormality

The 4 h SUV measurement was found to have a sensitivity and specificity of 100% and 76%, respectively [32]. In clinical practice, an uptake time of 4 h is impractical to efficiently keep up with patient throughput. A study by Al-Faham et al. studied the optimal uptake time for evaluating liver lesions in which they found that an uptake time of approximately 90 min significantly improves target-to-background ratio above that of an uptake time of 60 min [33].

In our practice of performing several thousand oncology FDG PET scans annually for almost 20 years, the uptake time of 60 min has worked out very well. An increased uptake time to 90 or 120 min could be considered in patient with blood glucose levels of higher than 200 mg/dL in an attempt to increase tumor and decrease background signal. This would be particularly important in sarcoma patients with high blood glucose levels. Other than that, the goal should be to keep the uptake time as close as possible to 60 min. This is important for intra-patient and inter-patient comparison of the findings.

References

1. Warburg O, Posener K, Negelein E. VIII. The metabolism of cancer cells. Biochem Z. 1924;152:129–69.
2. Weber G. Ezymology of cancer cells. N Engl J Med. 1977;296:486–93.
3. Carruthers A. Facilitated diffusion of glucose. Physiol Rev. 1990;70(4):1135–76.
4. Lizak B, Szarka A, Kim Y, Choi K, Nemeth C. Glucose transport and transporters in the endomembranes. Int J Mol Sci. 2019;20(23):5898.
5. Wagner S, Kopka K. Non-peptidyl 18F-labelled PET tracers as radioindicators for the noninvasive detection of cancer. In: Molecular imaging in oncology, vol. 187. Berlin/London: Springer; 2013. p. 106–32.

6. Swanson D, Chilton H, Thrall J, editors. Pharmaceuticals in medical imaging. New York: Macmillan Publishing Company; 1990.

7. Cole E, Stewart M, Littich R, Hoareau R, Scott P. Radiosyntheses using Fluorine-18: the art and science of late stage fluorination. Curr Top Med Chem. 2014;14(7):875–900.

8. Gallagher B, Fowler J, Gutterson N, MacGregor R, Wan C. Metabolic trapping as a principle of radiopharmaceutical design: some factors responsible for the biodistribution of [18F] 2-Deoxy-2-Fluoro-D--Glucose. J Nucl Med. 1978;19:1154–61.

9. The Feinstein Institute for Medical Research. Fludeoxyglucose F18 Injection (F-18 FDG) [package insert] U.S. Food and Drug Administration website. https://www.accessdata.fda.gov/drugsatfda_docs/label/2010/021870s004lbl.pdf. Revised July 2010. Accessed November 2019.

10. Qiao H, Bai J, Chen Y, Tian J. Kidney modeling for FDG excretion with PET. Int J Biomed Imaging. 2007;2007:63234.

11. Mettler FA, Guiberteau MJ. 18-F FDG PET/CT neoplasm imaging. In: Essentials of nuclear medicine imaging. 6th ed. Philadelphia: Elsevier Saunders; 2012. p. 361–95.

12. Wang Y, Chiu E, Rosenberg J, Gambhir S. Standardized uptake value atlas: characterization of physiological 2-Deoxy-2-[18F]fluoro-D-glucose uptake in normal tissue. Mol Imaging Biol. 2007;9:83–90.

13. Surasi DS, Bhambhvani P, Baldwin JA, Almodovar SE, O'Malley JP. 18F-FDG PET and PET/CT patient preparation: a review of the literature. J Nucl Med Technol. 2014;42:5–13.

14. Woerle HJ, Szoke E, Meyer J, Dostou JM, Wittlin SD, Gosmanov NR, Welle SL, Gerich JE. Mechanisms for abnormal postprandial glucose metabolism in type 2 diabetes. Am J Physiol Endocrinol Metab. 2005;290:E67–77.

15. Bantle JP, Laine DC, Castle GW, Thomas JW, Hoogwerf BJ, Goetz FC. Postprandial glucose and insulin responses to meals containing different carbohydrates in normal and diabetic subjects. N Engl J Med. 1983;309:7–12.

16. Wahl RL, Cody RL, Hutchins GD, Mudgett EE. Primary and metastatic breast carcinoma: initial clinical evaluation with PET with the radiolabeled glucose analogue 2-[F-18]-fluoro-2-deoxy-D-glucose. Radiology. 1991;179(3):765–70.

17. Wahl RL, Henry CA, Ethier SP. Serum glucose: effects on tumor and normal tissue accumulation of 2-[F-18]-fluoro-2-deoxy-D-glucose in rodents with mammary carcinoma. Radiology. 1992;183:643–7.

18. Lindholm P, Minn H, Leskinen-Kallio S, Bergman J, Ruotsalainen U, Joensuu H. Influence of the blood glucose concentration on FDG uptake in cancer: a PET study. J Nucl Med. 1993;34:1–6.

19. Nagaki A, Onoguchi M, Matsutomo N. Patient weight-based acquisition protocols to optimize 18F-FDG PET/CT image quality. J Nucl Med Technol. 2011;39(2):72–6.

20. Hamberg LM, Hunter GJ, Alpert NM, Choi NC, Babich JW, Fischman AJ. The dose uptake ratio as an index of glucose metabolism: useful parameter or oversimplification? J Nucl Med. 1994;35:1308–12.

21. Basu S, Kung J, Houseni M, Zhuang H, Tidmarsh GF, Alavi A. Temporal profile of fluorodeoxyglucose uptake in malignant lesions and normal organs over extended time periods in patients with lung carcinoma: implications for its utilization in assessing malignant lesions. Q J Nucl Med Mol Imaging. 2009;53:9–16.

22. Mirpour S, Meteesatien P, Khandani A. Dose hyperglycemia affect the diagnostic value of 18F-FDG PET/CT? Rev Esp Med Nucl Imagen Mol. 2012;31(2):71–7.

23. Rabkin Z, Israel O, Keidar Z. Do hyperglycemia and diabetes affect the incidence of false-negative 18F-FDG PET/CT studies in patients evaluated for infection or inflammation and cancer? A comparative analysis. J Nucl Med. 2010;51:1015–20.

24. Langen K, Braun U, Rota KE, Herzog H, Kuwert T. The influence of plasma glucose levels of Fluorine-18-Fluorodeoxyglucose uptake in bronchial carcinomas. J Nucl Med. 1993;34:355–9.

25. Khandani A, Bravo I, Patel P, Ivanovic KD. Frequency of high blood glucose prior to FDG PET. Abdom Radiol. 2016;42(5):1583–5.

26. Shephered P, Kahn B. Glucose transporters and insulin action – implications for insulin resistance and diabetes mellitus. N Engl J Med. 1999;341(4):248–57.

27. Iozzo P, Geisler F, Oikonen V, et al. Insulin stimulates liver glucose uptake in humans: an 18F-FDG PET study. J Nucl Med. 2003;44:682–9.

28. Lu Y, Grant C, Xie K, Sweiss N. Suppression of myocardial 18F-FDG uptake through prolonged high-fat, high-protein, and very-low-carbohydrate diet before FDG-PET/CT for evaluation of patients with suspected cardiac sarcoidosis. Clin Nucl Med. 2017;42:88–94.

29. Cusso L, Musteanu M, Mulero F, Barbacid M, Desco M. Effects of ketogenic diet on [18F]FDG-PET imaging in a mouse model of lung cancer. Mol Imaging Biol. 2018;21(2):279–85.

30. Baba S, Tatsumi M, Ishimori T, Lilien D, Engles J, Wahl R. Effect of nicotine and ephedrine on the accumulation of 18F-FDG in brown adipose tissue. J Nucl Med. 2007;48:981–6.

31. Delbeke D, Coleman RE, Guiberteau MJ, Brown ML, Royal HD, Siegel BA, et al. Procedure guideline for tumor imaging with 18F-FDGD PET/CT 1.0*. J Nucl Med. 2006;47(5):885–95.

32. Lodge MA, Lucas JD, Marsden PK, Cronin BF, O'Doherty MJ, Smith MA. A PET study of 18FDG uptake in soft tissue masses. Eur J Nucl Med. 1999;26:22–30.

33. Al-Faham Z, Jolepalem P, Rydberg J, Wong CYO. Optimizing 18-F-FDG uptake time before imaging improves the accuracy of PET/CT in liver lesions. J Nucl Med Technol. 2016;44(2):70–2.

PET/CT and PET/MR in Soft Tissue Sarcoma and Melanoma Patients: What to Image and How to Image It

Mitchel Muhleman, Marija Ivanovic, and Amir H. Khandani

PET/CT Imaging in Soft Tissue Sarcoma and Melanoma

In the era of hybrid imaging, the use of PET/CT, specifically fluorine-18 fluorodeoxy-glucose (F-18 FDG or FDG) PET/CT imaging, has been thoroughly investigated for its value in various malignancies, including sarcoma and melanoma. These investigations have highlighted its applicability and usefulness in staging, biopsy guidance, grading for several cancers, response to treatment, and surveillance.

Soft Tissue Sarcomas Imaging is an important tool in the evaluation and treatment planning for soft tissue sarcomas (STSs). The use of MRI and CT scans can characterize the anatomy of tumors extremely well, but may lack important information when attempting to stage, grade, select an optimal biopsy site, or evaluate a tumors' response to treatment (Figs. 3.1 and 3.2). This need for additional critical information has given molecular imaging, specifically FDG PET/CT imaging, an important role in the evaluation of STSs beyond that of anatomic detail. Unlike conventional imaging, FDG PET/CT assesses the metabolic status of tumors (Figs. 3.3 and 3.4). This gives PET/CT multiple advantages, including the ability to (1) distinguish benign to low-grade tumors from intermediate- to high-grade tumors, (2) identify the most metabolically active site for biopsies, (3) provide evidence suggesting local/regional or distant metastases, (4) evaluate response to treatment, and (5) allow opportunity for restaging patients with potential residual, recurrent, or metastatic disease (Figs. 3.5, 3.6, 3.7, and 3.8).

Malignant Melanoma FDG PET/CT plays a very important role in the staging of high-risk patients, evaluation of treatment response, and surveillance.

With regard to staging, FDG PET/CT is helpful in localizing potential biopsy sites (Fig. 3.9) and evaluation of distant visceral metastases. This allows for optimal tissue sampling and accurate staging for treatment planning (Figs. 3.10, 3.11, 3.12, and 3.13). It is important to note, however, that there is a limited utility of FDG PET/CT in the management of smaller early-stage melanoma, which includes stages I and II. This limited utility is due to the low likelihood of metastatic disease in this setting. FDG PET can potentially detect residual or recurrent local diseases, which are usually very mild on FDG PET due to their

M. Muhleman (✉) · M. Ivanovic · A. H. Khandani
Department of Radiology, Division of Molecular Imaging and Therapeutics, University of North Carolina, Chapel Hill School of Medicine, Chapel Hill, NC, USA
e-mail: mitchel_muhleman@med.unc.edu;
Marija.Ivanovic@unchealth.unc.edu;
khandani@med.unc.edu

© Springer Nature Switzerland AG 2021
A. H. Khandani (ed.), *PET/CT and PET/MR in Melanoma and Sarcoma*,
https://doi.org/10.1007/978-3-030-60429-5_3

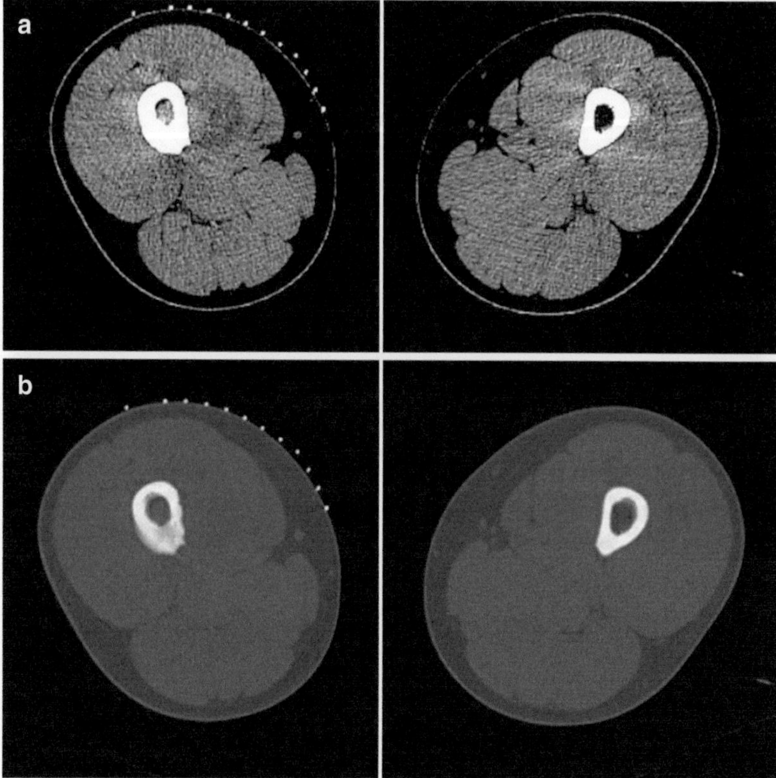

Fig. 3.1 Example of soft tissue sarcoma on non-contrast-enhanced CT. A 17-year-old male presenting with right mid-thigh mass. Non-contrast-enhanced CT for bone biopsy. (**a**) Soft tissue window: illustrating the hypoattenuating soft tissue mass along the medial cortex of the femur, along with ill-defined marrow enhancement. (**b**) Bone window: illustrating course cortical changes of the posterior and medial aspect of the proximal femur

size and effect of volume averaging (Fig. 3.14). Nonetheless, the use of PET/CT in the evaluation of treatment response is still important for melanoma, due to the resistance of melanoma to chemotherapy, and the introduction of new therapies, such as molecular target therapy and immunotherapy. Finally, the usefulness of PET/CTs in surveillance is in the ability to detect recurrence of disease early enough to treat when there is limited disease.

PET/CTs usefulness in STSs and malignant melanoma is the result of the combination of metabolic evaluation and anatomical localization and morphological detail, depending on use of a low-dose non-contrast CT versus standard-dose CT with or without contrast, to examine either a specific area of the patient or the entire patient in one scan. In utilizing this hybrid scan, it is important to know not only what to image but also how to image the patient to obtain the desired information.

Brief Basics of PET and PET/CT

Positron emission tomography (PET) is a specific form of imaging in nuclear medicine, utilizing a subset of radioactive elements which are proton-rich elements that have an excess energy of more than 1.022 MeV. These elements become stable either in the electron capture or beta plus (positron) decay process. The beta plus decay process produces a positron particle which has the same mass and magnitude of charge as a negatively charged electron, but with a positive charge. Positrons travel a short distance of up to few millimeters in tissue before it annihilates with an electron. This annihilation converts the mass of the two particles (positron and electron) into energy in the form of two 511 keV photons which are emitted in opposite directions in almost 180 degrees to each other. The distance that a positron travels in tissue is called positron range and depends on its energy. In case of 18F, the aver-

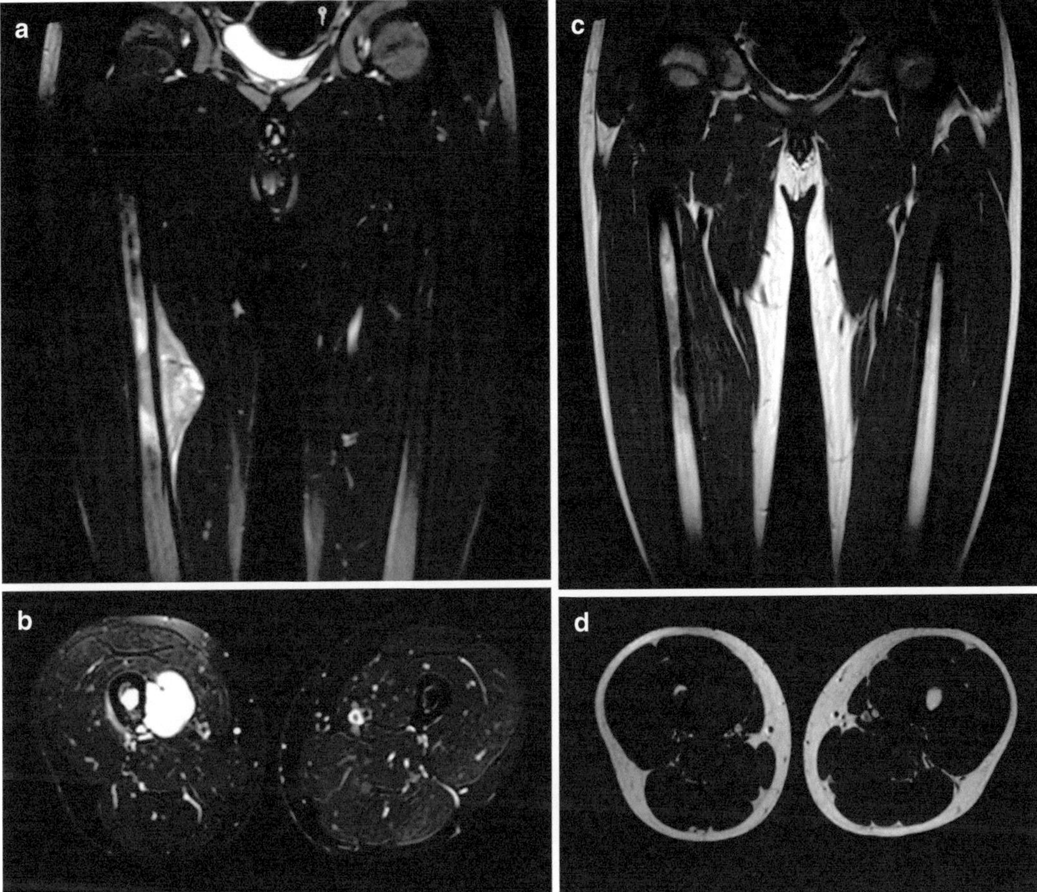

Fig. 3.2 Example of soft tissue sarcoma on contrast-enhanced MRI. A 17-year-old male presenting with right mid-thigh mass. (**a**) Coronal T2 w/ fat saturation: heterogenous predominantly exophytic soft tissue mass of the right femoral diaphysis. (**b**) Axial T2 w/ fat saturation: contrast enhancing predominantly exophytic soft tissue mass of the right femoral diaphysis with invasion of the vastus medialis. There is also ill-defined marrow enhancement centrally along with periosteal breakthrough centrally. (**c**) Coronal T1: non-enhancement of the central marrow enhancement on T2. (**d**) Axial T1: non-enhancement of the predominately exophytic right femoral diaphysis mass

age positron energy is 0.25 MeV and the average positron range 0.6 mm.

PET imaging uses a ring of scintillation detectors surrounding the patient to capture the paired annihilation photons. If the photons are detected within a coincidence window, approximately 4–6 nanoseconds, it is deemed that two photons are from the same annihilation event. A line joining the two detectors is drawn which creates a line of response (LOR), and it is assumed that the radioactive tracer is located somewhere along the LOR. However, the actual location of the annihilation along the line is ultimately unknown. This process is referred to as "coincidence detection" and has at least a 100-fold increase in sensitivity compared to conventional nuclear medicine imaging and higher image quality than single photon emission computed tomography (SPECT). The raw PET data is reconstructed into cross-sectional images with analytical image reconstruction methods such as filtered back projection (FBP) or iterative image reconstruction methods. Current PET systems use iterative reconstruction methods to reduce image noise and allow for incorporation of corrections for photon attenuation and scatter, random coincidences, dead

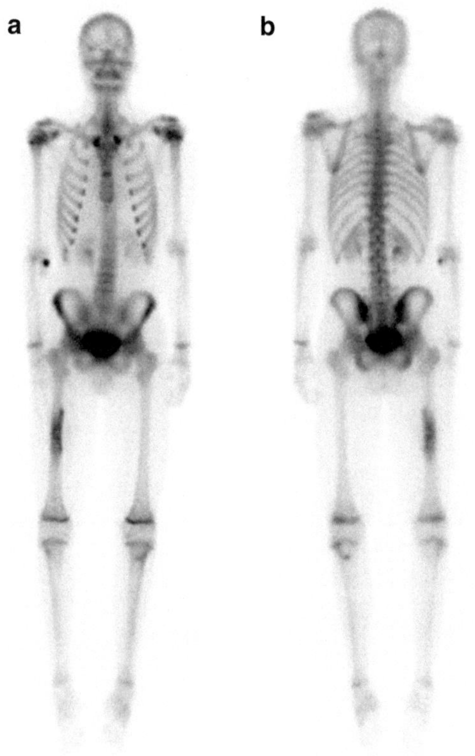

Fig. 3.3 Example of soft tissue sarcoma with skeletal involvement on Tc-99m HDP whole-body bone scan. ((**a**) Anterior planar, (**b**) posterior planar) Increased radiotracer uptake in the mid right femoral diaphysis corresponding to known lesion. No additional sites of abnormal uptake to suggest metastatic disease

time, and scanner-specific characteristics. With advances in technology such as faster computers and improved scintillation crystals, a new technique has been developed called time of flight (TOF). TOF can measure the relative differences in the arrival times of the two photons which allows for a more precise localization of the annihilation event. With TOF, the timing resolution is decreased to 500–600 ps, allowing for the annihilation event to be localized within 7–9 mm along the LOR. The use of newer silicon-based detectors allows for even further decrease in the timing resolution, to 200–400 ps, which improves the localization to within 3–5 mm along the LOR. These newer silicon-based detector materials are increasingly replacing the photomultiplier tubes in newer-generation PET scanners. This improved estimation of the origin of the annihila-

tion decreases image noise and improves spatial resolution [1].

The collected raw data from the PET scan includes random and scattered events in addition to the true coincident events. Photons can also be absorbed, or attenuated, before they reach the detectors, which results in the loss of true events. These components need to be accounted for and corrected in order to produce a more accurate scan.

Attenuation occurs as the photons pass through the different tissue densities. For example, photons emitted from tissues deep in the abdomen or pelvis are much more likely to be attenuated, absorbed, or deflected by the tissue they pass through, than photons emitted from tissues in the chest or superficial areas. To account for these differences in attenuation and resulting differences in photon detection, attenuation correction has to be applied. This was originally accomplished by rotating a Ge-68 source around the patient to measure the attenuation with an actual radioactive source of the same energy. Since the development of the hybrid PET/CT, a CT transmission scan is used to measure the attenuation in different tissues, by using averaged CT x-ray energy of approximately 70 keV. The measured attenuation is then scaled and applied to the PET data to correct for attenuation experienced by photons with an energy of 511 keV [1].

Instrumentation of PET Scanners

The photons are emitted from the site of annihilation of radiotracer in all directions. A conventional PET scanner is comprised of many, up to 35,000 in the current systems, individual detectors arranged in a circular geometry, creating a ring around the patient. Each detector is in a coincidence time window with multiple opposing detectors, creating a fan distribution of LORs. Early systems used a single ring to image one section at a time, approximately 2 cm in the axial length [2]. Subsequent systems used multiple detector rings coupled together to create a cylindrical geometry around the FOV, typically covering 15–22 cm in the axial length. Early

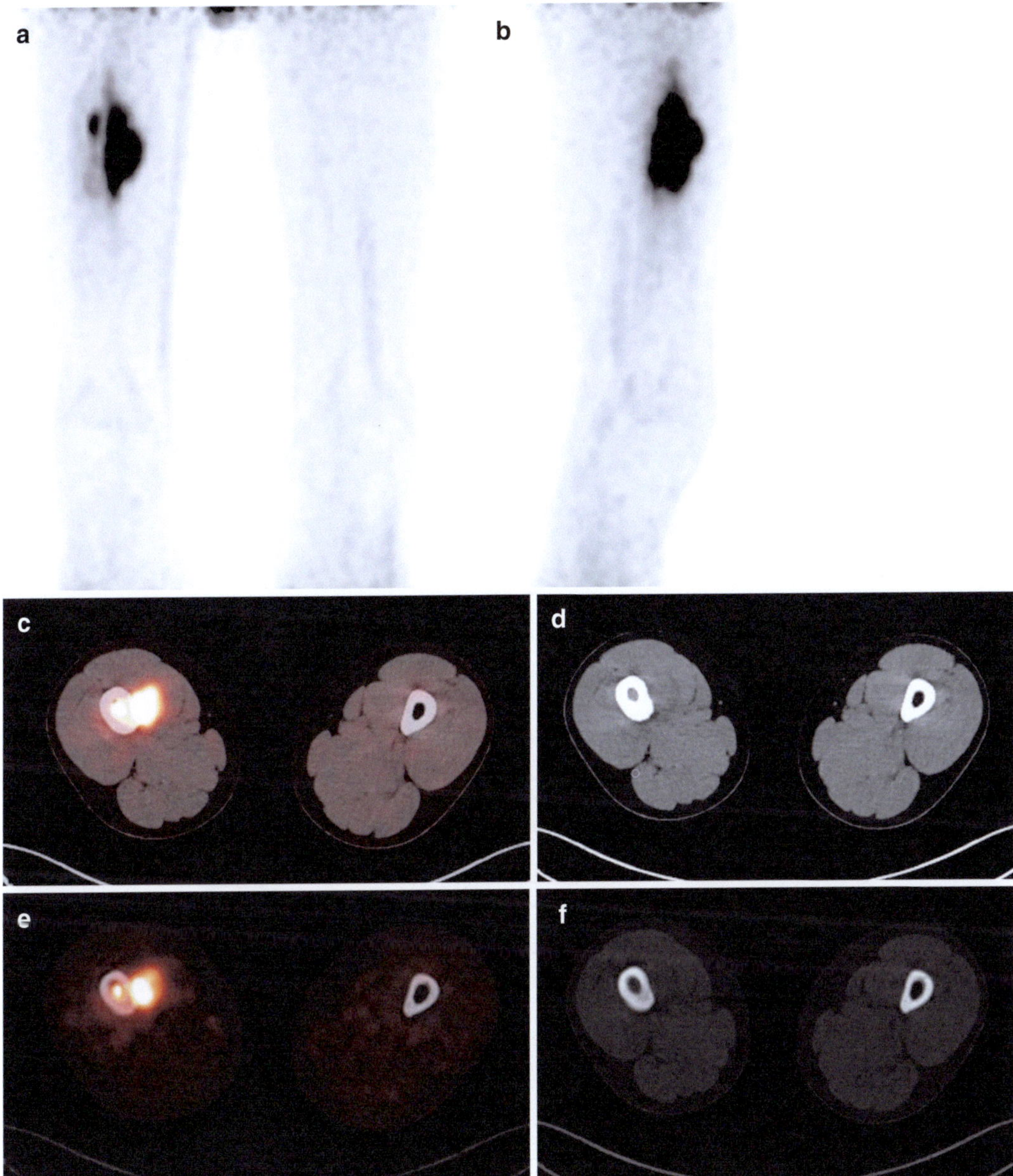

Fig. 3.4 Example of soft tissue sarcoma on F-18 FDG PET/CT. Limited field of view F-18 FDG PET/CT of previous patient showing right proximal femoral diaphyseal medial cortex with associated periosteal reaction and associated soft tissue component extending into the vastus medialis which is markedly FDG avid. (**a**) Anterior maximal intensity projection (MIP) image. (**b**) Right lateral (MIP). (**c**, **d**) Soft tissue window axial fused and axial CT images. (**e**, **f**) Bone window axial fused and axial CT images

forms of these subsequent systems used septa made of absorptive materials, such as tungsten or lead, between the rings to reduce errors caused by intraplane scatter and crosstalk. The systems that used septa were denoted as two-dimensional (2D) systems. Modern PET scanners do not use septa (denoted as 3D systems) and have increased the number of detector rings which cover approximately 25–30 cm in the axial length. An even newer model, the EXPLORER,

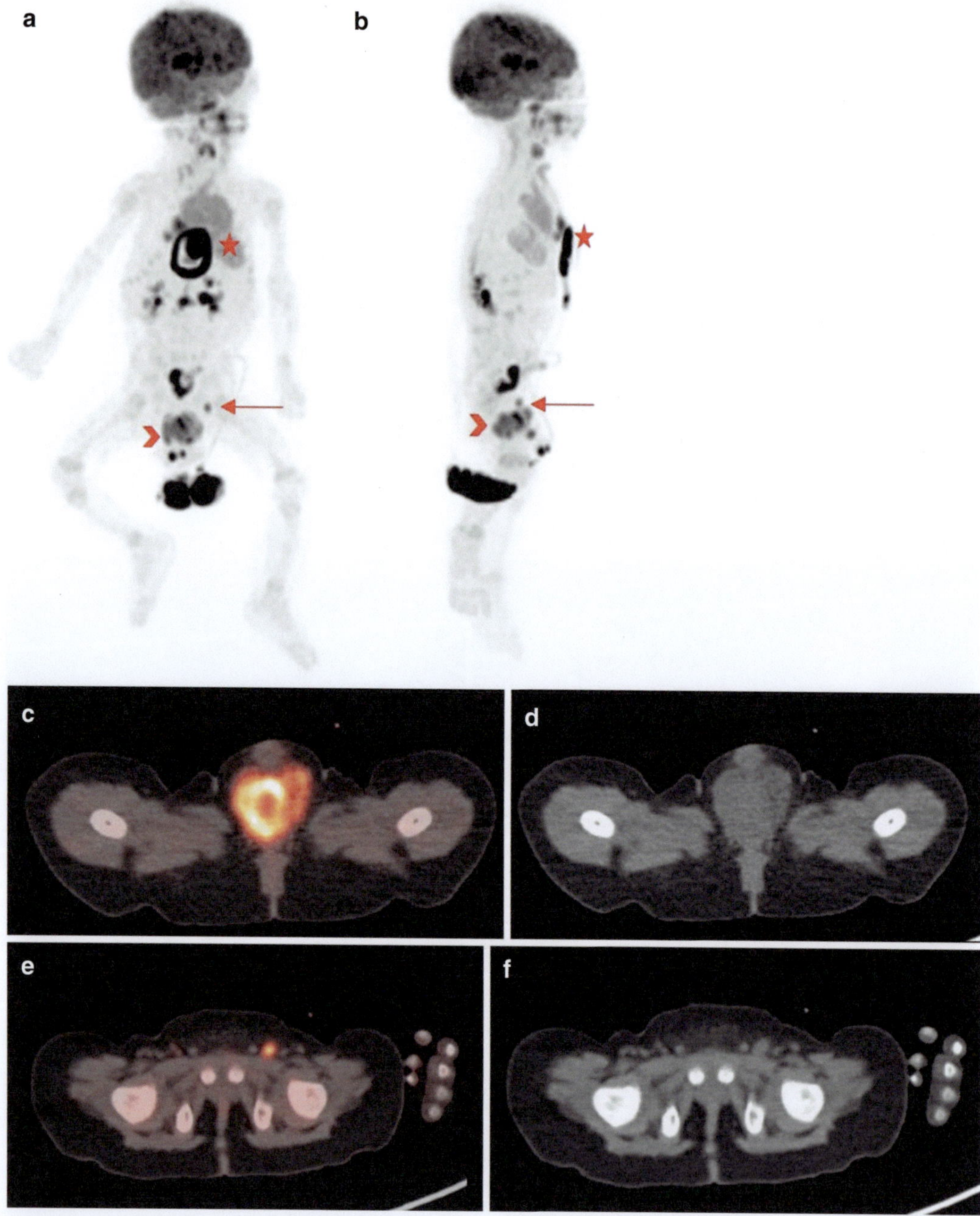

Fig. 3.5 Example of soft tissue sarcoma F-18 FDG PET/CT. A 4-month-old male with rhabdomyosarcoma. (**a, b**) MIP images anterior and right lateral illustrating heterogenous mass at the base of the penis (arrowhead) along with a hypermetabolic left inguinal lymph node suspicious for metastatic disease (arrow). The circular uptake overlying the anterior chest (star) is a port with injection tubing. (**c, d**) Axial fused and low-dose non-contrast CT images of the heterogenous soft tissue mass at the base of the penis. (**e, f**) Axial fused and low-dose non-contrast CT images of the hypermetabolic left inguinal lymph node

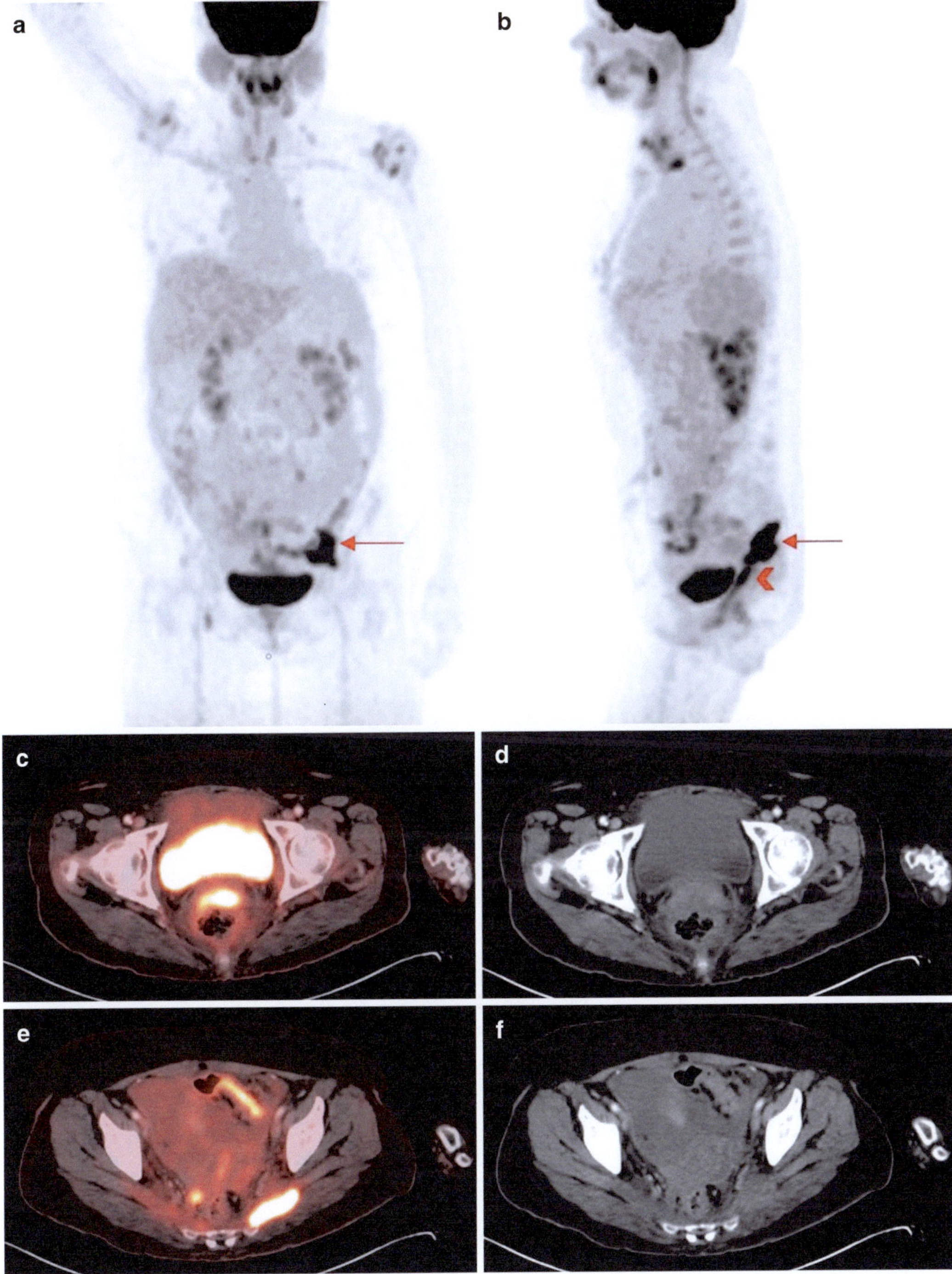

Fig. 3.6 Example of soft tissue sarcoma on F-18 FDG PET/CT. A 54-year-old female with angiosarcoma of the cervix. (**a**, **b**) Anterior and left lateral MIP images illustrating hypermetabolic focus posterior to the bladder (arrowhead) and hypermetabolic soft tissue mass in the left gluteal region (arrow). (**c**, **d**) Axial fused and low-dose non-contrast CT showing increased F-18 FDG uptake in the left aspect of the cervix, consistent with biopsy-proven angiosarcoma of the cervix. (**e**, **f**) Axial fused and low-dose non-contrast CT showing hypermetabolic soft tissue mass in the left gluteal musculature suspicious for metastatic disease

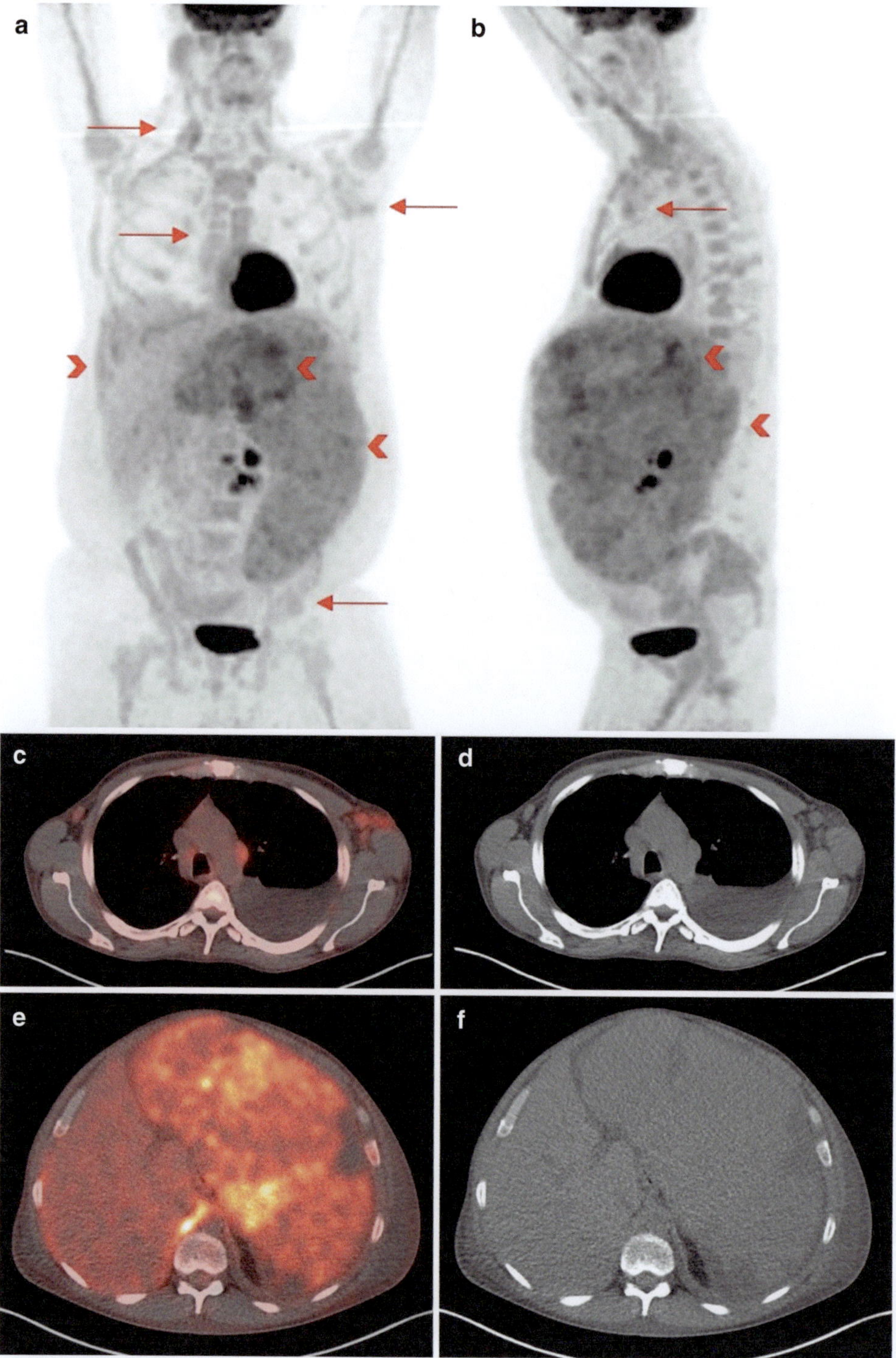

Fig. 3.7 Example of soft tissue sarcoma F-18 FDG PET/CT. A 47-year-old male with left axillary biopsy-proven myeloid sarcoma. (**a, b**) Anterior and left lateral MIP images illustrating mildly to moderately avid cervical, axillary, mediastinal, abdominopelvic, and inguinal adenopathy (arrow) and massive hepatosplenomegaly with multifocal increased uptake in the spleen (arrowhead). (**c, d**) Axial fused and low-dose non-contrast CT showing the mild to moderately avid axillary and mediastinal lymph nodes. Also non-FDG-avid left pleural effusion. (**e, f**) Axial fused and low-dose non-contrast CT showing massive hepatosplenomegaly with multifocal areas of increased FDG uptake in the spleen along with photopenic areas suggesting splenic infarcts

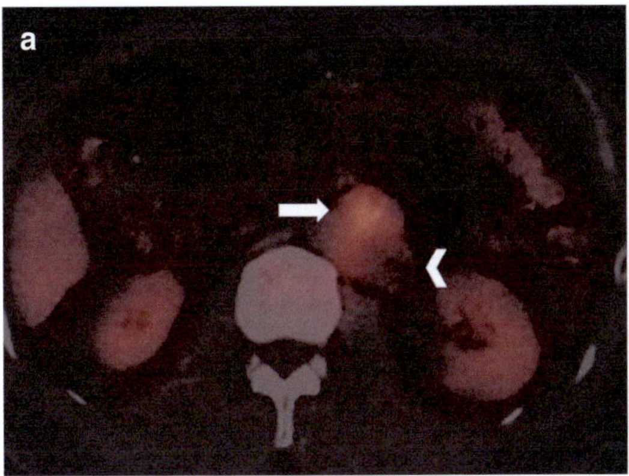

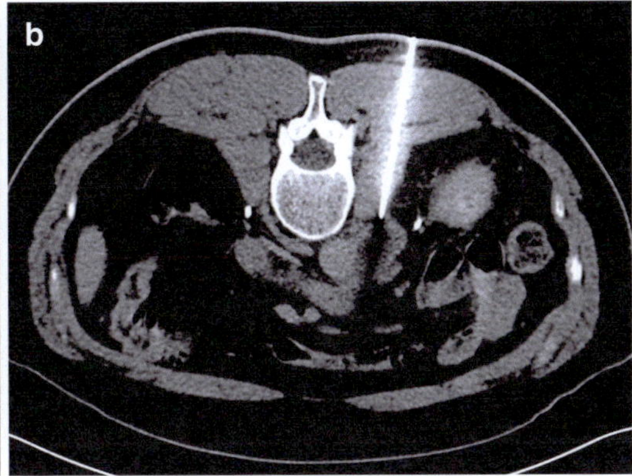

Fig. 3.8 Example of the utility of PET/CT in biopsy guidance. Patient with left flank pain. Malignancy in the left paraspinal mass was suspected based on CT. PET/CT was requested to assess any spread of the disease. On PET/CT, the anterior portion of the tumor was FDG-avid (arrow), while the posterior portion was not (arrowhead) (**a**). CT-guided core biopsy was negative for malignancy. Upon side-by-side review of PET and biopsy CT, it became apparent that the biopsy was taken from the non-FDG-avid portion (**b**). A repeat biopsy from the FDG-avid portion revealed malignant spindle call neoplasm, favoring sarcomatoid carcinoma. Patient underwent radiation followed by surgery

is comprised of 560,000 individual detectors covering an axial FoV of 2 m [3]. 3D systems have much higher sensitivity, approximately by a factor of 4–5, but also have a higher Compton scatter contribution (increased from approximately 10–15% to 30–40%) and random events [4]. With the improvement of computers, scatter correction algorithms, and newer and faster detectors, these increased errors can be corrected.

The detector components of a PET scanner have undergone evolution over time, particularly in the material of the scintillation crystals and the light-detecting component. The material used in the crystal impacts the image quality in the following ways: size of the individual crystal blocks, density for stopping power and thus sensitivity, light yield (number of light photons created per MeV), operating speed, and decay time. Early scintillation crystals were made of bismuth germanate oxide ($Bi_4Ge_3O_{12}$ or BGO) and cerium-doped gadolinium oxyorthosilicate ($Gd_2SiO_5(Ce)$ or GSO), which have high densities for stopping power but very low light yield and a long decay time specifically with the BGO crystals. Newer crystals comprised of cerium-doped lutetium oxyorthosilicate ($Lu_2SiO_5(Ce)$ or LSO) and cerium-doped lutetium yttrium orthosilicate ($Lu_2SiO_5(Ce)$ or LYSO) combine high density, significantly lower decay times, and increased light yield. These newer crystals allow for high counting rates and time-of-flight imaging. The size of the individual crystal blocks impacts the overall spatial resolution, for example, a $4 \times 4 \times 20$ mm LSO crystal has an axial resolution of 4.5 mm at 1 cm versus a $6.3 \times 6.3 \times 30$ mm BGO crystal with an axial resolution of 5.1 mm at 1 cm, both using photomultiplier tubes as the front-end interfaces.

Along with the improvements of the crystals in the detectors, there have also been improvements in the electronic interfaces with the crystals. More modern PET scanners use smaller silicon digital photomultipliers (SiPMs) or avalanche photodiodes and have been deemed "digital" PET scanners. The use of these new interfaces results in essentially a one-to-one interface between the photomultipliers and the crystals, in contrast to older PET scanners that have multiple crystals to one photomultiplier tube. The SiPMs also have a very good intrinsic timing resolution, approximately 44 ps, which is well suited for use with TOF, improving sensitivity, image resolution, and count rate. The spatial resolution is also improved to be less than 4 mm with the use of these new SiPMs when coupled with some of the smaller crystals such as the $4 \times 4 \times 20$–22 mm^3 LSO and LYSO crystals.

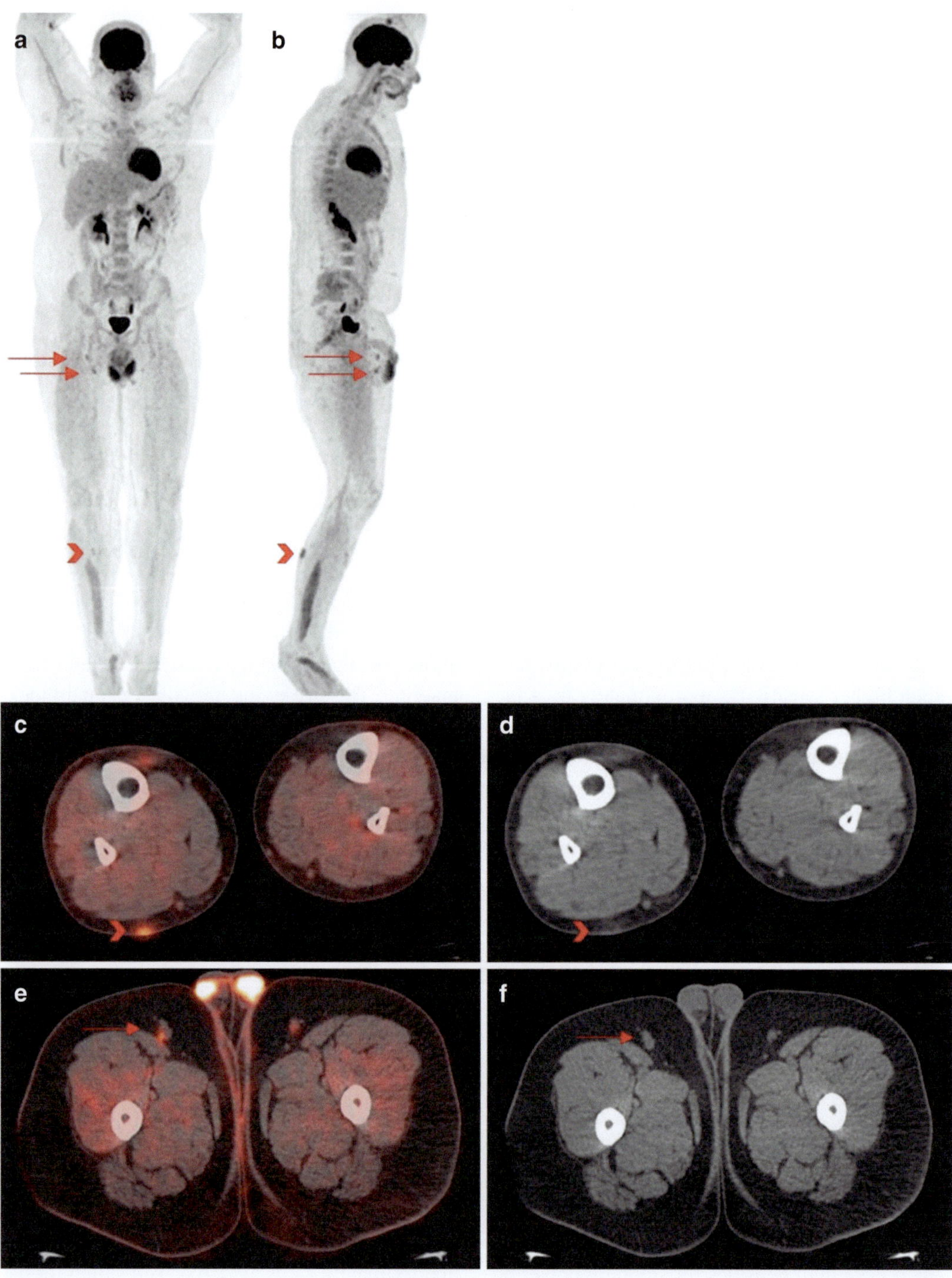

Fig. 3.9 Example of cutaneous malignant melanoma primary site in right lower extremity with lymph node metastasis. (**a, b**) Anterior and right lateral MIP images showing increased FDG uptake in the posterior right lower extremity (arrowhead) and two foci of increased FDG uptake in the right inguinal region (arrow). (**c, d**) Axial fused and low-dose non-contrast CT of the right lower extremity localizing the abnormal FDG uptake to thickening of the cutaneous right posterior calf (arrowhead), consistent with biopsy-proven malignancy. (**e, f**) Axial fused and low-dose non-contrast CT of the right inguinal region showing one of the two hypermetabolic right inguinal lymph nodes (arrow), which were excised and confirmed metastatic

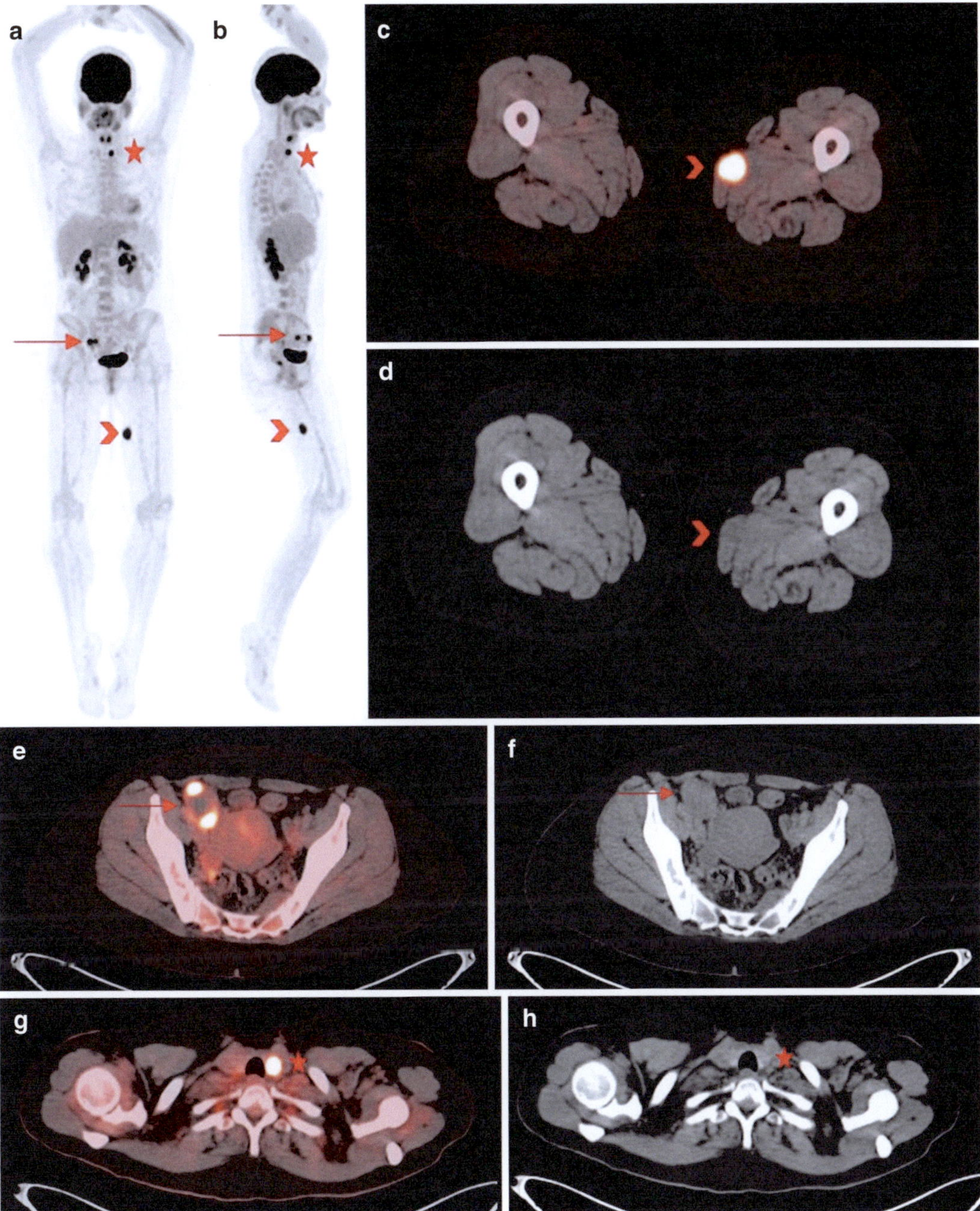

Fig. 3.10 Example of metastatic cutaneous melanoma status post surgical resection of primary site in the right lower calf 1 year prior. (**a**, **b**) Anterior and right lateral MIP images illustrating focal increase in FDG uptake in the left lower neck (star), right aspect of the pelvis (arrow), and medial aspect of the left lower extremity (arrowhead). (**c**, **d**) Axial fused and low-dose non-contrast CT of the left lower extremity focus corresponding to an ill-defined slightly hypodense lesion abutting the left abductor mus-cle of the left mid-thigh (arrowhead), proven metastatic disease from core biopsy. (**e**, **f**) Axial fused and low-dose non-contrast CT of the pelvis showing the hypermetabolic focus localizing to an enlarged centrally necrotic right external iliac lymph node (arrow), which was confirmed as metastatic after excision. (**g**, **h**) Axial fused and low-dose non-contrast CT of the lower neck localizing the focal uptake to a left lower thyroid lobe nodule (star), proven to be papillary thyroid cancer after excision

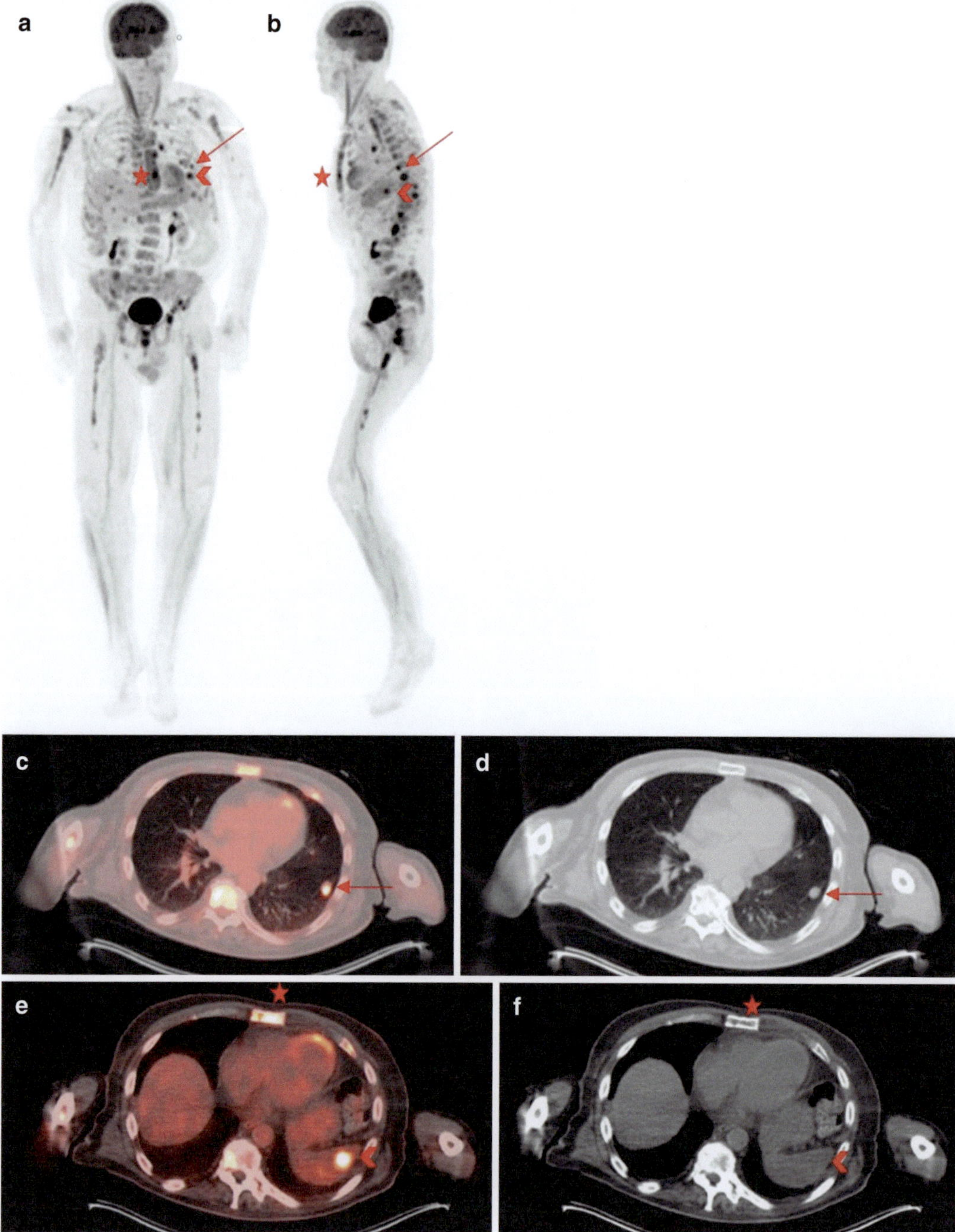

Fig. 3.11 Example of metastatic cutaneous melanoma status post excision of posterior right shoulder primary site 2 years prior. (**a**, **b**) Anterior and left lateral MIP images depicting widespread metastatic disease with abnormal focal FDG uptake throughout the appendicular/axial skeleton (star), mediastinum, lung (arrow), spleen (arrowhead), and liver. (**c**, **d**) Axial fused and low-dose non-contrast CT of the thorax illustrating a hypermetabolic left lower lobe metastatic pulmonary nodule (arrow). (**e**, **f**) Axial fused and low-dose non-contrast CT of the upper abdomen showing a hypermetabolic hypodense splenic lesion (arrowhead) and osseous lesion in the sternum (star)

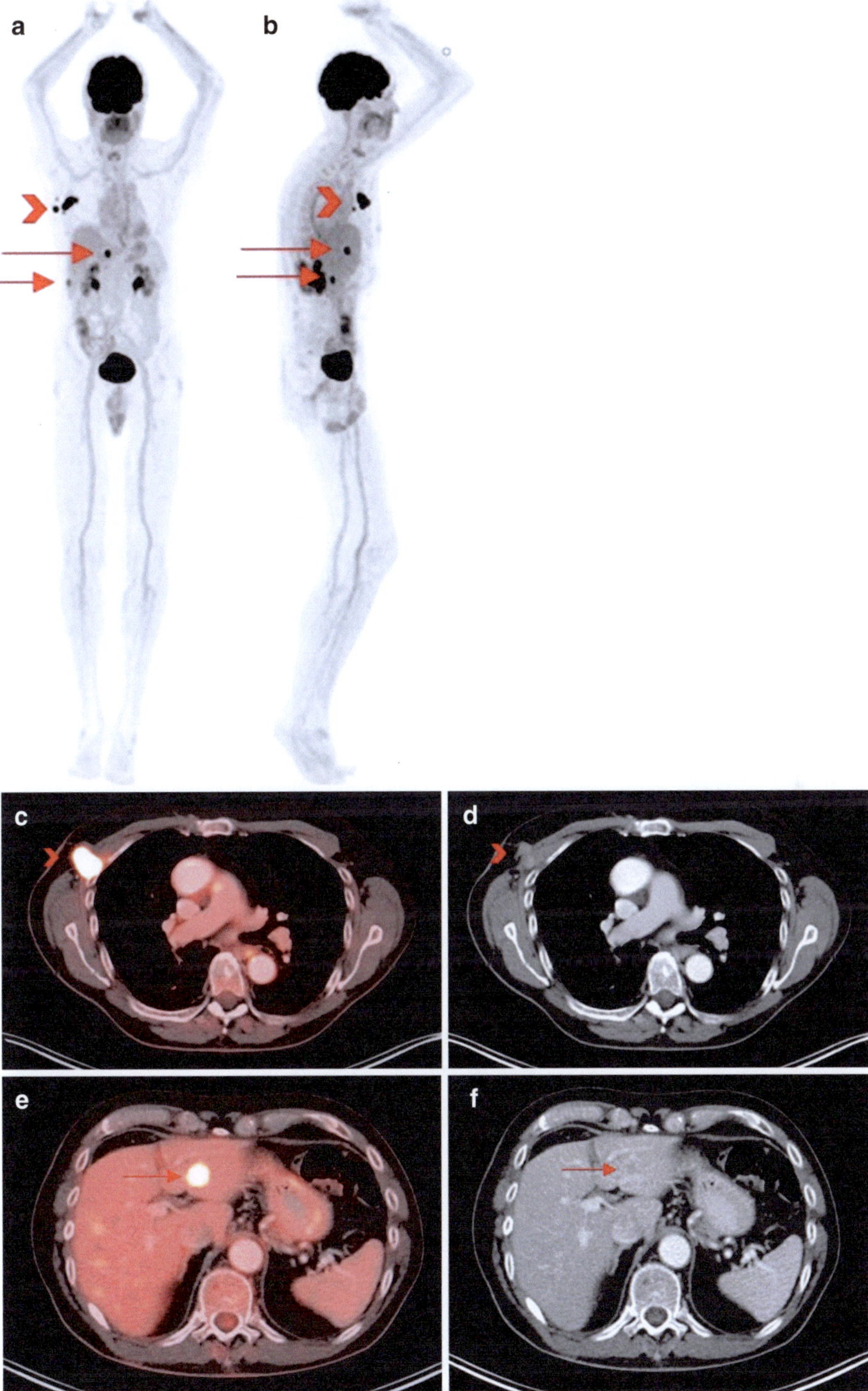

Fig. 3.12 Example of metastatic cutaneous malignant melanoma. (**a, b**) Anterior and right posterior oblique MIP images showing increased FDG uptake in the right axial/subpectoral region (arrowhead) and multiple foci in the right upper quadrant of the abdomen (arrows). (**c, d**) Axial fused and contrast-enhanced CT showing enlarged and hypermetabolic right axillary/subpectoral lymph nodes. (**e, f**) Axial fused and contrast-enhanced CT localizing one of the hypermetabolic foci in the right upper quadrant of the abdomen to a peripherally enhancing left hepatic lobe, biopsy-proven metastatic disease

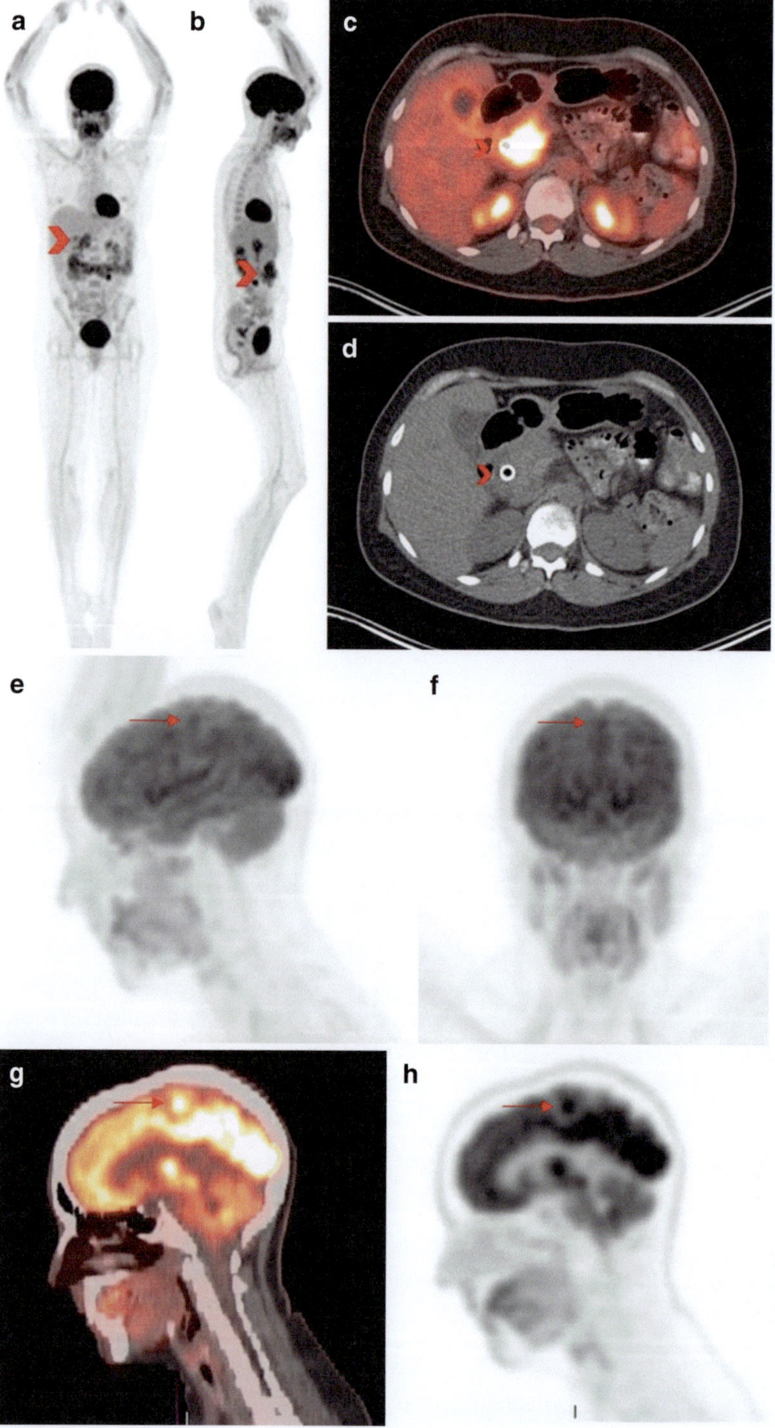

Fig. 3.13 Example of metastatic cutaneous malignant melanoma. (**a**, **b**) Anterior and right lateral MIP images illustrating abnormal increase in FDG uptake medial to the liver (arrowhead). (**c**, **d**) Axial fused and low-dose non-contrast CT showing hypermetabolic pancreatic head mass with biliary stent (arrowhead). (**e**, **f**) Left lateral and anterior MIP images showing a very subtle increased FDG uptake in the superior medial left frontal lobe (arrow). (**g**, **h**) Sagittal fused and PET-only images localizing subtle focus of increased FDG uptake to the left frontal lobe vertex (arrow), which corresponds to enhancing lesion on prior MRI

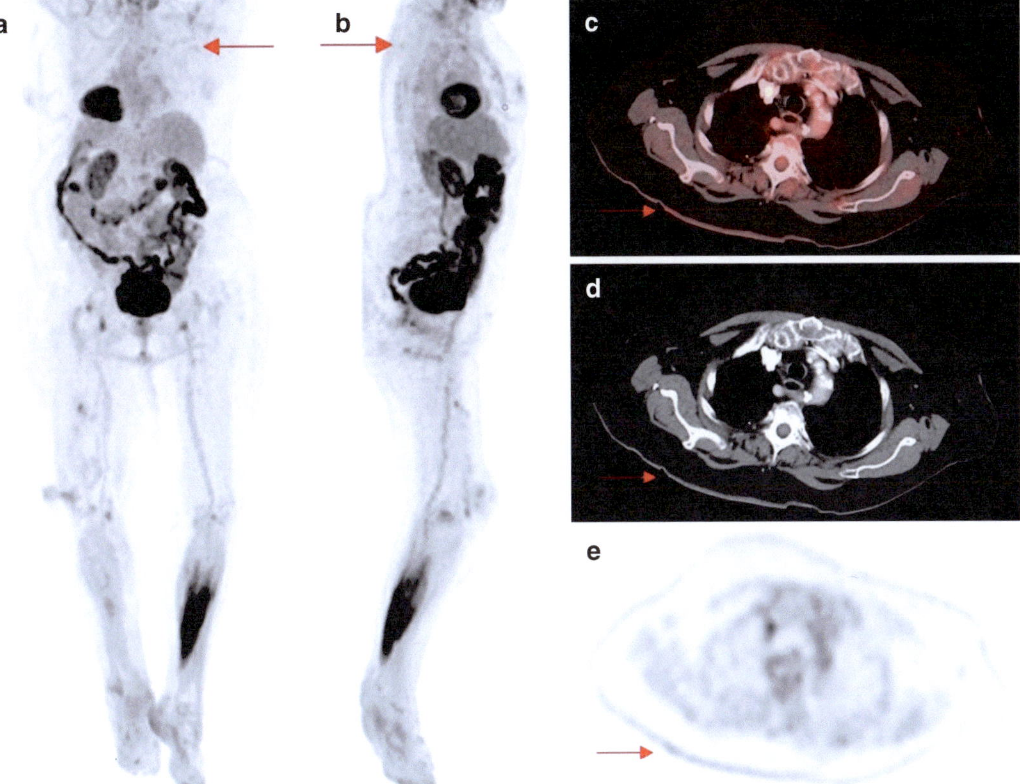

Fig. 3.14 Example of microscopic melanoma deposits on F-18 FDG PET/CT. (**a, b**) Posterior and right lateral MIP images showing F-18 FDG activity similar to surrounding cutaneous activity in the upper right back. (**c, d**) Axial fused and low-dose non-contrast CT of the upper right back showing the FDG activity similar to surrounding tissue and no abnormal CT correlation. (**e**) Axial PET-only image reillustrating similar FDG activity in this area to surrounding tissue. This area was proven to have microscopic malignant melanoma post-excisional biopsy

Computed Tomography Component of PET/CT

Attenuation correction (AC) has been incorporated into PET scanning since the development and use of the first scanners. The original AC used a radionuclide transmission rod source of Ge-68 to generate a photon attenuation map by directly mapping the attenuation of 511 keV photons from the Ge-68 source. More recently, CT scans have been used to generate linear attenuation coefficients (LACs). The LAC for 511 keV photons is generated by converting the measured LAC for 60–80 keV x-rays from the CT scan using a bilinear scaling to correspond to the LAC from PET 511 keV photons [5] (Fig. 3.15). The combination of modern CT with PET systems produced a hybrid system, which offered several advantages over the transmission rod source system – such as low-noise attenuation maps, quicker acquisitions, and removal of artifacts from contamination from post-injection transmission scans. With these advantages also came disadvantages, such as higher radiation doses, artifact from metallic implants, and misalignment artifacts from patient movement/respiration. Recent methods to address these new disadvantages include automatic registration of the CT to the PET and averaging the cine CT data acquisition over a respiration cycle [4].

The number of detector rows in a CT can vary from 16 to 320 slices. In the early 2000s, there was a trend to increase the number of detector rows, which, it was thought, would provide faster

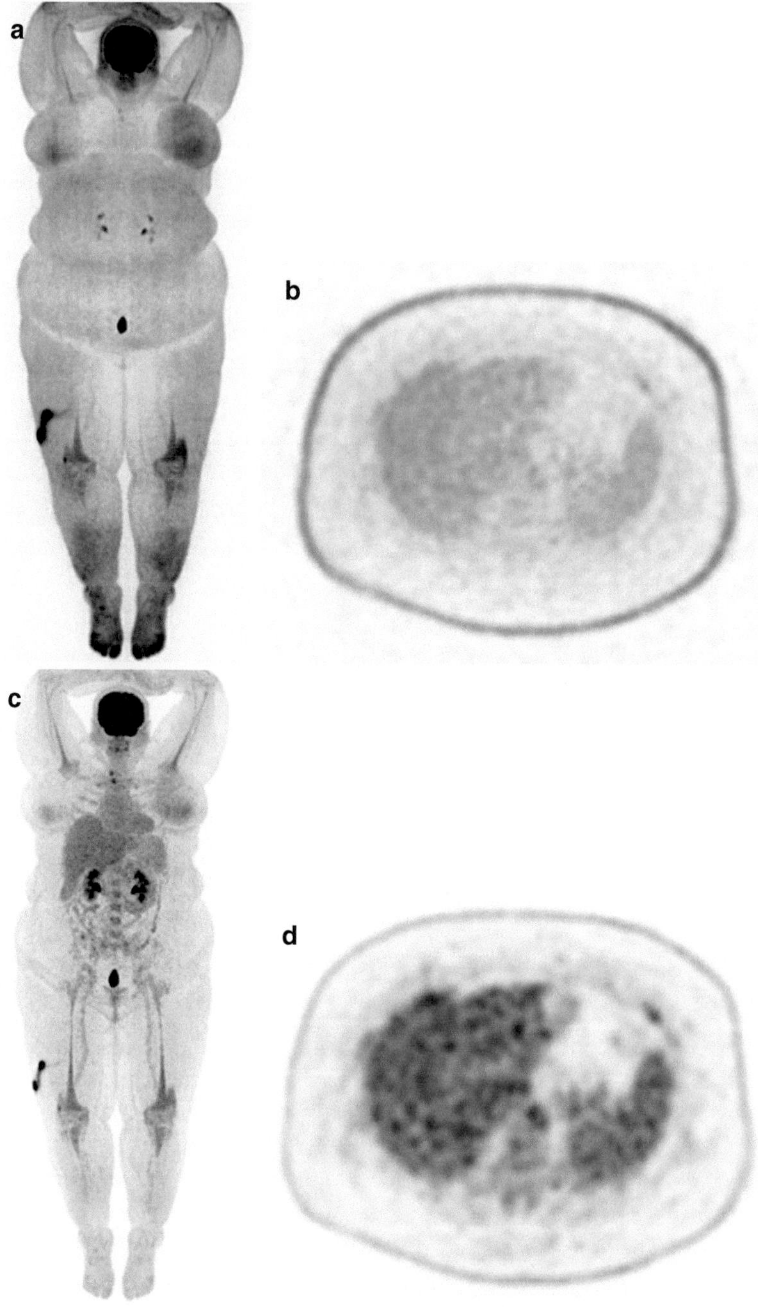

Fig. 3.15 Example of a non-attenuation-corrected PET acquisition: (**a**) anterior MIP image and (**b**) axial image at the level of the liver. This illustrates the increased radiotracer activity in the skin, diffuse mild uptake in the subcutaneous fat, and decreased resolution of the liver and spleen. Example of an attenuation-corrected PET acquisition: (**c**) anterior MIP image and (**d**) axial image at the level of the liver. This illustrates correction of the overestimated radiotracer activity in the skin and subcutaneous fat and improved resolution of the liver and spleen

scan times. However, it was found that with the increase in detector rows, there were also disadvantages, including increased scattered radiation exposure, decreased contrast, and potential artifacts. The number of detector rows in the CT component of modern PET/CT scanners can vary from 16 to 160 with a z-coverage of 9–60 mm, resulting in multi-slice CT/multi-detector CT (MSCT/MDCT). Today, the use of a 64–128-slice detectors is adequate for standard CT imaging studies.

It is well-known that diagnostic CT offers high diagnostic detail, but at the cost of using ionizing radiation. Early diagnostic CT scanners, introduced in the 1970s, delivered an average effective dose per examination of 1.3 mSv, mostly due to low x-ray tube power, and the scan was limited to the brain. This dose level increased through the 1980s and into the mid-1990s, with average effective dose per examination reaching up to 8.8 mSv. This increase was due to the introduction of whole-body scans, increased x-ray tube power, and spiral CT angiography [6]. In the late 1990s and early 2000s, decreasing the radiation dose levels to patients became an important focus, and many developments were implemented, such as tube current modulation, x-ray spectra optimization, x-ray beam collimation, iterative image reconstruction, more efficient x-ray detectors, and continuous bed motion. These implementations can decrease the dose to the patient by 5–60%, each.

The tube current modulation and tube voltage modulation have been an important aspect of diagnostic CT for many years and have also become an important component in modern PET/CT scanners. Tube current modulation automatically adapts the tube current to the size and shape of the patient and the density of the scanned region to minimize radiation exposure. A scout or topogram, image is acquired prior to the attenuation or diagnostic CT to allow the computer to determine the automatic exposure. With the use of automatic exposure controls, a low-dose non-enhanced CT from skull base to mid-thigh will expose a patient to an effective dose of approximately 2.9–7.2 mSv, with variance due to patient gender and size. This contrasts with a higher-dose diagnostic quality CT from skull base to mid-thigh performed with IV and oral contrast, in which the effective dose is approximately 5.4–27.8 mSv [7].

Utility of Diagnostic Quality CT with IV and/or Oral Contrast (CECT) in PET/CECT

The utility of a diagnostic quality standard-dose CT in PET/CT comes from the added morphological detail which improves detection of anatomical changes. The added morphological detail results in (1) improved delineation of anatomic structures, (2) increased sensitivity for detection of pathologic lesions, and (3) improved accuracy in lesion characterization [8]. The increased morphological detail from a diagnostic quality CT acquisition to a PET scan does not improve the resolution, sensitivity, or specificity of the PET portion of the exam. Today, most PET/CT studies use low-dose non-contrast-enhanced CT (NECT) for attenuation correction and limited anatomical information for localization of abnormalities found on the PET images.

With modern PET/CT scanners, a contrast-enhanced diagnostic quality standard-dose CT (CECT) can be acquired. The IV contrast is usually a nonionic iodine-based substance, and the oral contrast can also be an iodine- or barium-based substance. Both provide positive contrast by increasing the attenuation of the CT. Additionally, a negative contrast, water-based contrast agent can be used in oral contrast, which results in distension of the bowel and no changes in the attenuation of the CT [7]. The additional benefits from the use of IV and oral contrast in PET/CECT are (1) detection of isodense lesions on prior non-contrast studies, (2) distinguishing cystic from solid lesions, and (3) evaluation of internal vascularity and vascular invasion [9]. Lesions are detected and characterized by CT based on attenuation differences between the lesion and the adjacent structures. The use of IV contrast increases the attenuation differences between the normal and abnormal tissue allowing for increased detection [10]. Indications for a CECT in conjunction with a PET typically include initial staging studies and/or for a more accurate evaluation of prior incidental findings, such as pulmonary nodules and low-attenuation renal (Fig. 3.16), adrenal, and hepatic lesions [11]. The advantage of more accurate characteristic of prior incidental findings helps to make the proper recommendations and avoids further unnecessary studies or procedures (Fig. 3.17).

The addition of a CECT to a PET scan has its advantages; however, it also brings disadvantages. These disadvantages include the persistent issue of misregistration due to breathing and potential inaccurate attenuation correction due to different x-ray energies from the CT images and

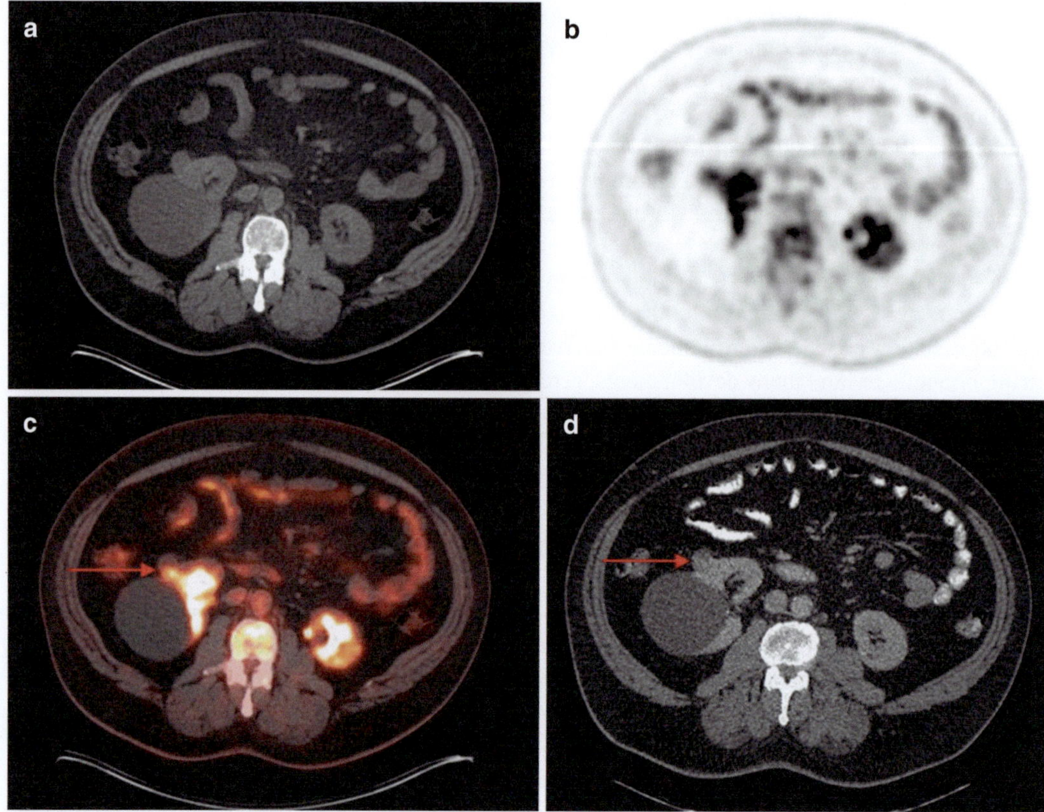

Fig. 3.16 Illustration of biopsy-proven renal cell carcinoma of the right kidney (arrow). (**a**) Axial low-dose non-contrast-enhanced CT showing mildly hypodense lesion. (**b**) Axial PET-only image showing no appreciable abnormal increased F-18 FDG uptake. (**c**) Axial fused F-18 FDG PET/CT image slightly misregistered but no appreciable abnormal uptake. (**d**) Axial standard-dose contrast-enhanced CT in the venous phase showing slight persistent enhancement

the use of high-density IV and oral contrast and contrast reaction from the iodine-based IV contrast [11]. With advancements in technology and software, these disadvantages have been eliminated or reduced and have no significant effects on the diagnostic quality. To reduce the misregistration artifact from breathing, PET/CECT scans can be acquired with suspended respiration at end-tidal volume or respiration gating or "4D PET/CT mode" [4]. The potential inaccurate attenuation correction error from the diagnostic CT images and high-density contrast is due to (1) the conversion difference of 120–140 kVp x-ray energies in the diagnostic CT and (2) overcorrection from the computer based off the increase in the tissue densities from the IV or oral contrast resulting in falsely elevated activity on the PET

images (Figs. 3.18 and 3.19). These errors have been reduced or corrected by new attenuation correction algorithms that can restrict the attenuation correction factor so as not to overcorrect at high radiodensity [11]. As for the potential iodine contrast reactions, patients are screened for prior reactions and premedicated if a prior reaction has occurred. If no prior reaction is documented, the patient is observed for any signs of a reaction, and appropriate steps are taken if the patient begins to show signs of a reaction.

PET/CECT in Soft Tissue Sarcomas The role of CECT for both the diagnosis and the local staging for preoperative planning of STSs has been incompletely assessed [12]. Currently, the utilization of CECT in the evaluation of STSs is reserved

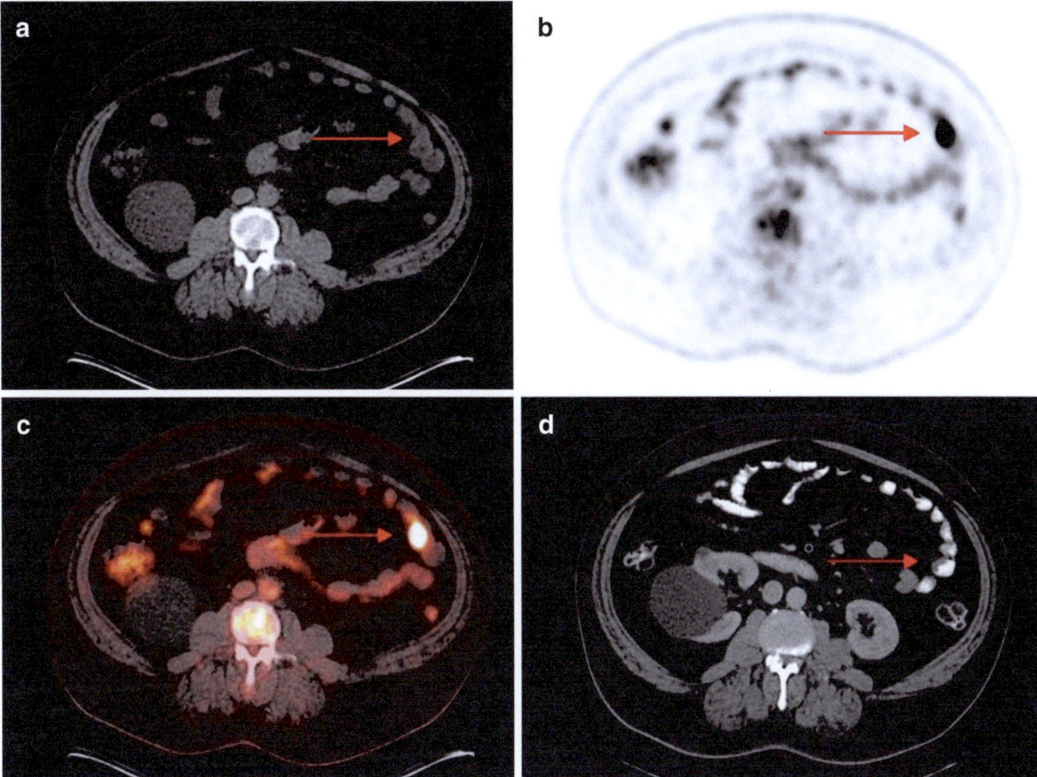

Fig. 3.17 Illustration of an abnormal focus of F-18 FDG uptake in a segment of jejunum biopsy-proven metastatic melanoma. (**a**) Axial low-dose non-contrast-enhanced CT with no evidence of soft tissue abnormality. (**b**) Axial PET-only image showing focal abnormal F-18 FDG uptake in the left aspect of the abdominal cavity. (**c**) Axial fused F-18 FDG PET/CT image localizing the abnormal focal uptake in a segment of jejunum. (**d**) Axial standard-dose contrast-enhanced CT of the abdomen identifying abnormal thickening of the wall in a segment of jejunum

for those who cannot obtain an MRI, which is the gold standard. Similar to the evaluation of metastatic melanoma with a PET/CECT scan, the benefits from the CECT would directly affect the anatomical characterization of the malignancy and not improve the PET portion. The major benefits of CECT in the evaluation of STSs come from the CECT's accuracy in detecting calcification of soft tissue masses, bone details, enhancement patterns along with vascular patterns, and involvement of major vessels from the use of CT angiography. These are all important in diagnosis, in differentiating benign from malignant masses, and in surgical planning, particularly in the pelvis and extremities [12]. However, there is currently a lack of information in the literature evaluating the diagnostic utility of PET/CECT over PET/NECT in the diagnosis and surgical planning of STSs.

PET/CECT in Metastatic Melanoma The use of CT imaging in the evaluation of metastatic melanoma is an important and established modality, especially in the detection of lung metastases. This modality has been proven to be superior to other imaging modalities, such as FDG PET-only scans, and prevents unnecessary surgical procedures. The diagnostic value of combining full-dose contrast-enhanced CT to a PET scan in the evaluation of metastatic melanoma was studied by Pfluger et al. This study compared the sensitivity and specificity of full-dose contrast-enhanced CT (CECT – 145mAs, 120 kV), low-dose non-enhanced CT (NECT – 20 mAs, 140 kV), FDG PET only, PET/NECT, and PET/CECT in metastatic melanoma. This study found that both PET/CECT and PET/NECT outperformed F-18 FDG PET only, CECT, and NECT

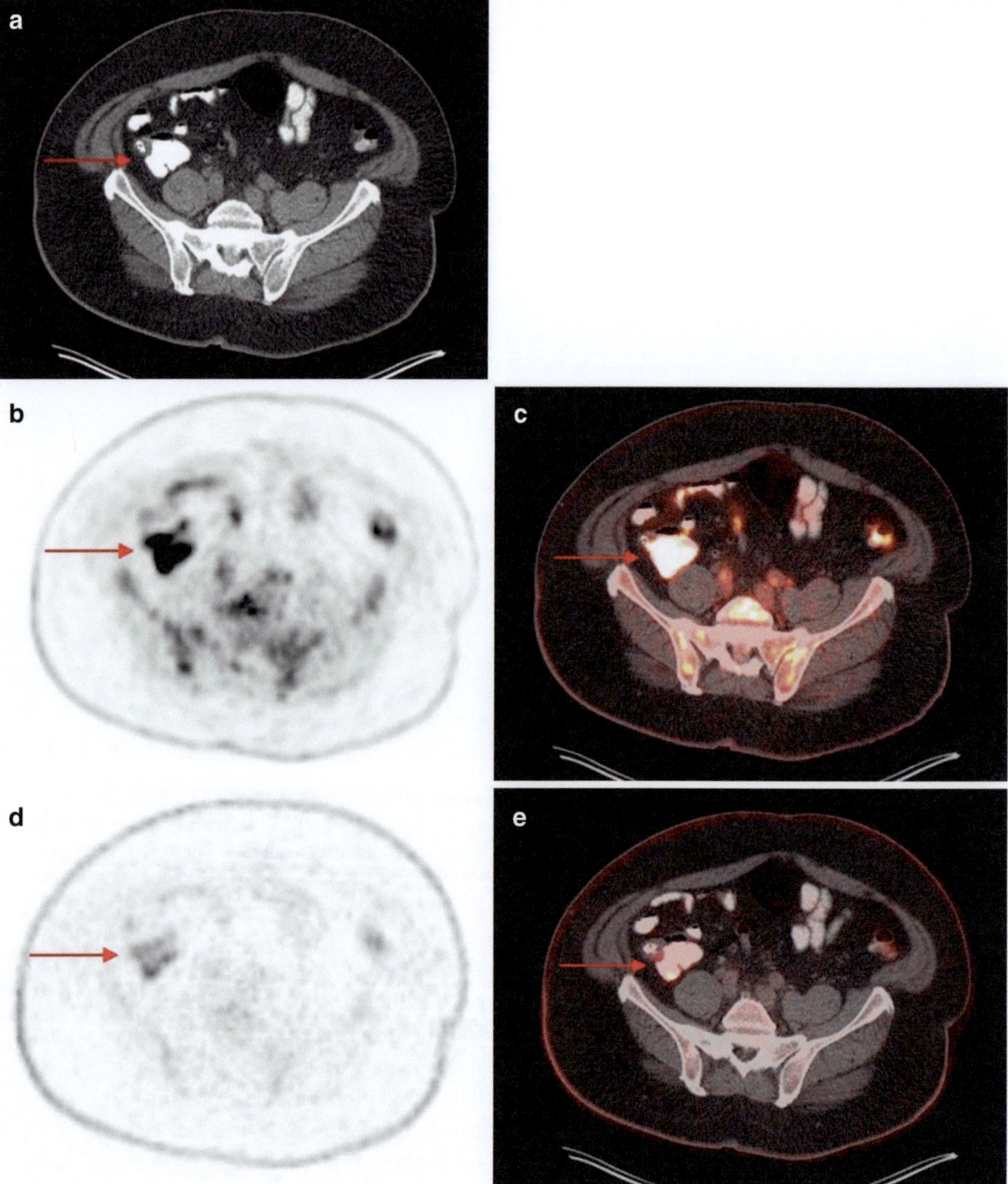

Fig. 3.18 Illustration of computer-generated artifact of attenuation overcorrection due to oral contrast. (**a**) Axial low-dose CT with oral contrast, specifically in the cecum. (**b**) Axial attenuation-corrected PET image showing increased F-18 FDG uptake in the region of the cecum. (**c**) Axial fused PET/CT image localizing the increased F-18 FDG uptake to the cecum. (**d**) Axial non-attenuation-corrected PET image showing minimal F-18 FDG in the region of the cecum. (**e**) Axial fused PET/CT image localizing the minimal F-18 FDG uptake to the cecum

in the detection of lung metastasis. In the evaluation of lymph node metastases, CECT and NECT rely on visible morphological changes and size criteria. This results in an increase in false-negatives in small lymph nodes and false-positives in enlarged lymph nodes. In parenchymal organs such as the liver, NECT has shown significant limitation in detecting lesions, due to a lack of significant attenuation changes which could be accentuated with IV contrast (Figs. 3.20

Fig. 3.19 Example of a F-18 FDG PET/CT with oral contrast. (**a**) Coronal view of an attenuation-corrected PET/CT illustrating an increased FDG activity in the transverse colon with presence of oral contrast. (**b**) Coronal view of a non-attenuation-corrected PET/CT illustrating no increased FDG activity in the transverse colon confirming the computer-generated artifact due to the increased density of the oral contrast

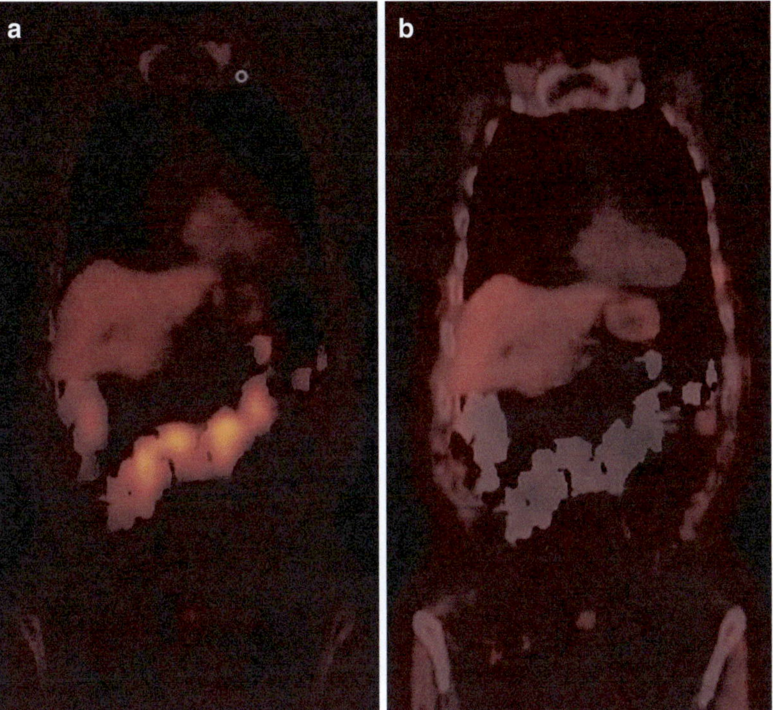

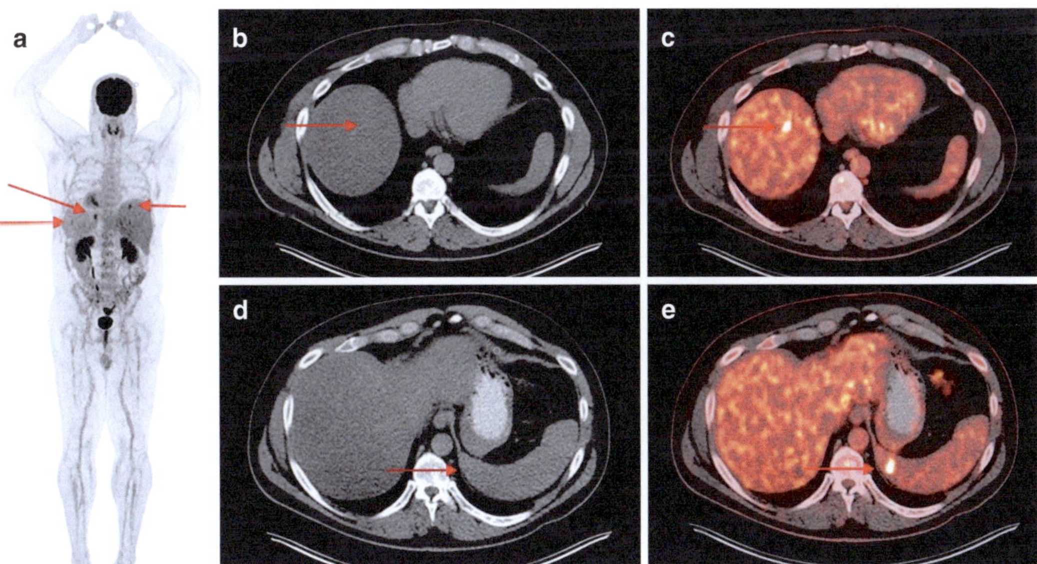

Fig. 3.20 Example of metastatic lesions to the liver and the spleen (arrows). (**a**) Posterior coronal MIP image with abnormal foci of radiotracer uptake in the liver and spleen. (**b**) Axial low-dose non-contrast-enhanced CT showing no appreciable lesion in the liver. (**c**) Axial fused PET/CT image localizing the foci of abnormal uptake in the region of the liver with no CT abnormality. (**d**) Axial low-dose non-contrast-enhanced CT showing no appreciable lesion in the spleen. (**e**) Axial fused PET/CT image localizing the focal radiotracer uptake in the region of the spleen with no abnormal CT findings

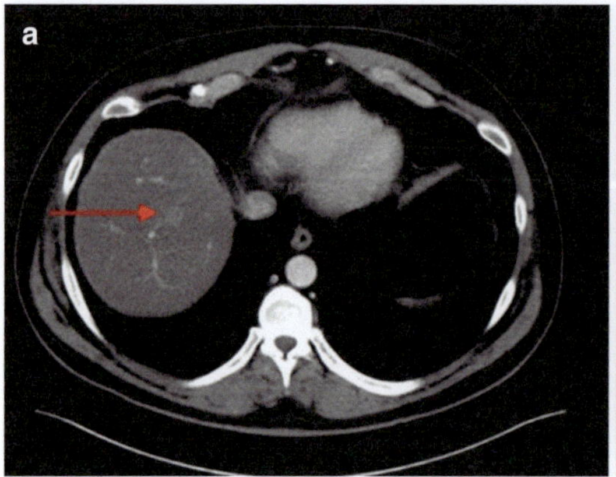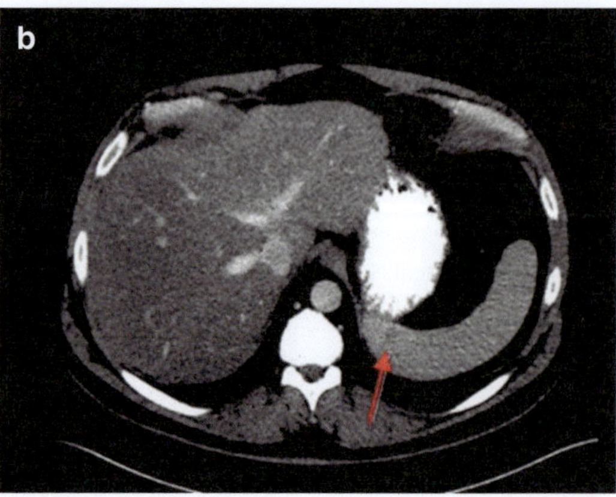

Fig. 3.21 Follow-up contrast-enhanced CT of the previous patient. (**a**) Axial contrast-enhanced standard-dose CT arterial phase identifying the enhancing right hepatic lesion. (**b**) Axial contrast-enhanced standard-dose CT venous phase identifying splenic lesion with mild persistent contrast enhancement

and 3.21). The comparison between PET/NECT and PET/CECT showed a difference in sensitivity of only 3% and no difference in specificity. This difference in sensitivity did not affect the TNM classification. Furthermore, an important advantage of low-dose PET/NECT over PET/CECT is an approximate 60% reduction in radiation exposure. The study concluded that due to the small increase in sensitivity, and no change in the TNM scores, it is justifiable to perform PET/NECT over PET/CECT for the staging of malignant melanoma [13].

Dose of F-18 FDG

In PET/CT the computed tomography component is not the only aspect that delivers radiation to the patient. The radiopharmaceuticals, such as FDG, also contribute to the overall radiation dose to the patient per scan. Consistent with the focus on the reduction of the radiation dose delivered by the CT component, there has also been focus on reducing the administered dose of FDG as well.

Initially, a standardized dose of FDG ranging from 10 to 20 mCi (350–740 MBq) was administered to the patient, which resulted in an effective dose of 0.1 rem per mCi (0.027 mSv per MBq) [14, 15]. As the concern for the effects of the radiation delivered per dose grew, facilities and societies began to develop dose equations

to incorporate factors to help reduce the amount of activity administered. These factors included recommended FDG activity (MBq), bed overlap, time per bed position, and patients' weight. The weight-based dosing algorithm was first initiated to help decrease the radiation doses to the pediatric population but is now used in adult studies by a few societies such as the EANM, SNMMI, and Japanese Society of Nuclear Medicine [16, 17]. In comparison to that of standardized doses, the use of weight-based doses reduced the administered dose by approximately 36.3% [18]. The EANM has adopted weight-based dosing for both adult and pediatric patients.

The EANM suggests using a linear or quadratic relationship weight-based approach and also taking into consideration percentage of bed overlap for the different PET systems.

Linear formulas accounting for bed overlap:

1. Bed overlap <30%: FDG (MBq) = 14 (MBq·min·bed^{-1}·kg^{-1}) × patient weight (kg)/ emission acquisition duration per bed position (min·bed^{-1}).
2. Bed overlap >30%: FDG (MBq) = 14 (MBq·min·bed^{-1}·kg^{-1}) × patient weight (kg)/ emission acquisition duration per bed position (min·bed^{-1}).

Quadratic formulas accounting for bed overlap:

1. Bed overlap <30%: FDG (MBq) = 1050 (MBq·min·bed^{-1}·kg^{-2}) × (patient weight (kg)/75)^2/emission acquisition duration per bed position (min·bed^{-1}).
2. Bed overlap >30%: FDG (MBq) = 525 (MBq·min·bed^{-1}·kg^{-2}) × (patient weight (kg)/75)^2/emission acquisition duration per bed position (min·bed^{-1}) [19].

In the pediatric population, the EANM suggests using the formula 3 MBq/kg for brain and 6 MBq/kg for whole-body imaging [20].

In the United States, the SNMMI has adopted the North American Guidelines for pediatric nuclear medicine imaging which suggests using a dose of 3.7 MBq/kg (0.10 mCi/kg) for brain imaging and 3.7–5.2 MBq/kg (0.10–0.14 mCi/kg) for whole-body oncology studies [21]. As for the adult population in the United States, the SNMMI suggests a dose range of 370–740 MBq (10–20 mCi) [22]. The Japanese Society of Nuclear Medicine suggests a dosing of 3.7 MBq/kg (0.10 mCi/kg) in their adult oncology scans [23]. In our institution we have implemented a weight-based dose of 0.15 mCi/kg in our adult oncology patients. With our pediatric patients, we have implemented the body mass (straight weight basis) formula of FDG = {[weight (kg)/70 (kg)]^0.7}*Adult dose.

Recently, with the development of new hardware and software, there have been investigations into using a body mass index (BMI) formula to further decrease the administered dose of F-18 FDG. In a study conducted by Sanchez-Jurado et al., researchers compared the diagnostic quality and the radiation dose reduction (to both patient and imaging staff) of a BMI-based dosing to that of a weight-based dosing algorithm. The study showed that it is achievable to further reduce the administered FDG dose with a BMI-based dose algorithm without increasing time per bed position. The study calculated a 56.4% and a 12.5% reduction in radiation dose per patient and imaging staff, respectively [24]. However, a BMI-based dose algorithm has not been implemented as the standard protocol to date.

F-18-FDG Dosing in STSs and Malignant Melanoma In the evaluation of malignancies, specifically soft tissue sarcoma and malignant melanoma, there is no indication that an increase in the administered dose will increase the resolution, sensitivity, or specificity of the study. An increase in the administered dose would only increase the overall radiation dose to the patient. For this reason, the current weight-based dose algorithm is the standard of care.

Field of View

Currently, there is no true consensus on a standardized field of view (FOV) in terms of limited whole-body (WB) PET/CT, or on which imaging protocol to implement when evaluating for certain types of cancer. In 2006, the Society of Nuclear Medicine and Molecular Imaging (SNMMI) released their consensus, which illustrated three FOVs. These FOVs included (1) WB, vertex to toes (Fig. 3.22); (2) limited WB, skull base to mid-thigh (Fig. 3.23); and (3) limited area, such as cardiac PET (Fig. 3.24). A similar consensus of FOVs was also released by the European Association of Nuclear Medicine in 2010. Even though the SNM illustrated what they deemed as limited WB FOV, there are many other FOVs used in clinical practice that are identified as limited WB imaging. These other limited FOVs often exclude portions of the head and upper and lower extremities due to presumed lack of clinical benefit, reduction in time, and radiation exposure [25] (Fig. 3.25). The most common versions of limited WB are the skull base to mid-thigh and vertex to upper thighs. Within these versions, various portions of the upper extremities are imaged due to placement of the arms during acquisition. The lower extremities also show variation in the extent of imaging from as proximal as the lesser trochanter to as distal as the knees. The use of whole-body versus limited whole-body PET/CT does have several disadvantages, which include increased radiation exposure, increased acquisition time, patient movement, increased interpretation time, and decreased efficiency of the imaging center.

There have been multiple studies to evaluate for the added benefits of whole-body versus limited whole-body PET/CT. A study conducted by

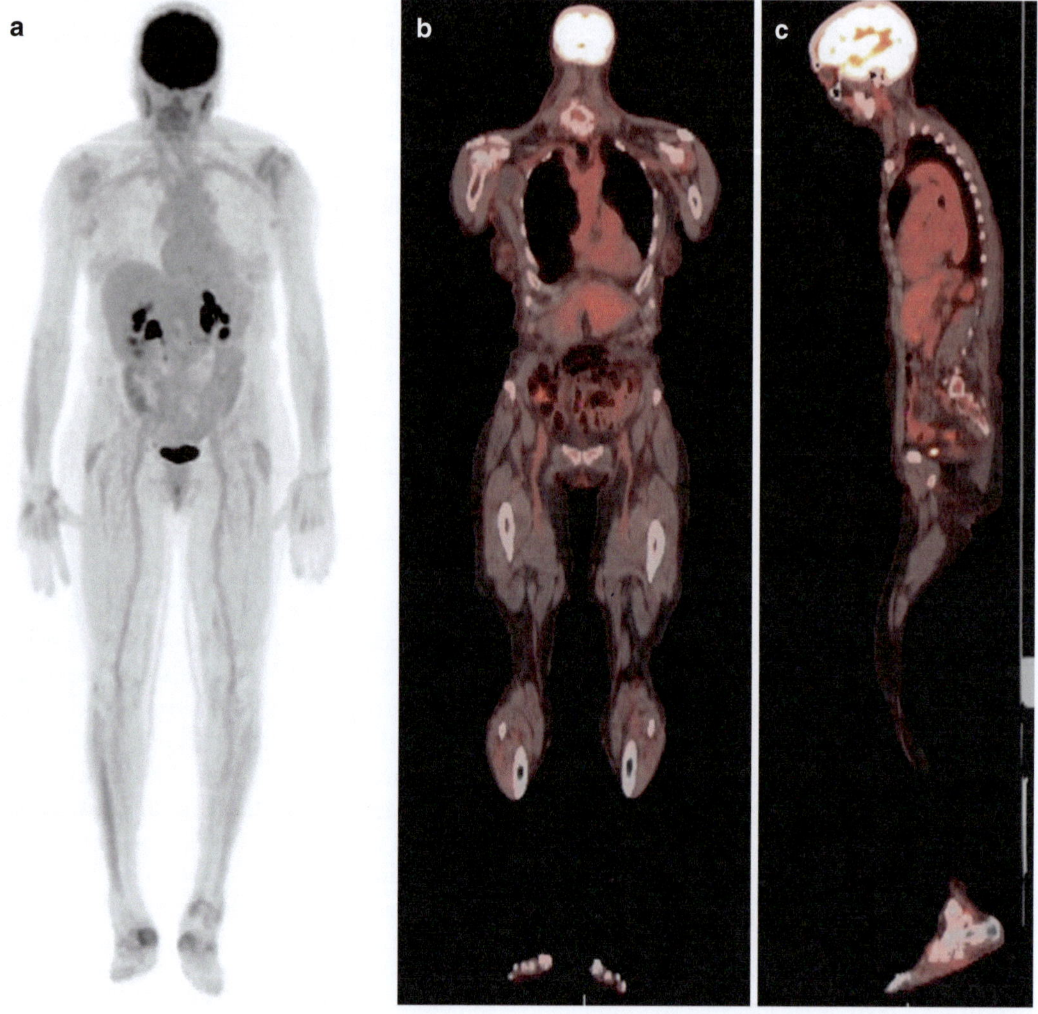

Fig. 3.22 Example of a true whole-body F-18 FDG PET/CT. (**a**) Anterior MIP image. (**b, c**) Coronal and sagittal fused images

Sebro et al. retrospectively looked at 556 oncology patients (14 (2.5%) melanoma and 5 (0.9%) sarcoma patients) which included 804 PET/CTs to evaluate how often the use of WB PET/CT changed the stage and management of patients compared to limited WB PET/CT. The study found that 47/556 (8.5%) of the patients had abnormal findings outside the most limited WB FOV (skull base to upper thighs). Of these, there were more abnormal findings in the proximal lower extremities than in the upper extremities (proximal and distal) and distal lower extremities. There was only one patient in whom there was an upstaging (0.2%), but six patients (1.1%)

had a change in management due to brain metastasis. The study also found that the cancers more likely to have findings outside the most limited WB (skull base to upper thighs) were melanoma, lymphoma, multiple myeloma, sarcomas, and stage IV lung, breast, prostate, bladder, testicular, and renal malignancies [25] (Fig. 3.26).

A more specific study was conducted by Webb et al. to evaluate the performance of true whole-body versus limited whole-body PET/CT in melanoma and sarcoma patients. This study retrospectively examined 352 PET/CTs in 194 melanoma patients and 75 PET/CTs in 44 sarcoma patients, to evaluate for the benefit of

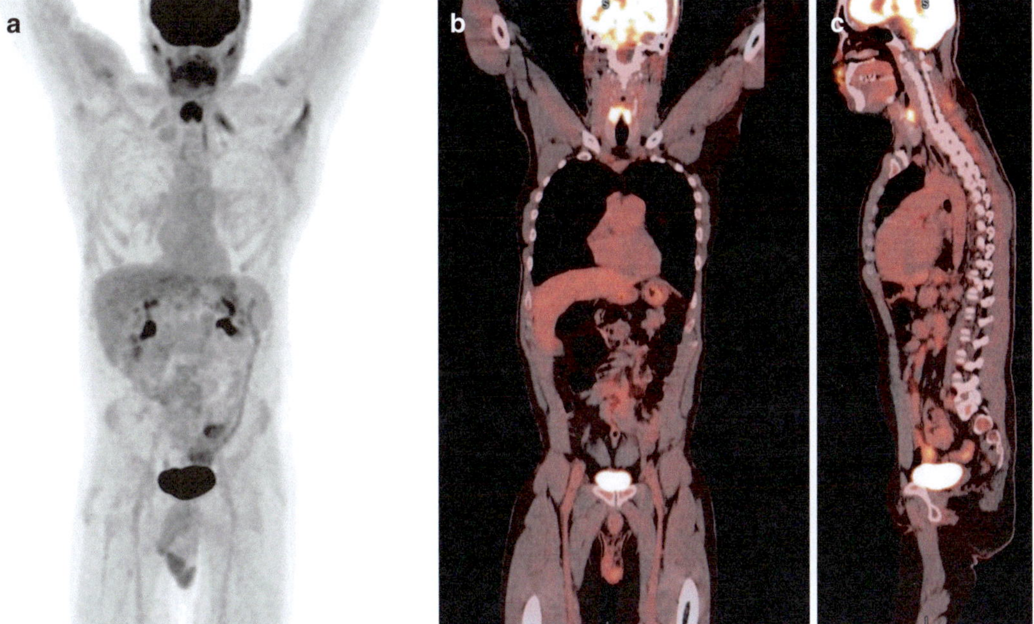

Fig. 3.23 Example of a limited whole-body (skull base to mid-thigh). (**a**) Anterior MIP image. (**b, c**) Coronal and sagittal fused images

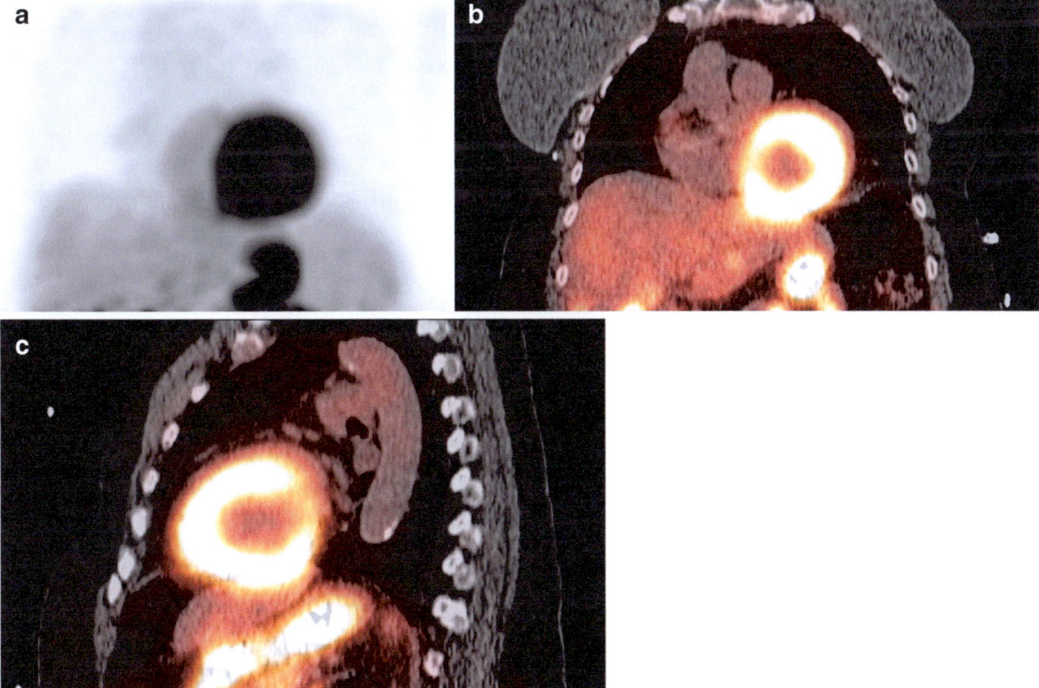

Fig. 3.24 Example of a limited Rb-82 myocardial PET/CT. (**a**) Anterior MIP image. (**b, c**) Coronal and sagittal fused images

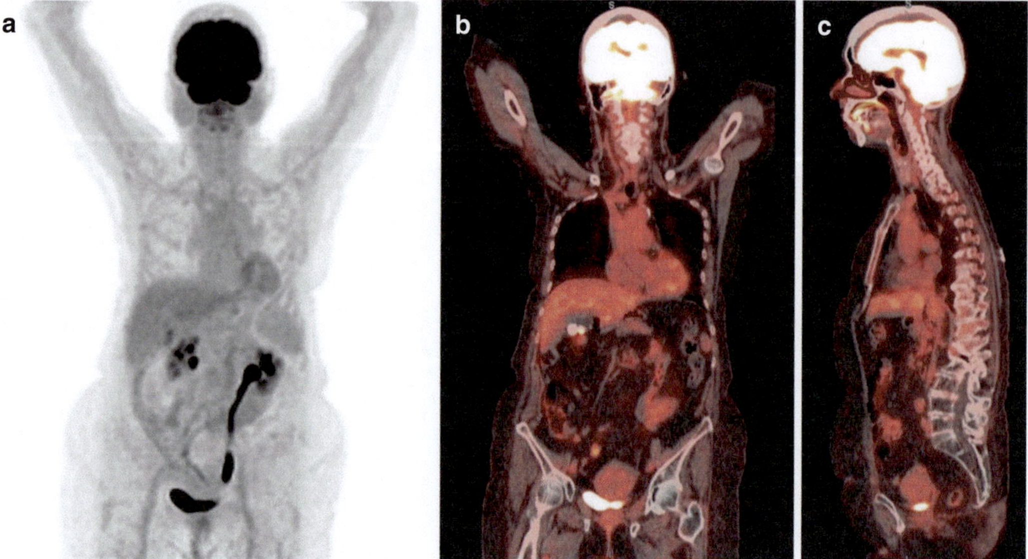

Fig. 3.25 Example of a variation of a limited whole-body F-18 FDG PET/CT, vertex to mid-thigh. (**a**) Anterior MIP image. (**b**, **c**) Coronal and sagittal fused images

whole-body versus limited whole-body "eye-to-thighs." Through their evaluation, they found 13 brain metastases (5 were unknown) and 27 lower extremity metastases in melanoma patients, but all were in the setting of other metastatic diseases. In the sarcoma patients, one patient had an unexpected brain metastasis and six patients had leg metastasis, which were not isolated. The study concluded that the addition of the lower extremities in patients in whom the primary lesion was not in the lower extremities added little value to the study. The study also concluded that the addition of whole-brain imaging may have added value, given that the presence of brain metastasis changes the clinical management [26].

Field of View (FOV) Selection in STSs The selection of the FOV in the evaluation of STSs should take into consideration the location of the primary tumor and potential for brain metastasis. Typically, a limited whole-body FOV is selected for STS evaluation. However, if the tumor is in an extremity, it is recommended that the entire extremity should be included in the imaging. In the cases where there is potential for brain metastasis, inclusion of whole brain imaging should be considered – although, in these cases, a brain MRI is usually obtained due to MRI's superior high resolution and contrast.

FOV Selection in Metastatic Melanoma Typically, the FOV of choice in the evaluation of metastatic melanoma is the whole-body (vertex to toes) FOV. This FOV is selected to image the entire patient for accurate staging, primarily due to melanoma's ability to metastasize to several different locations by lymphatic or hematogenous means.

Patient Positioning

Prior to the scan, all patients should remove metallic objects (e.g., jewelry, removable dental implants, belts, clothing with zippers and bras with metal wires, etc.) to avoid creating streak artifacts from the CT transmission scan (Figs. 3.27 and 3.28). The patient should be positioned comfortably on the table due to the length of the time of the scan and with sufficient positioning aids such as arm, head, and knee support. These supports help with the comfort of the patient and reduce the incidence of involuntary motion which may cause misregistration during fusion of the PET and CT images [27].

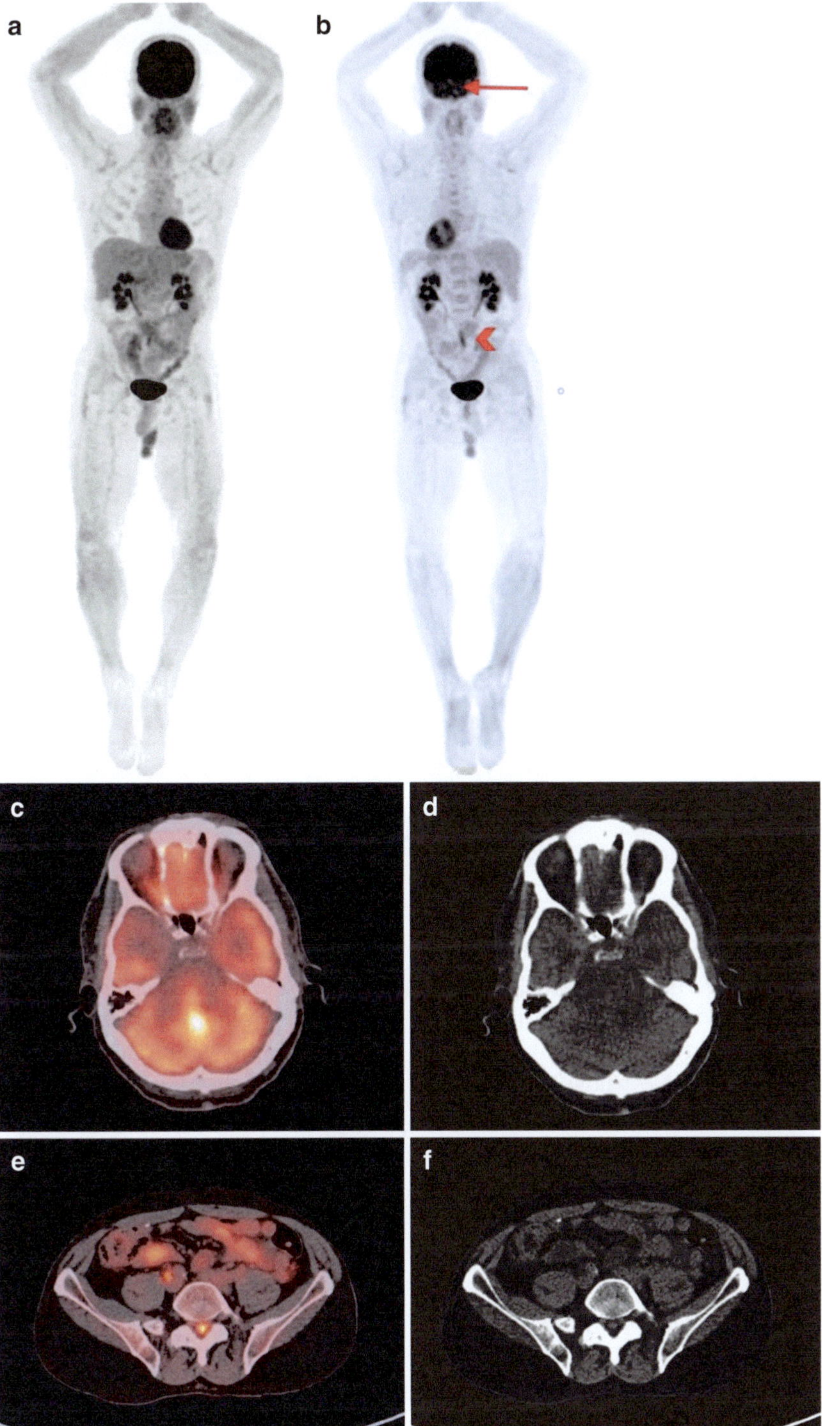

Fig. 3.26 A 57-year-old male with a history of malignant melanoma of the right lower extremity, now presenting with metastatic disease to the brain and spinal cord. (**a, b**) Anterior and posterior MIP images showing abnormal F-18 FDG uptake in the region of the base of the brain (arrow) and in the lower lumbar upper sacral region (arrowhead). (**c, d**) Axial fused and low-dose non-contrast CT showing focal increase in F-18 FDG uptake in the fourth ventricle without definite CT correlation. (**e, f**) Axial fused and low-dose non-contrast CT showing focal increase in F-18 FDG uptake in the spinal cord at the level of L5-S1 with a soft tissue correlation on CT

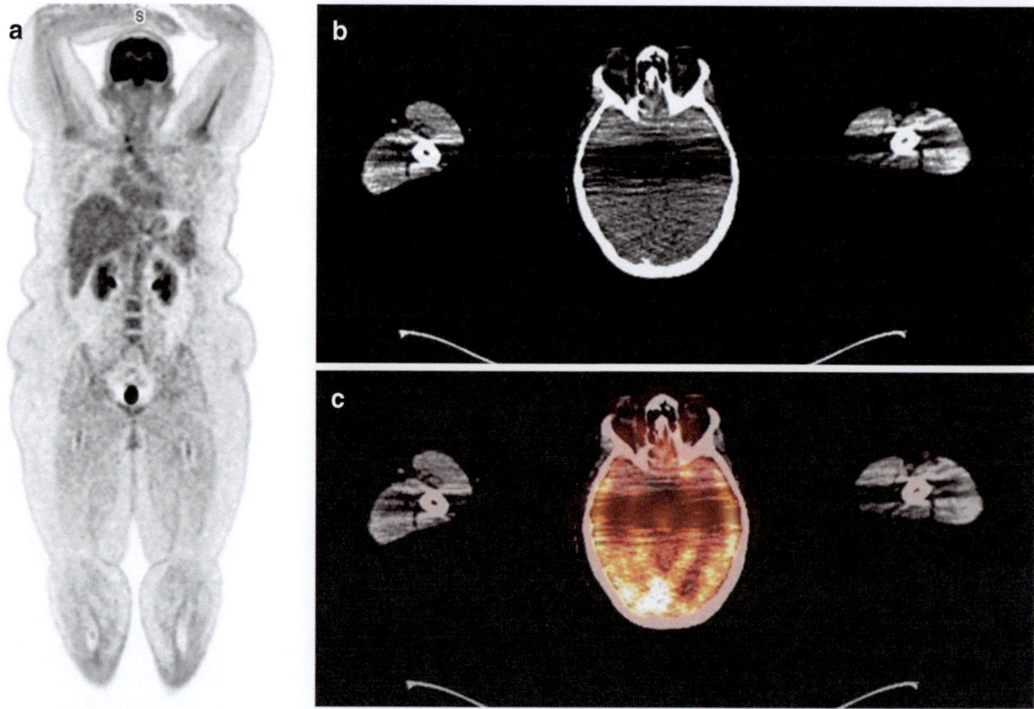

Fig. 3.27 Example of a whole-body F-18 FDG PET/CT with the arms up showing beam-hardening artifact and its effect on attenuation correction in the skull. (**a**) Coronal attenuation-corrected PET illustrating the arms above the head. (**b**) Axial low-dose non-contrast-enhanced CT illustrating beam-hardening artifact coursing through the skull. (**c**) Axial fused F-18 FDG PET/CT showing decreased radiotracer uptake correlating to the course of the beam-hardening artifact through the skull

The positioning of the arms is variable based on the type of scan FOV (true whole-body, limited whole-body with or without dedicated images, or limited area) required for the region of interest. In the acquisition of a true whole-body (vertex to toes), it is preferred that the patient be imaged with arms raised above his or her heads. This reduces beam-hardening artifacts in the abdomen and pelvis. This also avoids artifacts caused by truncation of the FOV. Not all patients will be able to complete the scan with their arms raised for the extended period. In these cases, one arm can be raised while one arm is positioned beside the body or both arms can be positioned beside the body. The arms should be positioned so truncation of the CT is avoided, and when using systems that have extended CT FOVs, this is easily accomplished [28].

In cases of head and neck tumor evaluation, a two-step approach may potentially be useful. This approach acquires the scan in two different acquisitions. First, the head and neck regions are imaged with the arms at the patients' side, to avoid beam-hardening artifact of the head and neck region. Second, the patient is imaged from the apex of the lungs through the mid-thigh with the arms raised [28]. This repositioning of the arms out of the FOV helps to prevent artifacts from beam-hardening and attenuation (Fig. 3.29).

Arm Positioning in STSs Evaluation Arm positioning for limited whole-body scans, with or without dedicated images, in the evaluation of STSs is variable and dependent on the region of interest. The goal of the arm positioning is to reduce any beam-hardening artifact within the field of view. If the tumor resides in a portion of an upper extremity, it is important that the entire limb be in the field of view for evaluation. This is usually best accomplished by placing the

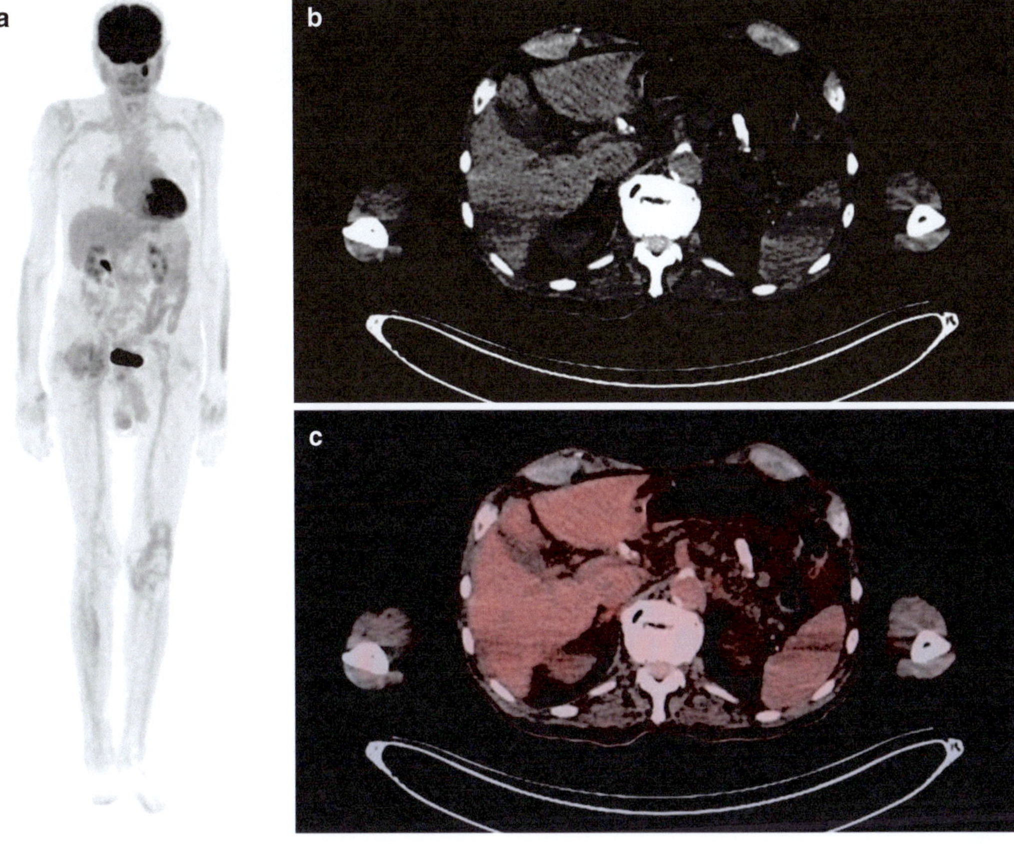

Fig. 3.28 Example of a whole-body F-18 FDG PET/CT with the arms down resulting in beam-hardening artifact and its effects on attenuation correction in the abdomen. (**a**) Anterior MIP of F-18 FDG PET/CT with the arms down at the side. (**b**) Axial low-dose non-contrast-enhanced CT with beam-hardening artifact coursing through the liver and spleen. (**c**) Axial fused F-18 FDG PET/CT illustrating decreased radiotracer uptake corresponding to the course of beam-hardening artifact

arms at the side of the patient. If the tumor is in the head and neck region, the previously mentioned two-step approach, resulting in two scans with alternating placement of the arms, may be preferred. If the location of the tumor is in the thorax, abdomen, or pelvis, it would potentially be beneficial to have the arms raised, in order to avoid a beam-hardening artifact in the region of the tumor location.

Arm Positioning in Metastatic Melanoma Evaluation The arm positioning for limited whole-body scans in the evaluation of metastatic melanoma is also dependent on the region of inter-est. Consistent with the evaluation of STSs, the goal of arm positioning is to reduce any beam-hardening artifact within the field of view. If the region of interest of the scan is the head and neck, the arms are placed at the patients' side. If the region of interest involves the extremities, thorax, abdomen, or pelvis, the arms are positioned above the head. These arm positions minimize the potential for any beam-hardening artifact. It is important to note that when a whole-body (vertex to toes) scan is indicated, rather than a limited whole-body with or without dedicated images, the indications for arm positioning to keep a field of view free of hardening artifacts are slightly different.

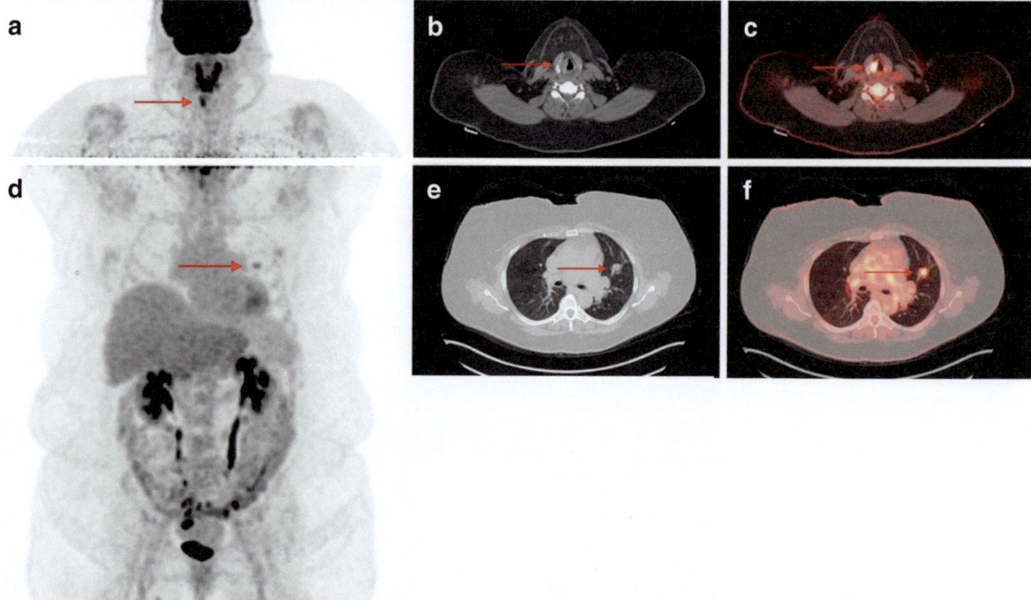

Fig. 3.29 Example of a dedicated head and neck acquisition with the arms down to avoid beam-hardening artifact during evaluation of right vocal cord lesion (arrows). (**a**) Anterior MIP image with the arms down showing focal uptake in the mid neck just right of midline. (**b**) Axial low-dose non-contrast-enhanced CT showing soft tissue thickening of the right vocal cord. (**c**) Axial fused F-18 FDG PET/CT localizing the abnormal focal uptake to the soft tissue thickening of the right vocal cord. Subsequent whole-body F-18 FDG PET/CT with the arms raised to avoid beam-hardening artifact in the thorax, abdomen, and pelvis. (**d**) Anterior MIP imaging illustrating abnormal focal uptake in the left thorax. (**e**) Axial low-dose non-contrast CT in lung window identifying a lobulated pulmonary nodule in the left upper lobe. (**f**) Axial fused F-18 FDG PET/CT localizing the abnormal focal uptake in the left thorax to the left upper lobe pulmonary nodule

PET/CT Imaging Workflows

Similar to the FOV protocols, the workflows of PET/CT can vary due to indication, type of scan desired, and institution/user preference. Once the type of PET/CT scan (i.e., whole-body vs limited whole-body vs whole-body with dedicated area, low-dose CT vs diagnostic grade CT with or without contrast) has been determined, the workflow of obtaining the scan can also be determined. All workflows, whether they are for whole-body, limited whole-body, or limited area PET/CT, are comprised of the same elements – a "scout" or topogram data, CT images, and PET emission scan.

The scan is started following the uptake time of 60–90 min, with the initial CT image called a "scout" or topogram image. This "scout" image covers the desired image region, dedicated and/or whole-body, in order to plan for the subsequent CT and PET emission acquisitions and to calculate the tube current modulation and voltage control. Following the "scout" image, the attenuation correction or diagnostic CT with or without contrast is acquired of the same region. Once the CT is acquired, the PET emission scan is acquired of the same region. When performing a whole-body, limited whole-body with or without dedicated images, and limited area PET/CT, these elements are acquired in the same order for each region of interest [22].

Examples of the workflows for the different PET FOVs, AC/CT, or Diag/CT with or without contrast enhancement are as follows: limited whole-body PET/NECT (Fig. 3.30), whole-body PET/NECT (Fig. 3.31), limited whole-body

Fig. 3.30 Limited whole-body F-18 FDG PET/NECT. NECT Non-enhanced computed tomography, AC attenuation correction, BP bed position

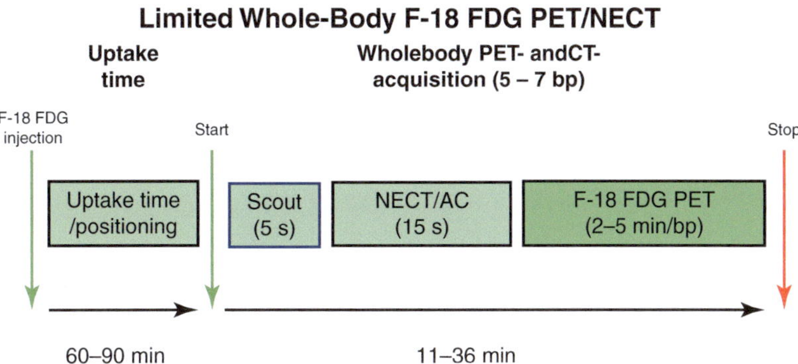

Fig. 3.31 Whole-body F-18 FDG PET/NECT. NECT Non-enhanced computed tomography, AC attenuation correction, BP bed position

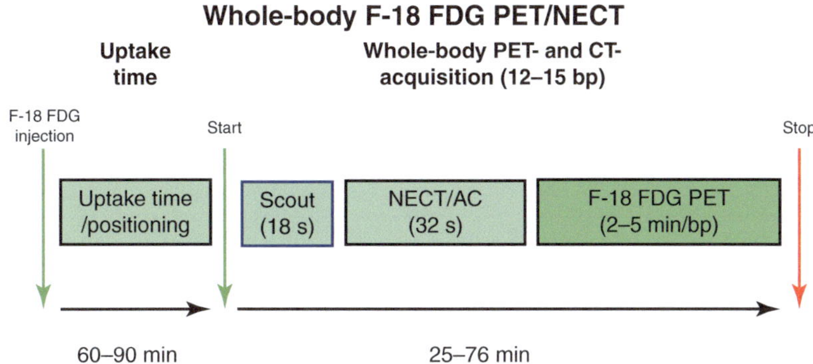

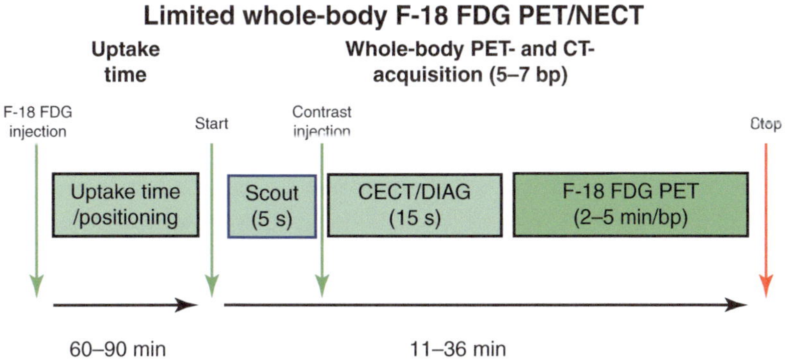

Fig. 3.32 Limited whole-body F-18 FDG PET/CECT. CECT Contrast-enhanced computed tomography, DIAG diagnostic CT, BP bed position

PET/CECT (Fig. 3.32), whole-body PET/CECT (Fig. 3.33), and limited whole-body PET/CECT with dedicated images (Fig. 3.34).

There are different scan strategies that have been used from institution to institution in relation to the order in which the CT and PET emission scans are acquired when IV contrast is used [29]. One strategy is to acquire the PET emission scan first, followed by the CECT. This strategy is an attempt to avoid any effects that IV contrast may have on the SUV measurements. The second strategy is to acquire the CECT prior to the PET emission scan in the same way that a NECT is acquired. Most institutions continue to acquire the CECT prior to the PET emission scan, since the effects of IV contrast on SUV measurements are negligible.

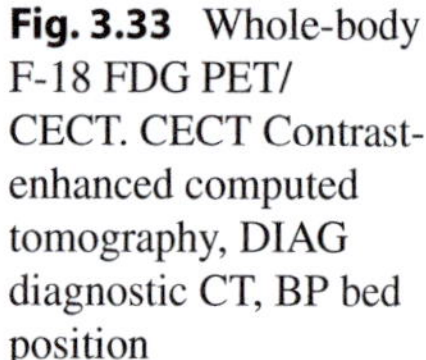

Fig. 3.33 Whole-body F-18 FDG PET/CECT. CECT Contrast-enhanced computed tomography, DIAG diagnostic CT, BP bed position

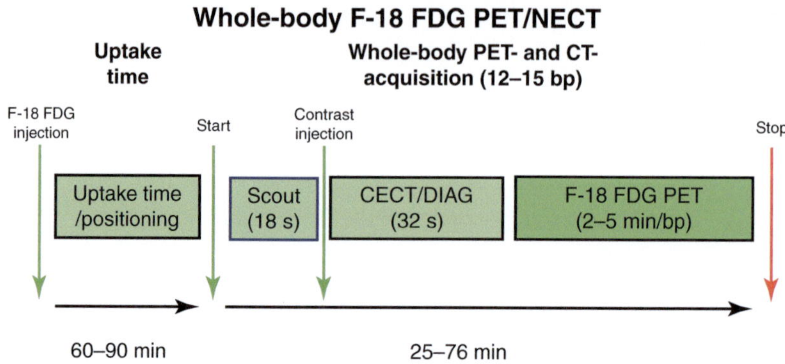

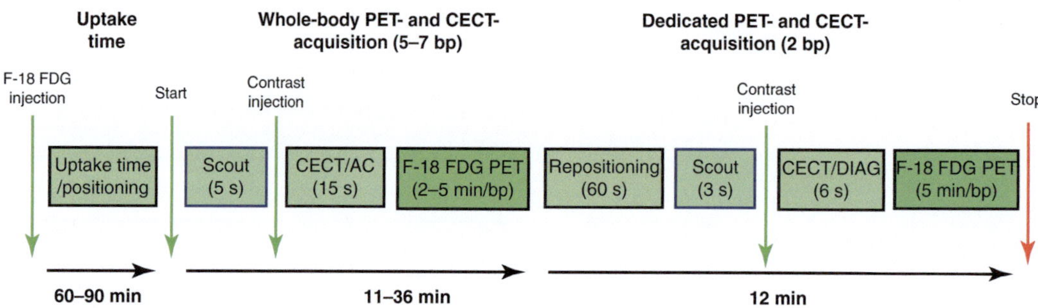

Fig. 3.34 Limited whole-body F-18 FDG PET/CECT w/ dedicated images. CECT Contrast-enhanced computed tomography, DIAG diagnostic CT, BP bed position

Utility of PET/MRI in Soft Tissue Sarcomas and Malignant Melanoma

The integration of PET with MR imaging into a single imaging unit has been of interest for decades, long before the development of integrated PET/CT scanners. This interest has arisen out of the potential combination of advantages from both imaging modalities – such as MRI's high-contrast, high-resolution anatomical images and PET's biological process evaluations. Additionally, more advanced MR sequences allow for evaluation of physiology, function, and metabolism using endogenous contrast and further enhancement of anatomical structures with exogenous contrast materials [30]. Typical indications for whole-body PET/MRI in oncological examinations include staging/restaging of known tumors, detection/exclusion of tumor recurrence, therapy monitoring, detection of a cancer of unknown primary (CUP), evaluation of indeterminate findings of conventional exams, and biopsy/radiation/surgical planning [31].

The high soft tissue contrast and high resolution from MR imaging is ideal for pre-surgical planning, given that it allows for an accurate assessment of the tumor margins and potential nearby structures involved. Along with the high soft tissue contrast and high-resolution anatomical images, there are multiple different MRI sequences that can be used – not only in conventional images but in combined PET/MRI. These potentially helpful sequences include short tau inversion recovery (STIR), diffusion-weighted imaging (DWI) with apparent diffusion coefficient (ADC) maps, dynamic contrast-enhanced

(DCE), and blood oxygen level-dependent (BOLD) imaging sequences. These sequences allow for further evaluation of aspects of tumor tissue, like fat suppression for improved contrast, cellular density, diffusion to potentially predict responses to chemotherapy, vascular density for assessment of early antiangiogenic treatment, and hypoxia for radiation therapy [32]. Another advantage is seen in patients who will need multiple follow-up imaging studies, like those in the pediatric population. In these populations there is a significant reduction in radiation exposure when using PET/MRI versus PET/CT. These advantages have been evaluated and demonstrated in multiple oncology cases dealing with head and neck, lung, and breast cancer. Currently, the data, although limited, on the performance of PET/MRI in the evaluation of both soft tissue sarcoma and malignant melanoma show mixed results. The mixed results are most likely due to the limited number and size of the studies.

MRI Evaluation of Soft Tissue Sarcomas

MRI is the most heavily depended upon imaging modality when evaluating STSs. This is due to the superior high contrast and high resolution of soft tissue in the preoperative evaluation, as well as the evaluation of malignancy response to treatment and recurrence seen in MRI. Along with the use of MRI, the use of CT and PET is also important. CT is used in screening for potential lung metastasis prior to surgery. In the case of high-grade sarcomas, PET is used for the metabolic evaluation of the primary site of disease, potential metastatic disease, response to treatment, and residual or recurrent disease. The use of anatomical imaging such as MRI, no matter how detailed, does, however, in some instances lack important information needed for diagnostic and/or therapeutic decisions – for example, in cases where there is consideration of neoadjuvant chemotherapy or reinitiating chemotherapy or when morphological changes mimic progression. It is in these individual cases that the combination of metabolic functionality and the superior

high soft tissue contrast of PET/MRI may be extremely beneficial [33].

MRI Evaluation of Metastatic Malignant Melanoma

The initial staging of melanoma relies heavily on the TNM staging criteria, in which imaging has a major role in only one of the three separate stages.

The T-staging of melanoma is based on clinical exam and full-thickness biopsy, where findings are classified using the classification system set forth by the American Joint Committee on Cancer (AJCC). This classification system identifies the stage of the tumor, determining which tumors are low-, intermediate-, or high-risk based on the depth of the tumor margins. Currently, anatomical and functional imaging does not have a major role to play in the diagnosis or T-staging of melanoma. This is due to the variability in the sensitivity and specificity of anatomical and functional imaging, which correlates to the size, depth, and location of the tumor. However, it is important to note that to date there has been no prospective study conducted to evaluate the performance of PET/MRI in the T-staging of melanoma.

In terms of N-staging of melanoma, the current standard is sentinel lymph node sampling. This is usually done with Tc-99m sulfur colloid lymphoscintigraphy in order to identify the sentinel lymph node for excision. A recent study conducted by Schaarschmidt et al. evaluated the performance of FDG PET/CT, FDG PET/MRI, and FDG PET/MRI-DWI for detecting sentinel lymph node metastasis in melanoma. The study found that F-18 FDG PET/MRI with or without DWI was not able to reliably distinguish node-positive from node-negative patients [34]. Thus, the current standard of sentinel lymph node sampling cannot be replaced by current imaging techniques.

Despite imaging currently not having a pivotal role to play in the T- or N-staging of melanoma, it does have a role to play in the M-staging and restaging of patients with a high risk of metastasis (AJCC ≥3). Melanoma tends to develop distant metastasis due to the simultaneous lymphatic and hematogenous spread. For example, patients with uveal melanomas have shown a tendency for early metastasis to the liver. In this subtype of melanoma, the FDG uptake of the liver metastasis tends to be poor or non-existent, which is different than the abnormal increase in FDG uptake in metastasis from cutaneous malignant melanoma. The use of FDG PET/MRI to evaluate the liver in patients with uveal melanoma may provide an increase in sensitivity for detection, due to the superior anatomical imaging characteristics of MRI. Another example is patients with cutaneous melanoma stage IV – these patients develop brain metastasis approximately 40–50% of the time. In this group, FDG PET/MRI potentially has an advantage in early diagnosis of brain metastasis. However, this may be due mostly to the anatomical information from the MRI, rather than the F-18 FDG PET portion, due to high physiologic brain uptake that limits the distinction of tumor from normal brain tissue [35].

In the practical application of PET/MRI's hybrid combination of the biological processes from PET and the high-contrast, high-resolution anatomical detail from MRI in the evaluation of soft tissue sarcoma, melanoma, or another form of malignancy, it is important to know what to image and how to image it.

Basics of MR Imaging

MRI is a noninvasive imaging modality based on the evaluation of nuclei with magnetic momentum changes, using an external magnetic field and electromagnetic radiofrequency (RF) pulses. When introduced into an external static magnetic field, most of the nuclei will align with the external magnetic field. The application of an electromagnetic radiofrequency pulse to the nuclei can excite them and change their rotational alignment to precess around instead of aligning with the external magnetic field [36].

The nuclei of hydrogen atoms are the nuclei of interest in MR imaging. External radiofrequency coils can measure the precession of the hydrogen nuclei as their magnetic momentum changes. The application of additional magnetic gradient fields changes the magnetic field in the MRI scanner. The changes in the magnetic field measured by the external RF coils can be placed spatially within the field of view and are proportional to the number and density of nuclei. The nuclei that are excited by the RF pulses realign to be parallel with the static external magnetic field once the RF pulse is turned off. The realigning process is called "relaxation," and the time it takes is dependent on the chemical surroundings, resulting in a signal that is tissue dependent. Furthermore, adjusting the time points of the measurements results in multiple different soft tissue contrasts. These measurements are repeated several times in order to achieve the desired spatial resolution [36].

Integration of PET with MRI

PET Component Issues

The integration of PET with MR imaging required addressing multiple technical issues around hardware challenges. The major hardware challenge was the inability of PET detectors to operate within a magnetic field. Many older and even newer PET detectors are composed of a scintillation material and a photomultiplier tube (PMT). The scintillation material converts the 511 keV gamma photons to visible light which is then converted to an electrical signal via the PMT. The type of scintillation material and the mechanism of the PMT, based on the acceleration of electrons, are susceptible to magnetic fields and are unable to operate within an MRI scanner [36].

The initial solution to the incompatible hardware components was to spatially separate the two imaging units. It was not until the advent of magnetic field-insensitive detectors, such as avalanche photodiodes which replaced PMTs, that a truly integrated PET/MRI scanner was created. However, due to low gain, excess noise, and time variations, APDs are restricted from use in TOF imaging [37]. Since then additional detectors such as solid-state photomultipliers (SSPM), silicon photomultipliers (SiPMs), or multi-photon pixel counters (MPPC) have been developed to potentially replace avalanche photodiodes. Extra shielding was also added around the PET detectors to help block interference with the MRI scanner and control temperature variations created by the switching of the magnetic field by the MRI scanner.

Additionally, the material of the scintillation crystals needs to be considered. Certain scintillator materials show a magnetic susceptibility close to that of human tissue, in which a degree of magnetization of the material results from an applied magnetic field. The scintillation material used in bismuth germanium oxide (BGO), lutetium oxyorthosilicate (LSO), and lutetium yttrium oxyorthosilicate (LYSO) has been found to have a lower magnetic susceptibility. Conversely, crystals made from gadolinium orthosilicate (GSO) and lutetium gadolinium orthosilicate (LGSO) are not compatible with magnetic fields and cause MRI artifacts. The current crystal material of choice is LSO, due to its inherent high light output, efficiency, and short decay time allowing for TOF [38].

MRI Component Issues

To fully integrate PET and MR imaging to achieve simultaneous acquisitions, the components of both separate imaging modalities must be combined in a particular way. First the components of the PET unit (photon detectors, electronics, shielding and cooling mechanism) are required to be placed within the bore of the MR unit. In doing this, there needs to be attention to maintaining the homogeneity of the static primary magnetic field for proper MR function. As a result, the components for the PET unit need to be comprised of non-magnetic materials.

Second, any electromagnetic interference in the radiofrequency spectrum needs to be minimized to avoid creating artifacts in the MR images. This is challenging since the photon detectors and electronics from the PET unit have radiofrequency-radiating processes. Additionally,

the shielding implemented to minimize the photon detectors interference with the MRI can also cause artifacts and spatial distortions from eddy currents created from magnetic field switching.

Lastly, the MR radiofrequency coils need to be placed within the PET field of view for accurate measurements. Careful consideration is needed in the materials and design selected for the RF coils in order to minimize photon attenuation, since the RF coils are placed inside the PET FOV.

Early MR scanners were constructed with bore sizes of approximately 60 cm. The sizes of the earlier scanners left minimal space for the placement of the PET components. Newer scanners have been developed with an increase in bore size to 70 cm and allow for more space allocated for placement of the PET components.

MRI-Based Attenuation Correction

The fundamental principle that a percentage of the 511 keV gamma photons are attenuated from positron emission tomography is no different between stand-alone PET, PET/CT, and PET/MRI. The difference between these imaging modalities comes in the way that an attenuation map is generated. PET imaging has used two methods to generate the attenuation maps, originally a transmission source with early stand-alone PET scanners and then a CT with integrated PET/CT cameras. These two methods, transmission source and HU conversion from the CT acquisition, are not applicable to PET/MRI [36].

MRI measures the densities and relaxation times of tissues using magnetic field changes, which is dependent on proton density via the nuclei and the chemical environment. The measurements from MRI, specifically the proton density and relaxation times, are not related to the electron density that causes the attenuation of the 511 keV gamma photons and thus cannot be used directly in the calculation of attenuation correction. Due to the lack of a direct correlation, three concepts were developed to address MRI-based attenuation correction: segmentation-based, atlas-based, and reconstruction-based methods [36].

Segmentation-Based The MRI acquisition is segmented into different tissue types based on their image-based gray scale. The different tissue types are compartmentalized into background air, fat, soft tissue, and lung tissue, which then are assigned a predetermined linear attenuation coefficient (LAC) [36].

Atlas-Based This method is based on a database of matching MRI and CT images and supplied by the vendor of the PET/MRI. MR images of the current patient are compared to MR images from the database that correspond to matched CT images and LACs, resulting in assigning LACs to the current MR images. Once the LACs are assigned, there is still a need to use photon energy conversion [36].

Reconstruction-Based This method uses an algorithm called maximum likelihood esti-mation of attenuation and activity (MLAA). This algorithm is present on all current PET/MRI systems and used in the overall attenuation correction calculations in conjunction with the segmentation method. The segmentation method is used for much of the attenuation correction calculation, while the MLAA algorithm is used to construct the contours of the patient from non-AC PET data. The data created by the MLAA algorithm is used to supplement missing attenuation data from the MRI truncation artifact (Fig. 3.35). This method has obvious known limitations since it relies on the accumulation of F-18 FDG in the skin where other radiotracers do not. Other applications of MLAA are in investigation to resolve the missing data from the truncation artifact and also from bone and air cavities from the MRI-based LAC data [36].

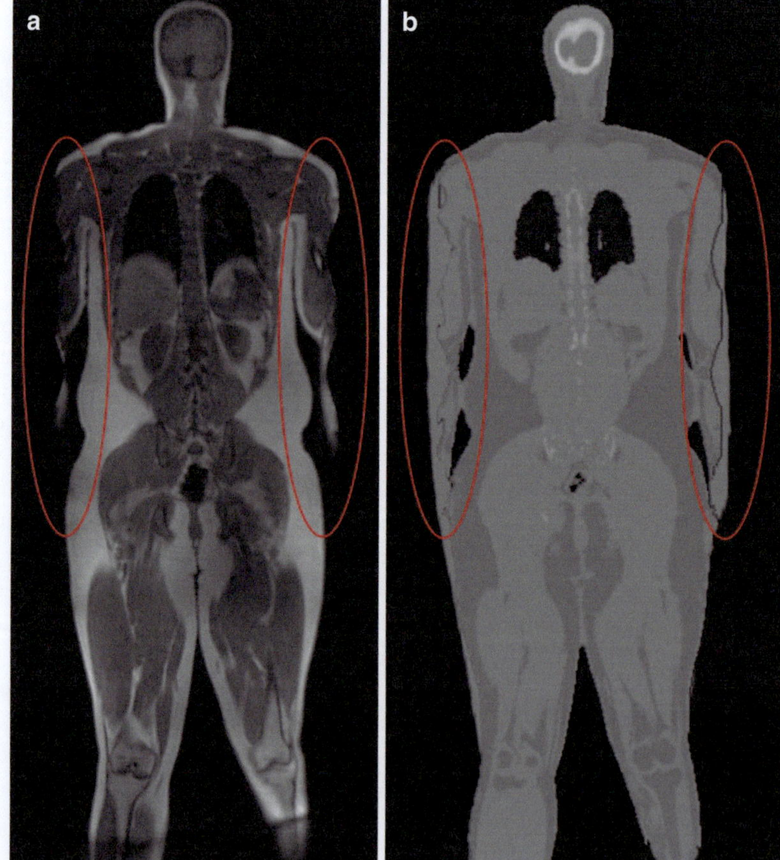

Fig. 3.35 Example of truncation artifact from MRI field of view and reconstruction. (**a**) Coronal view of MR Dixon in-phase sequence illustrating truncation artifact. (**b**) Coronal MR Dixon in-phase sequence with maximum likelihood estimation of attenuation and activity (MLAA) applied

PET/MRI Artifacts and Technical Issues

The majority of PET/MRI today utilize the segmentation method using T1-weighted MR images and Dixon sequences, which allows for fast acquisition and processing times that are reproducible. However, studies have been conducted that show an underestimation of PET quantification in PET/MRI compared to PET/CT when T1-weighted and Dixon sequence-based AC methods are used. This underestimation is credited to three MRI-based AC flaws. These flaws are (1) lack of information of bone from MR images, (2) truncation of MR images due to small FOV, and (3) the presence of RF coils in the PET FOV.

Solution of Bone AC The implications of not considering bone attenuation in PET/MRI have been shown to have a negative impact on PET quantification. When cortical bone is treated as soft tissue, there is an underestimation of PET quantification of soft tissue lesions adjacent to bone and bone lesions by 0.2–4% and 1.5–30.8%, respectively [39]. Multiple solutions to the lack of bone information from MRI data have been proposed, including using special sequences, such as ultrashort echo and zero echo times, or applying a CT-based 3D bone model to the actual MRI-based AC data in order to create a bone segment.

MRI Truncation Issues A limitation of MRI-based AC is that the transaxial FOV for MRI is approximately 50 cm. Once outside the 50 cm FOV, there are geometric distortions and voids which result in truncation and potential PET quantification artifacts. A solution to the truncation issue is the implementation of the MLAA algorithm, which, as previously discussed, generates non-AC PET data in the outer contours of the imaged patient to replace missing data, thus correcting the truncation artifact. However, this method is still limited by the fact that radiotracers other than F-18 FDG do not accumulate at an appropriate level in the skin. An alternative solution to the truncation issue, called homogenization, was developed by Blumhagen et al.

using gradient enhancement (HUGE), which can extend the lateral MRI-based FOV to 60 cm to incorporate the arms [37].

Hardware AC With the integration of PET and MR units, components of the MR system are placed into the FOV of the PET. Placement of these elements inside the PET FOV creates an additional source of attenuation and affects the PET quantification. To compensate for the hardware attenuation, a CT-based map of LACs for each hardware component is generated and applied to each specific PET/MRI system.

Lung Artifact Correction

MR imaging of the lung poses many challenges not only from the fundamental that LACs are generated from electron density and MRI measures proton density but also from characteristics of the lung tissue and motion. The characteristics of the lungs which make the images susceptible to artifacts are air within the lung, low signal-to-noise ratio of aerated lung, and motion artifacts from breathing during image acquisition [40]. The air within the lung causes difficulty in the segmentation process, as air has very low signal-to-noise ratio (similar to bone) but with very different attenuation properties. The low signal to-noise ratio of aerated lungs is due to lungs having a low tissue density (approximately 10% of other tissues throughout the body).

To address the issue of no direct conversion of proton density measurements to electron density measurements to create attenuation correction maps, PET/MR imaging of the lungs utilizes the previously mentioned techniques such as segmentation, atlas, and emission-based techniques. The segmentation method is the most widely used. This method varies from vendor to vendor and can include three (air, lung, and soft tissue) or four (air, lung, soft tissue, and fat) (Fig. 3.36) tissue classes with or without the addition of a major bone atlas (Fig. 3.37). Most of these segmentations use the non-breath-hold T1-weighted MR Half-Fourier Acquisition Single-shot Turbo spin Echo (HASTE) sequence (Fig. 3.38), but

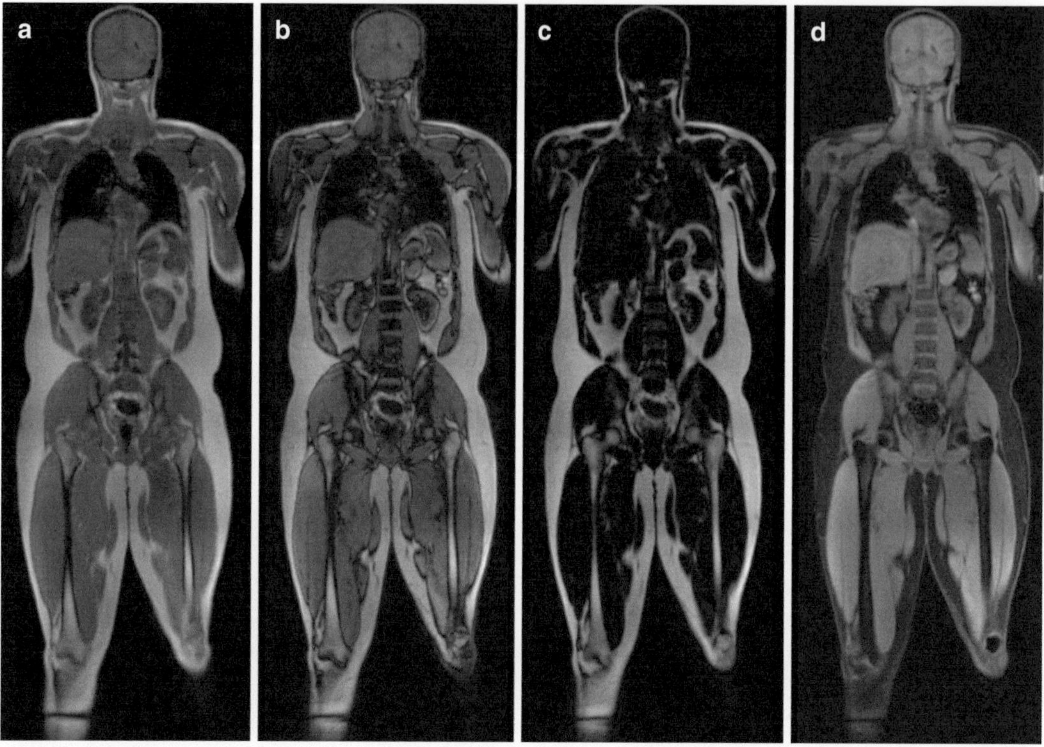

Fig. 3.36 Example of tissue classification using a Dixon four-class segmentation method from a F-18 FDG PET/MR study. Coronal Dixon: (**a**) in-phase, (**b**) out-of-phase, (**c**) fat, and (**d**) water sequences

additional, more advanced sequences are starting to be utilized – such as a T1-weighted Dixon two-point 3D volume-interpolated breath-hold (VIBE) (Fig. 3.39), free-breathing 3D spoiled T1 w/ gradient echo (FLASH or MPSPGR), and dual-echo RF spoiled gradient echo (LAVA-FLEX) sequences, in order to improve on the low signal-to-noise effects.

Following the acquisition of the MRI using the vendor dictated sequences, a single-valued population-based LAC is applied to each individual tissue class segment. In the literature, the LAC for lung varies from 0.018 to 0.027 cm^{-1}. The use of a single-valued LAC for lungs and variation of the LAC among various vendors has introduced a problem. It has been found that there is a significant change in the quantification of radiotracer activity in reconstruction of the lung. Multiple studies have investigated this and have uncovered evidence that there is a deviation of 8–15% in the lung SUVs. The significant differences in results from various studies suggest a need for improvement in the attenuation correction of the lung [5].

An additional problem encountered with the use of the segmentation-derived LAC method is errors resulting in mis-segmentation. This error typically occurs from bone mis-segmentation and the combination of air in the stomach or bowel with respiratory and cardiac motion. Bone is often misclassified due to its low relaxation signal. The combination of air in the stomach and bowel with respiratory and cardiac motion can lead to poor separation of the lungs at the bases. These errors result in PET quantification errors, but the errors are significantly less compared to techniques that ignore bone attenuation, resulting in up to 15% PET quantification errors in lesions. To address these errors, multiple techniques have been investigated to improve segmentation of the lungs that include application of the intensity threshold region growing model, atlas-based susceptibility artifact correction algorithm, and patient-specific mean whole-lung LAC based from total lung volumes [5]. These techniques have shown improvements of varying degree.

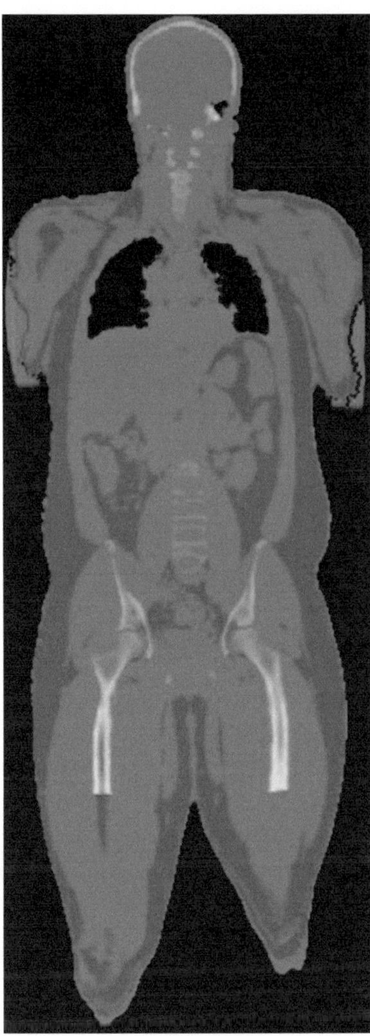

Fig. 3.37 Example of a coronal view of an MR attenuation correction map with MLAA and a bone atlas applied resulting in an MR-derived pseudo-CT

Motion Correction

In PET imaging, motion causes significant decrease in image quality and quantification. The image may become blurred or smeared, and, as a result, the measured activity will be inaccurate. The motion causing image degradation can be voluntary, such as patient repositioning, or involuntary, such as respiration, cardiac cycle, swallowing, or intestinal peristalsis.

The motion from respiration and the cardiac cycle can cause misregistration artifacts in the PET data in PET/MRI, as they do in PET/CT. In the case of PET/MR, this is due to the different acquisition techniques between PET, which is not acquired during breath-hold, versus MR, which can be acquired during breath-hold (Fig. 3.40). It has been reported that on average there is 15–20 mm of movement from respiration and 8–23 mm of movement from the cardiac cycle. To reduce the motion artifact from respiration or the cardiac cycle, gating can be performed. For gating, the PET raw data is divided into subsets corresponding to the different phases of the respiratory or cardiac cycle. The phases can be determined by MRI navigators tracking the diaphragm movement in respiration, or cine-/tagged-MRI imaging for the cardiac cycle [36].

A more advanced technique has been developed to simultaneously model and correct for respiration and cardiac cycle motion. This technique uses a 3D cine-MRI, which allows for real-time self-gating of respiration combined with ECG-gating for the cardiac cycle. In a simultaneous PET/MRI unit, this technique allows for motion correction of both the PET and MR acquisitions at the same time [26].

Gadolinium-Based Contrast-enhanced MRI (CE-MRI)

The first clinically approved contrast agent for MRI was launched in 1988, based on the results of clinical trials using gadolinium-based contrast complexes. All gadolinium-based contrast agents (GBCAs) contain the paramagnetic ion of gadolinium (Gd^{3+}), which is a rare earth metal. This element is effective in enhancing proton relaxation due to its seven unpaired electrons, resulting in shorter T1 and T2 relaxation times of surrounding water molecules. This ability to shorten relaxation time is called relaxivity, and its main effect is on the T1 signal, which yields bright contrast [41].

The majority of GBCAs are administered in the amount of 0.1–0.3 mmol/kg and are renally excreted. A few GBACs are taken up by the hepatocytes and excreted through the biliary system. The Gd^{3+} ions are toxic to the body alone and

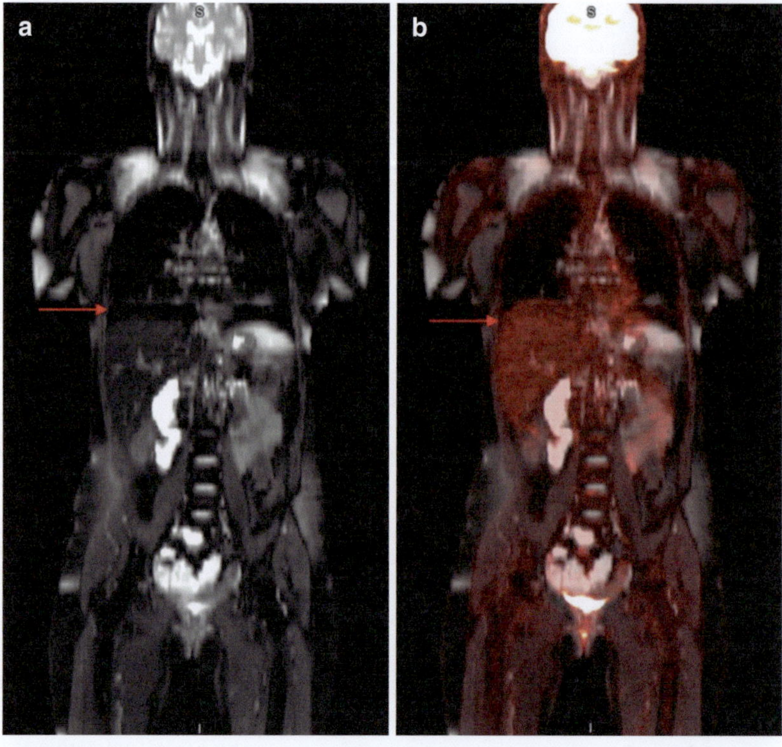

Fig. 3.38 Example of non-breath-hold HASTE sequence PET/MR exam, illustrating low signal-to-noise ratio of the lungs and significant movement of the diaphragm and liver (arrow). (**a**) Coronal view of a PET/MR non-breath-hold HASTE sequence. (**b**) Coronal fused F-18 FDG PET/MR non-breath-hold HASTE sequence

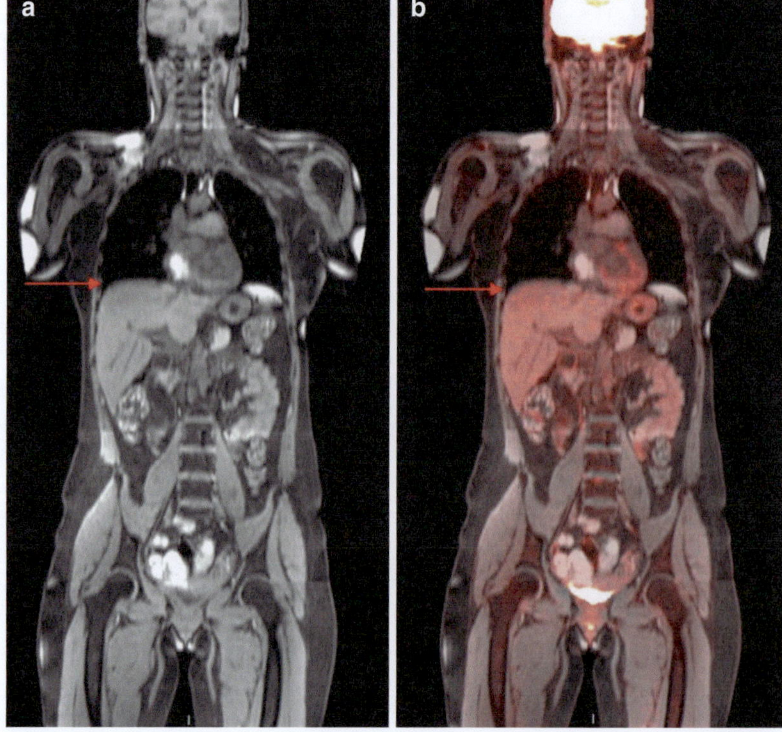

Fig. 3.39 Example of a breath-hold VIBE sequence PET/MR exam, illustrating improved signal-to-noise ratio in the lung and no significant movement of the diaphragm and liver (arrow). (**a**) Coronal view of a PET/MR breath-hold VIBE sequence. (**b**) Coronal fused F-18 FDG PET/MR VIBE sequence

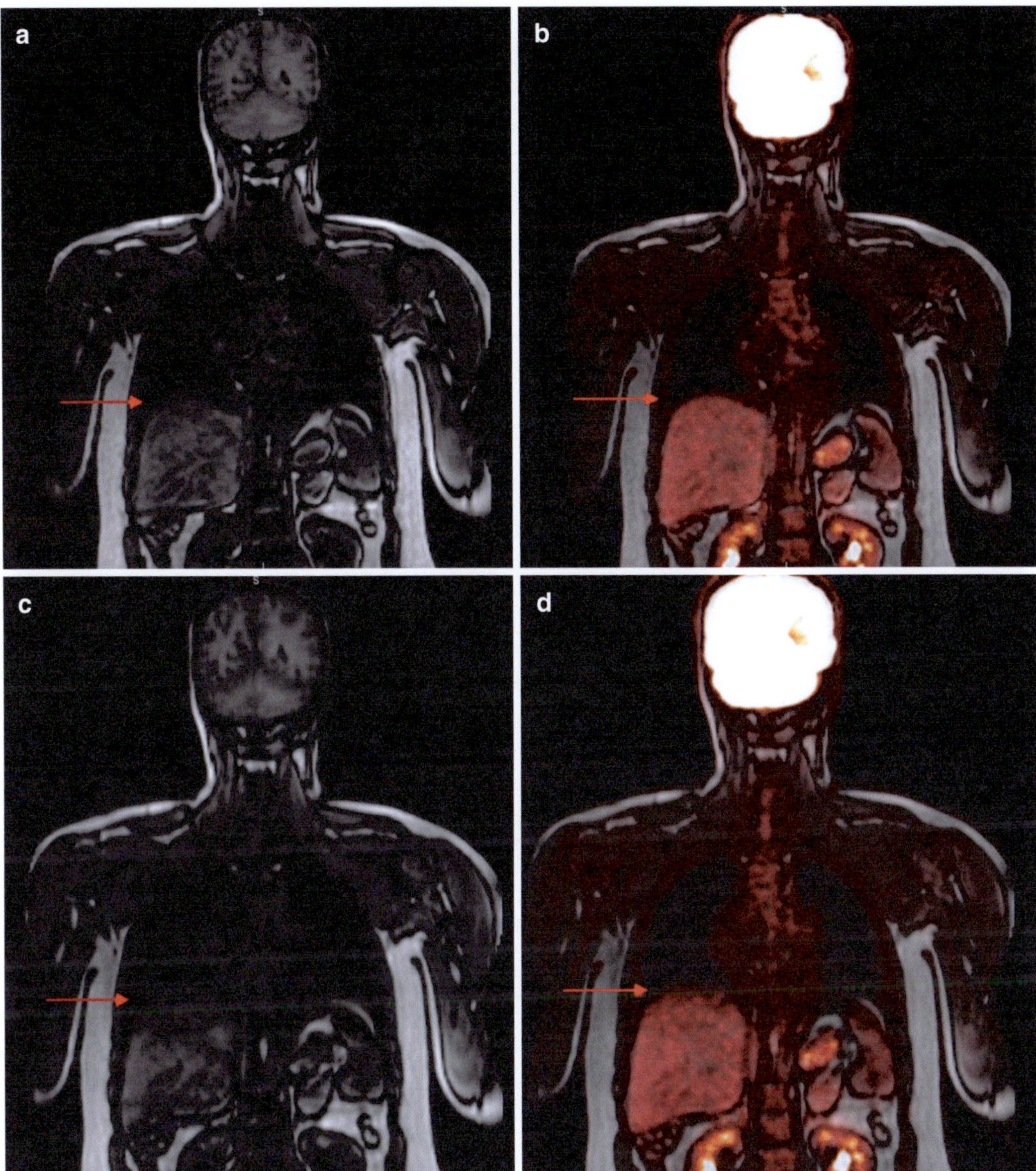

Fig. 3.40 Example of breath-hold versus non-breath-hold PET/MR exam, illustrating significant movement of the diaphragm and liver (arrow). Coronal view (**a**) breath-hold Dixon out-of-phase MR sequence, (**b**) fused breath-hold PET/MR Dixon out-of-phase MR sequence, (**c**) non-breath-hold Dixon out-of-phase MR sequence, and (**d**) fused non-breath-hold PET/MR Dixon out-of-phase MR sequence

thus are bonded to organic compounds in either a linear or macrocyclic structure. The configuration of the bonded organic structure determines the stability of the compound. An in vitro study was conducted to simulate the release of Gd^{3+} into the body of renally impaired patients, which found that a significant amount of Gd^{3+} was detected when using linear agents versus undetectable amounts from macrocyclic compounds over a 15-day period. However, in vivo, GBCAs are excreted within a few days from injection even in the renally impaired patients [31].

The utility of GBCAs has been evaluated in the imaging of multiple anatomical regions and structures and has been found to be useful in multiple areas, such as CNS, angiography, cardiac, abdominal, breast, and MSK evaluations. In the area of abdominal imaging, CE-MRI has particularly excelled in the evaluation of the liver. This is due to development of hepato-specific GBCAs, such as gadobenate and gadoxetic acid, which allow for delayed imaging with gadobenate due to decreased excretion from the liver and early hepato-specific imaging with gadoxetic acid. Gadoxetic acid has also been found useful in the imaging of cirrhotic livers, cholangiopancreatography, biliary imaging, and pre- and posttreatment follow-up. In the area of MSK imaging, CE-MRI has been utilized early in the modality's clinical implementation. The use in MSK is separated into three categories: tumor, infection, and joint evaluation [41]. In the case of tumors, CE-MRI offers several advantages, resulting from its high soft tissue contrast, high-resolution, multi-planar capabilities, and advanced sequences – which allow for optimal contrast between neurovascular, muscle, bone marrow, and abnormal tissue.

Use of CE-MRI in the Evaluation of STSs: Preoperative Planning The primary utility of gadolinium contrast-enhanced MRI in the evaluation of STSs is in the preoperative planning and workup, in which gadolinium contrast-enhanced MRI is the gold standard for imaging. This is due to the improvement of the already excellent high contrast and high resolution in soft tissue. However, there are concerns in the limitations of gadolinium CE-MRI's ability to exactly define the tumor boarders in adjacent structures and into peritumoral edema. Even with gadolinium CE-MRI's superior soft tissue contrast, the edge detection is impacted by inflammation and edema. The effect may lead to overestimation of the tumor volume and extension, which, if there are major structures nearby (such as vessels, nerve bundles, or bone) may result in major surgery or amputation. The addition of the metabolic information that FDG PET can provide to the information provided by the CE-MRI has been found to be valuable regarding possible tumor invasion of adjacent structures. This benefit is particularly helpful in tumors with heterogenous signals and ill-defined edges.

Use of CE-MRI in the Evaluation of STSs: Posttreatment In the evaluation for residual or recurrent STSs in the posttreatment setting (surgical, radiation, or chemotherapy), the use of gadolinium contrast enhancement of the MRI is valuable. The use of contrast increases the already high contrast of soft tissue in MR imaging. The presence of soft tissue enhancement post-contrast injection is suggestive of residual or recurrence disease. However, the drawbacks are consistent with those discussed in the preoperative planning section above. CE-MRI can be affected by edema and inflammation, which is very common in the postsurgical and post-radiation setting. It is important that this is taken into account in the image interpretation.

CE-MRI in the Evaluation of Metastatic Melanoma Gadolinium contrast enhancement to MRI in the evaluation of metastatic melanoma is best utilized in the setting of visceral metastasis. CE-MRI has been found to be particularly helpful in the CNS and liver, which are common sites of melanoma metastasis. The use of contrast can potentially improve the identification of malignant versus benign lesions and assist in treatment planning. The addition of contrast increases the anatomical detail of the MRI, helping to delineate edges of the lesion, which is important in preoperative or pre-radiation planning. Along with the increase in anatomical detail, there are certain patterns of enhancement from the contrast that may be beneficial in identifying malignant versus benign etiologies.

PET/MR Imaging Workflows

As with PET/CT, the imaging protocols of PET/MRI can vary widely based on the type of scanner, vendor, desired sequences, and indication for the examination. Use of PET/MRI in oncology cases is similar to that of PET/CT, in that the scan is performed in whole-body, limited whole-body, and limited area mode, scanning the patient from vertex to toes, vertex/base of skull to mid-thigh, or limited area over multiple bed positions, respectively. Depending on the MR scanner type and sequences, a whole-body

PET/MR scan can take considerably longer than PET/CT scans. Due to this, there was a movement to standardize the PET/MRI workflows [31].

The sequence of acquisitions for a PET/MRI is not unlike that of a PET/CT scan. The image acquisition of a PET/MRI starts with a localization sequence, which is comparable to the "scout" image for a PET/CT. This sequence covers the entire desired area and is needed to plan the following acquisitions and to define the axial range for the PET/MRI. Following the localization sequence, each bed position requires an attenuation sequence – usually using a T1-weighted or Dixon sequence. Once the AC sequence is acquired, additional sequences, such as HASTE and VIBE or other special sequences, are then acquired at each bed position. The sequence of MR acquisitions is acquired either prior to the PET acquisition or simultaneously, depending on the type of scanner being used.

Early PET/MRI scanners were not fully integrated. The two systems were located either in the same room or in close proximity to each other. The two modalities were acquired in a sequential order, with the MRI sequences acquired first, followed by the PET data. In order to reduce the overall imaging time, the MRI acquisitions are started during the uptake time, approximately 25 min after injection of the radiotracer. One advantage of the sequential systems is that it allowed for more flexibility in the combination of MRI sequences that were acquired, since the timeframe of each bed position was not as strictly regulated as with simultaneous PET/MRI systems (Fig. 3.41). The sequential PET/MRI acquisition could also be done with IV contrast, if desired (Fig. 3.42).

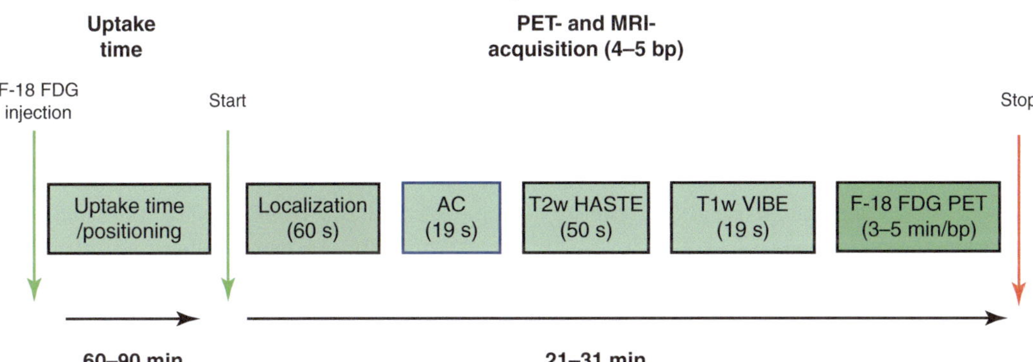

Fig. 3.41 Sequential limited whole-body F-18 FDG PET/MRI. AC attenuation correction, HASTE Half-Fourier Acquisition Single-shot Turbo spin Echo, VIBE volume-interpolated breath-hold, BP bed position

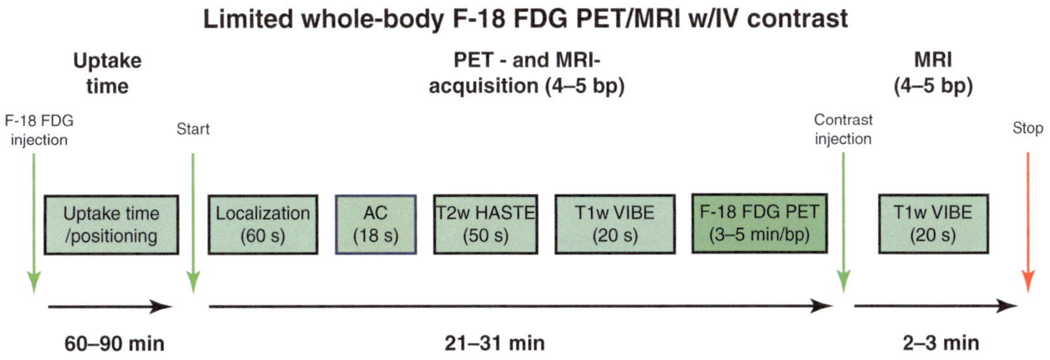

Fig. 3.42 Sequential limited whole-body F-18 FDG PET/MRI w/ IV contrast. AC Attenuation correction, HASTE Half-Fourier Acquisition Single-shot Turbo spin Echo, VIBE volume-interpolated breath-hold, BP bed position

Newer PET/MRI hybrid systems allow for simultaneous acquisition of both the MR sequences and PET data. This form of imaging takes some prior planning on which MR sequences to acquire per bed position, due to PET's timed step and shoot method. The simultaneous PET/MR acquisition starts following the 60–90 min uptake period. As with the sequential systems, a localization sequence is first acquired. This is followed by an attenuation correction sequence, additional MR sequences, and the PET data at the same time for each bed position.

Depending on the indication for the study, oncology PET/MRI protocols can be classified in a few different ways. These classifications are organ-based, basic whole-body, or advanced whole-body protocols. Of these protocols, the organ-based protocol is used for localized disease and is the easiest and most straightforward. The organ-based protocol does not require prior planning or a complicated workflow since it is acquired over 1–2 bed positions. The basic whole-body and advanced whole-body protocols are indicated when evaluation of the primary tumor and staging is required. These protocols are more complicated and take prior planning in selecting specific sequences, regions for dedicated images, and potential use of IV contrast.

Basic whole-body and advanced whole-body protocols can be further classified. Umutlu et al. proposed the further classification of the whole-body protocols which includes ultra-fast PET/MRI, fast PET/MRI, and dedicated local and whole-body PET/MRI. Each of the workflows has its advantages and indications, due to acquisition duration, specific sequences, dedicated images, and tumor type [31].

Ultra-Fast PET/MRI This workflow sets out the protocols for a PET/CT scan in that it is acquired in just under 20 min and is based off 2 min per bed positions. This ultra-fast protocol is aimed to be used with "low compliance" patients, such as elderly and pediatric patients, and in combination with local dedicated imaging. The indications with ultra-fast PET/MRI include imaging for whole-body staging for such malignancies as lymphoma or for evaluation of recurrence. The sequences utilized in this protocol include fast T2-weighted spin echo (HASTE) and non-enhanced fast fat-saturated T1-weighted gradient echo (VIBE). GBCA can be used, and post-contrast T1-weighted fat-saturated images can be acquired in addition to the non-contrast sequences [31] (Fig. 3.43).

Fast PET/MRI This protocol is similar in structure to the ultra-fast protocol, in terms of the order of steps and use of HASTE and VIBE sequences. However, this protocol does increase the overall time of the scan by increasing the acquisition time to 4 min per bed position and incorporation of a diffusion-weighted imaging (DWI) sequence, resulting in an overall time of approximately 30 min. The addition of DWI offers additional information on the cellularity of tissue in

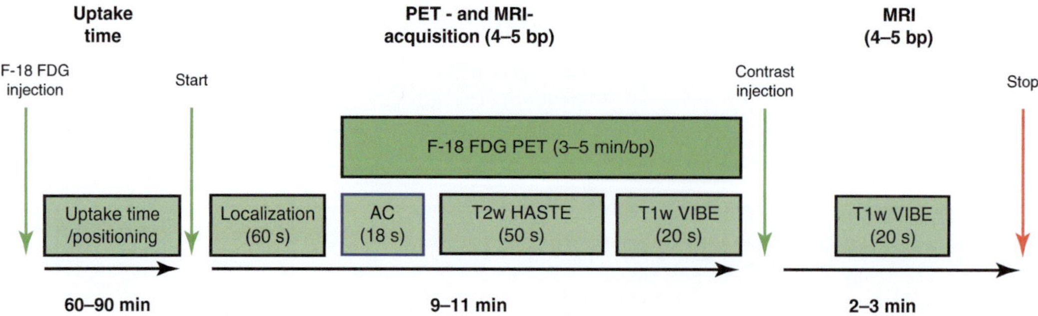

Fig. 3.43 Simultaneous ultra-fast limited whole-body F-18 FDG PET/MRI w/ IV contrast. AC Attenuation correction, HASTE Half-Fourier Acquisition Single-shot Turbo spin Echo, VIBE volume-interpolated breath-hold, BP bed position. (Reproduced with permission from Umutlu et al. [31])

question. This added information is useful in the detection of small lesions that would potentially be undetected by PET alone [31] (Fig. 3.44).

Dedicated and Whole-Body PET/MRI This protocol combines the dedicated imaging of a local region and whole-body coverage. The dedicated imaging is useful in malignancies involving the head and neck, pelvis, and extremities. The whole-body imaging portion can be performed using the ultra-fast or fat protocol depending on the state of patient compliance, length of the scan time, and usefulness of DWI [31] (Fig. 3.45).

PET/MRI Workflows in STSs Selecting the workflow for PET/MRI in evaluating STSs depends on the stage of the evaluation, specifically the initial staging, preoperative evaluation,

or treatment response. In the initial staging of STSs using PET/MRI, the most common workflow is the limited whole-body FOV, without contrast enhancement or any dedicated imaging. This workflow allows for the primary site to be evaluated, along with evaluation of the remainder of the body for metastatic disease. In the preoperative setting, the use of whole-body PET/CE-MRI with dedicated images of the region of interest provides the most information. The contrast enhancement allows for increased soft tissue evaluation, and the dedicated imaging of the specific region allows for improved target-to-noise ratio from the added PET acquisition time. In the setting of treatment response, including with regard to postoperative, post-radiation, or post-chemotherapy, a standard whole-body image acquisition is justified. The standard whole-body

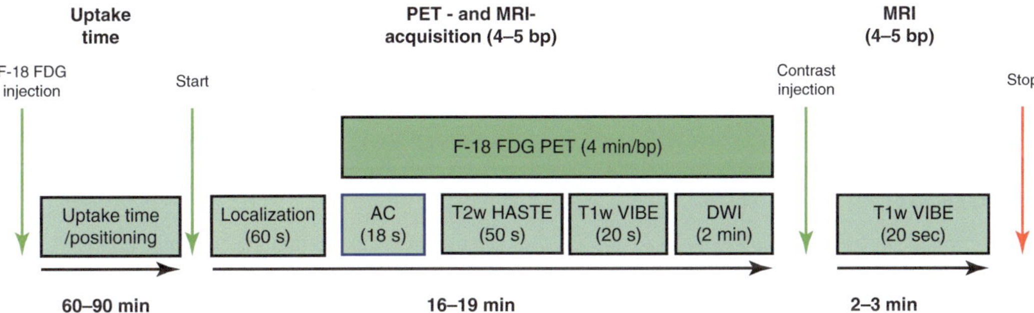

Fig. 3.44 Simultaneous fast limited whole-body F-18 FDG PET/MRI w/ IV contrast. AC Attenuation correction, HASTE Half-Fourier Acquisition Single-shot Turbo spin Echo, VIBE volume-interpolated breath-hold, DWI diffusion-weighted imaging, BP bed position. (Reproduced with permission from Umutlu et al. [31])

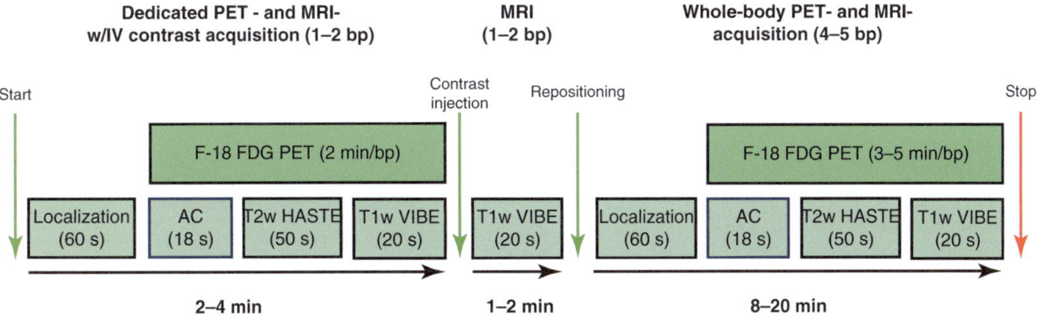

Fig. 3.45 Simultaneous limited whole-body F-18 FDG PET/MRI w/ IV contrast and dedicated images. AC Attenuation correction, HASTE Half-Fourier Acquisition Single-shot Turbo spin Echo, VIBE volume-interpolated breath-hold, BP bed position. (Reproduced with permission from Umutlu et al. [31])

PET/MRI allows for evaluation of the site of treatment for residual or recurrent disease and for potential metastatic disease.

PET/MRI Workflows in Metastatic Melanoma As stated previously, imaging is not currently indicated in the T- or N-staging in metastatic melanoma. The role that imaging plays in the evaluation of metastatic melanoma is in the M-staging. In the initial evaluation for metastatic disease, PET/CT tends to be the hybrid imaging method of choice. However, PET/MRI has the potential to excel in the evaluation of metastatic melanoma when there is visceral metastasis, such as brain or liver. In the evaluation of visceral metastasis, the workflow of choice would be the whole-body PET/CE-MRI with dedicated imaging. The whole-body portion of the exam would potentially detect metastatic disease from vertex to toes. The dedicated images with contrast enhancement allow for a more detailed evaluation of potential lesions, particularly when evaluating the brain and liver.

References

1. Schafferkoettter J, Townsend D. PET scanning: principles and instrumentation. In: von Schulthess GK, editor. Molecular anatomic imaging: PET/CT, PET/MR and SPECT/CT. Philadelphia: Wolters Kluwer; 2016. p. 16–25.
2. Jones T, Townsend D. History and future technical innovation in positron emission tomography. J Med Imaging. 2017;4(1):011013.
3. Cherry S, Jones T, Karp J, Qi J, Moses W, et al. Total-body PET: maximizing sensitivity to create new opportunities for clinical research and patient care. J Nucl Med. 2018;59:3–12.
4. Slomka PJ, Pan T, Germano G. Recent advances and future progress in PET instrumentation. Semin Nucl Med. 2016;46(1):5–19.
5. Lillington J, Brusaferri L, Klaser K, Shmueli K, Neji R, Hutton R, et al. PET/MRI attenuation estimation in the lung: a review of past, present, and potential techniques. Med Phys. 2020;47(2):790–811.
6. Kalender WA. Dose in x-ray computed tomography. Phys Med Biol. 2014;59(3):R129–50.
7. Quinn B, Dauer Z, Pandit-Taskar N, Schoder H, Dauer LT. Radiation dosimetry of 18F-FDG PET/CT: incorporating exam-specific parameters in dose estimates. BMC Med Imaging. 2016;16(1):41.
8. Antoch G, Freudenberg LS, Beyer T, Bockisch A, Debatin JF. To enhance or not to enhance? 18F-FDG and CT contrast agents in dual-modality 18F-FDG PET/CT. J Nucl Med. 2004;45:56S–65S.
9. Patel DB, Matcuk GR Jr. Imaging of soft tissue sarcomas. Chin Clin Oncol. 2018;7(4):35.
10. Cronin CG, Prakash P, Blake MA. Oral and IV contrast agents for the CT portion of PET/CT. AJR Am J Roentgenol. 2010;195(1):W5–W13.
11. Wong TZ, Paulson EK, Nelson RC, Patz EF Jr, Coleman RE. Practical approach to diagnostic CT combined with PET. AJR Am J Roentgenol. 2007;188:622–9.
12. Verga L, Brach del Prever EM, Linari A, Robiati S, De Marchi A, Martorano D, et al. Accuracy and role of contrast-enhanced CT in diagnosis and surgical planning in 88 soft tissue tumours of extremities. Eur Radiol. 2016;26:2400–8.
13. Pfluger T, Melzer HI, Schneider V, La Fougere C, Coppenrath E, Berking C, et al. PET/CT in malignant melanoma: contrast-enhanced CT versus plain low-dose CT. Eur J Nucl Med Mol Imaging. 2011;38:822–31.
14. Schelbert HR, Hoh CK, Royal HD, Brown M, Dahlbom MN, Dehdashti F, et al. Procedure guideline for tumor imaging using fluorine-18-FDG. J Nucl Med. 1998;39:1302–5.
15. Waxman AD, Herholz K, Lewis DH, Herscovitch P, Minoshima S, Ichise M, et al. Society of nuclear medicine procedure guideline for FDG PET brain imaging v1.0. SNMMI February 8, 2009. https://s3.amazonaws.com/rdcms-snmmi/files/production/public/docs/Society%20of%20Nuclear%20Medicine%20Procedure%20Guideline%20for%20FDG%20PET%20Brain%20Imaging.pdf.
16. Wahl RL, Henry CA, Ethier SP. Serum glucose: effects on tumor and normal tissue accumulation of 2-[F-18]-fluoro-2-deoxy-D-glucose in rodents with mammary carcinoma. Radiology. 1992;183:643–7.
17. Nagaki A, Onoguchi M, Matsutomo N. Patient weight-based acquisition protocols to optimize 18F-FDG PET/CT image quality. J Nucl Med Technol. 2011;39(2):72–6.
18. Del Sole A, Lecchi M, Gaito S, Lucignani G. An international multi-center comparison of [18F]FDG injection protocols and radioactive dose administered to patients undergoing [18F]FDG-PET examinations. J Nucl Med. 2013;54(2):372.
19. Boellaard R. Standards for PET image acquisition and quantitative data analysis. J Nucl Med. 2009;50(suppl 1):11S–20S.
20. Holm S, Borgwardt L, Loft A, Graff J, Law I. Pediatric doses—acritical appraisal of the EANM paediatric dosage card. Eur J Nucl Med Mol Imaging. 2007;34:1713–8.
21. Lassmann M, Treves S. Pediatric radiopharmaceutical administration: harmonization of the 2007 EANM paediatric dosage card (version 1.5.2008) and the 2010 North American Consensus guideline. Eur J Nucl Med Mol Imaging. 2014;41:1636.

22. Delbeke D, Coleman RE, Guiberteau MJ, Brown ML, Royal HD, Siegel BA, et al. Procedure guideline for tumor imaging with 18F-FDGD PET/CT 1.0*. J Nucl Med. 2006;47(5):885–95.
23. Fukukita H, Suzuki K, Matsumoto K, Terauchi T, Daisaki H. Japanese guideline for the oncology FDG-PET/CT data acquisition protocol: synopsis of version 2.0. Ann Nucl Med. 2014;28:693–705.
24. Sanchez-Jurado R, Devis M, Sanz R, Aguilar JE, del Puig CM, Ferrer-Rebolleda J. Whole-body PET/CT studies with lowered 18F-FDG doses: the influence of body mass index in dose reduction. J Nucl Med Technol. 2014;42:62–7.
25. Sebro R, Mari-Aparici C, Hernandez-Pampaloni M. Value of true whole-body FDG-PET/CT scanning protocol in oncology: optimization of its use based on primary diagnosis. Acta Radiol. 2013;54:534–9.
26. Webb H, Latifi H, Griffeth L. Utility of whole-body (head-to-toe) PET/CT in the evaluation of melanoma and sarcoma patients. Nucl Med Commun. 2018;39(1):68–73.
27. Beyer T, Antoch G, Muller S, Egelhof T, Freudenberg LS, Debatin J, et al. Acquisition protocol considerations for combined PET/CT imaging. J Nucl Med. 2004;45:25S–35S.
28. Boellaard R, Delgado-Bolton R, Oyen WJG, Giammarile F, Tatsch K, Eschner W, et al. FDG PET/CT: EANM procedure guidelines for tumour imaging: version 2.0. Eur J Nucl Med Mol Imaging. 2015;42:328–54.
29. Graham MM, Wahl RL, Hoffman JM, Yap JT, Sunderland JL, Boellaard R, et al. Summary of the UPICT protocol for 18F-FDG PET/CT imaging in oncology clinical trials. J Nucl Med. 2015;56(6):955–61.
30. Catana C. Principles of simultaneous PET/MR imaging. Magn Reason Imaging Clin N Am. 2017;25(2):231 43.
31. Umutlu L, Beyer T, Grueneisen JS, Rischpler C, Quick HH, Veit-Haibach P, et al. Whole-body [18F]-FDG-PET/MRI for oncology: a consensus recommendation. Nuklearmedizin. 2019;58(2):68–76.
32. Partovi S, Kohan A, Zipp L, Faulhaber P, Kosmas C, Ros P, Robbin M. Hybrid PET/MR imaging in two sarcoma patients – clinical benefits and implications for future trials. Int J Clin Exp Med. 2014;7(3):640–8.
33. Schuler MK, Richer S, Beuthien-Baumann B, Platzek I, Kotzerke J, van den Hoff J, Ehninger G, Reichardt P. PET/MRI imaging in high-risk sarcoma: first findings and solving clinical problems. Case Rep Oncol Med. 2013;2013:793927. https://doi.org/10.1155/2013/793927.
34. Schaarschmidt B, Grueneisen J, Stebner V, Klode J, Stoffels I, Umutlu L, Schadendorf D, Heusch P, Antoch G, Poppel T. Can integrated 18F-FDG PET/MR replace lymph node resection in malignant melanoma? Eur J Nucl Med Mol Imaging. 2018;45:2093–102.
35. Nguyen N, Yee M, Tuchay A, Kirkwood J, Hussein T, Mountz J. Targeted therapy and immunotherapy response assessment with F-18 fluorothymidine positron-emission tomography/magnetic resonance imaging in melanoma brain metastasis: a pilot study. Front Oncol. 2018;8:1–9.
36. Rausch I, Quick HH, Cal-Gonzalez J, Sattler B, Boellaard R, Beyer T. Technical and instrumentational foundations of PET/MRI. Eur J Radiol. 2017;94:A3–A13.
37. Blumhagen J, Ladebeck R, Fenchel M, Scheffler K. MR-based field-of-view extension in MR/PET: B_0 homogenization using gradient enhancement (HUGE). Magn Reason Med. 2013;70(4):1047–57.
38. Khalil MM. Basic science of PET imaging. Part III PET physics and instrumentation. In: Chapter 9 PET/MR: basics and new developments. Heidelberg: Springer; 2017. p. 207.
39. Samarin A, Burger C, Wollenweber SD, Crook DW, Burger IA, Schmid DT, et al. PET/MR imaging of bone lesions – implications for PET quantification from imperfect attenuation correction. Eur J Nucl Med Mol Imaging. 2012;39(7):1154–60.
40. Rice SL, Friedman KP. Clinical PET-MR imaging in breast cancer and lung cancer. PET Clin. 2016;11(4):387–402.
41. Lohrke J, Frenzel T, Endrikat J, Alves FC, Grist TM, Law M, et al. 25 years of contrast-enhanced MRI: developments, current challenges and future perspectives. Adv Ther. 2016;33:1–28.

Systematic Approach to Evaluation of Melanoma and Sarcoma with PET

4

Jorge Daniel Oldan

Introduction

Positron emission tomography (PET), combined with CT (PET/CT) and MR (PET/MR), using fluorodeoxyglucose (FDG) as radiotracer, is often used for diagnosing, staging, assessing response to therapy, and follow-up for recurrence of a variety of malignancies. Other chapters in this book outline the utility of FDG-PET in melanoma and sarcoma. While both of these can spread throughout the body, they nonetheless have some important differences—melanoma (Fig. 4.1) is almost always very intense on FDG-PET and is notorious for spreading to unusual organs, whereas sarcomas (Fig. 4.2) are variably intense. A systematic approach is needed in each on these malignancies for proper evaluation of a patient's PET-CT scan for minimizing the chances a potential metastasis is missed.

Systematic Approach: Looking at the Whole Body

As with chest radiographs, a variety of systems may be used, and each reader must use the

method they personally find most useful. Similarly, in FDG-PET, there is disagreement on the proper windowing, the use of fused images, and the utility of the standardized uptake value (SUV), to name a few key issues. We will describe the method we use at our institution, keeping in mind that other orders of operations and methodologies may prove just as effective.

Before even opening the study, it is worthwhile to investigate the purpose of the study and narrow down the question to be answered. Is the patient being staged initially, in which case one must look first at the initial site of disease and the expected location of the draining nodes? Are we assessing response to therapy, in which case it would be useful to know how conspicuous the prior disease was and where it was located? Or are we doing investigation of a suspected recurrence, in which case the results of other imaging and non-imaging studies would be crucial to focus on one area? Or are we doing surveillance scan in which case, the entire scanned area could conceivably hide a recurrence?

It is also good to know what prior surgeries the patient has had and even if there are any other malignancies. A mildly avid axillary node may become much more concerning if near the site of recurrence or less so if the patient has been recently operated on in this area. A history of radiation therapy is also a potentially relevant fact to be aware of, as post-radiation change and scarring may persist and even be mildly FDG

J. D. Oldan (✉)
Department of Radiology, Division of Molecular Imaging and Therapeutics, University of North Carolina, Chapel Hill School of Medicine, Chapel Hill, NC, USA
e-mail: jorge_oldan@med.unc.edu

© Springer Nature Switzerland AG 2021
A. H. Khandani (ed.), *PET/CT and PET/MR in Melanoma and Sarcoma*,
https://doi.org/10.1007/978-3-030-60429-5_4

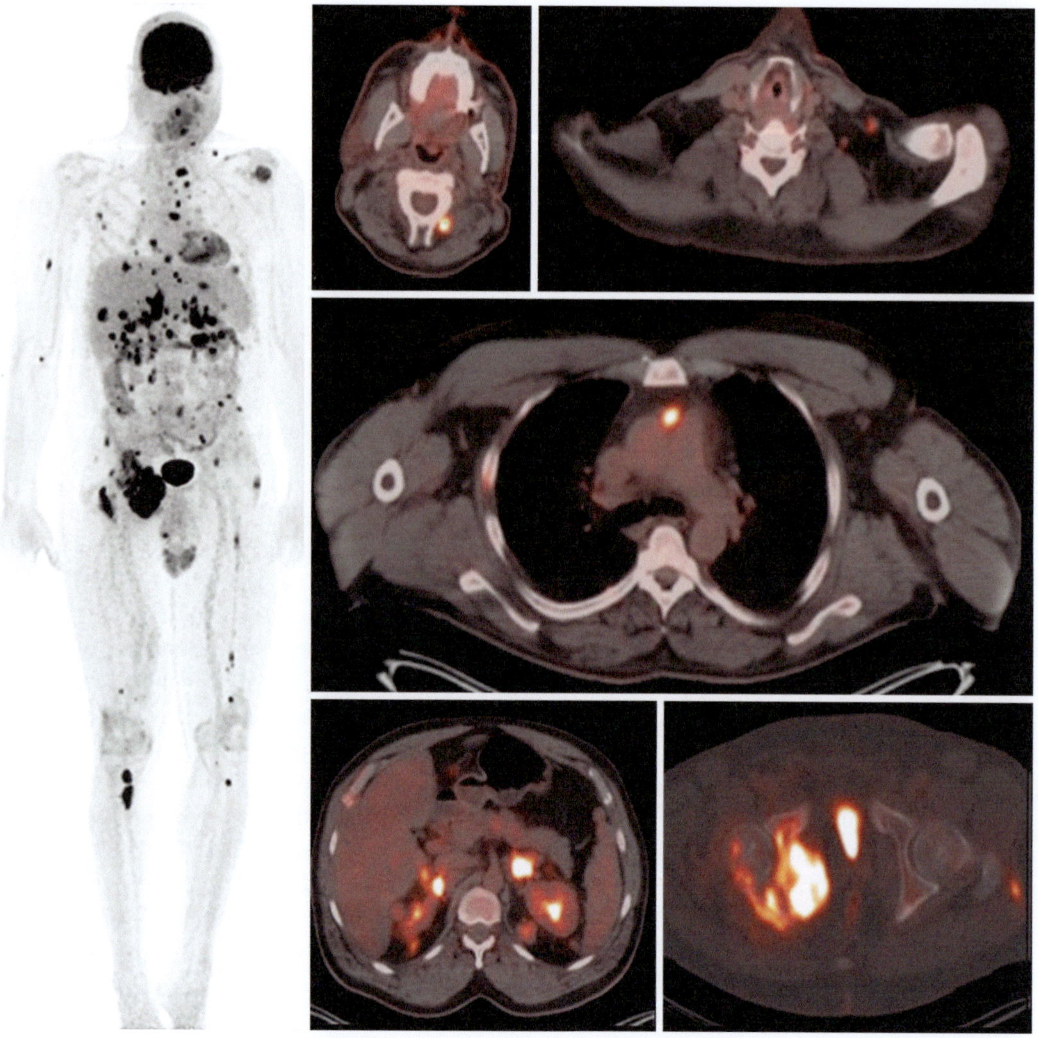

Fig. 4.1 MIP (maximum intensity projection) shows multiple metastases throughout the body, with individual axial fused images showing intense metastases throughout the body

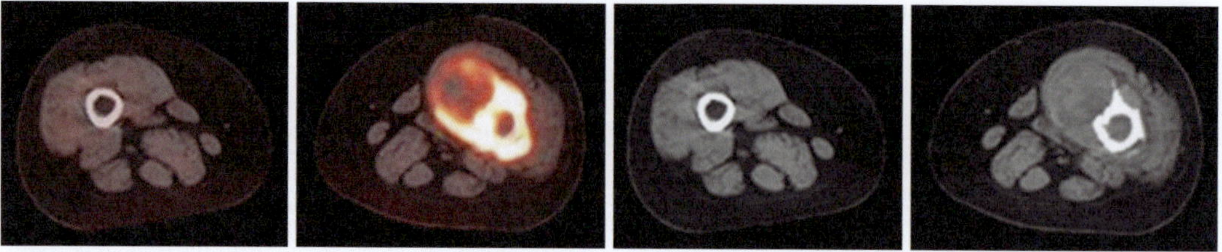

Fig. 4.2 Heterogeneous osteosarcoma in distal femur of adolescent. Note the wide variation in FDG uptake in different parts of the tumor. SUV ranges from 0.4 (in the necrotic core) to 10.2 in the mass. At the same time, due to lack of IV contrast, the CT appearance of the mass lacks the heterogeneous appearance often seen in sarcoma on contrasted CT

avid. Finally, recent chemotherapy can cause activity in bone marrow and occasionally spleen, and this should not be confused with diffuse metastatic disease.

Once the history is known, one way we start is to look at the maximum intensity projection (MIP) images (example in Fig. 4.1). These are a series of projection images obtained at a range of angles around the patient in the axial plane, which when viewed as a movie give the effect of the patient's scan spinning around; as a result this has also been referred to as the "spinning person" view.

Apart from the always intense brain and bladder activity and, frequently, intense and sometimes heterogeneous heart activity, metastases will stand out as intense foci. For the remainder of this discussion, we will assume a gray-scale MIP display where higher intensities appear "dark" and the principal locations of metastases can be assessed. Are they in the lung, liver, bones, muscles, or other locations? The overall metastatic burden (if any) can be assessed—if there were plenty of metastases throughout the body last time, are they more or less numerous and/or more or less metabolically active now?

A word on overall intensity is in order. PET images usually have a window, where a particular set of values in the source data set (usually an SUV) is mapped to a gray scale, ranging from black to white, or to a color scale. Numbers below the lower limit appear white on gray scale (e.g., MIP), and those above the upper limit appear black. Display protocols may reverse black and white or use color scales for fused PET/CT images, but the principle remains the same. The lower limit is set to 0, indicating no activity, and negative numbers are meaningless as there cannot be negative amounts of radioactivity. Note that this is different from CT, where 0 indicates pure water and tissues with negative numbers exist and include less dense materials like fat and air. The upper limit varies depending on user preference, but is usually set to 5–6 when beginning to read. Usually the intensity increases roughly linear to SUV, but this depends on the specific program and thus depends on the software developer.

It should be noted that while majority of malignant lesions independent of their intensity are usually visualized and detectable, using this SUV-derived default display of images, there are circumstances, where the intensity of images have to be increased or decreased in order to visualize malignant lesions. The two extreme ends of the spectrum are brain metastases on one hand and small soft tissue metastases on the other hand. In order to visualize brain metastases, the intensity of the image has to be "decreased" in order to decrease physiologic brain FDG uptake and give the metastases the opportunity to "come through." On the other hand, in order to visualize the subtle soft tissue metastases, the intensity of the image has to be "increased," in order to increase their target-to-background ratio and conspicuity (Fig. 4.3). With the SUV-derived display, the liver, which has an SUV of 2–3, is used as a background reference. However, this reference activity is empiric and other factors such as size of a lesion and its FDG avidity at cell level, and resulting count density has to be taken into account, when assessing a lesions, particularly smaller ones, for malignancy, as detailed in Chap. 1.

While maximum standard uptake value (SUV_{max}) is generally not useful for assessing benign versus malignant tumors [1], the mean SUV (SUV_{mean}) of the liver should be about 2–3, and if it is much higher or lower, an error in dose, weight, or uptake time may be present. The liver should appear as a light to intermediate shade of gray (with the upper SUVmax window around 5–6)—an excessively dark or bright liver may suggest a window that is too narrow, in which case noise will appear bright and produce many false positives and a grainy appearance making the image difficult to read, or too bright, in which case many smaller or less avid metastases may be missed (Fig. 4.4).

Using more than one window may also be wise—it is worthwhile to use a window with a higher maximum, for example, to look for brain metastases (Fig. 4.2, above). PET is not sensitive for brain metastases due to the intense physiologic uptake in the brain, which uses a lot of glucose. However, particularly large and avid

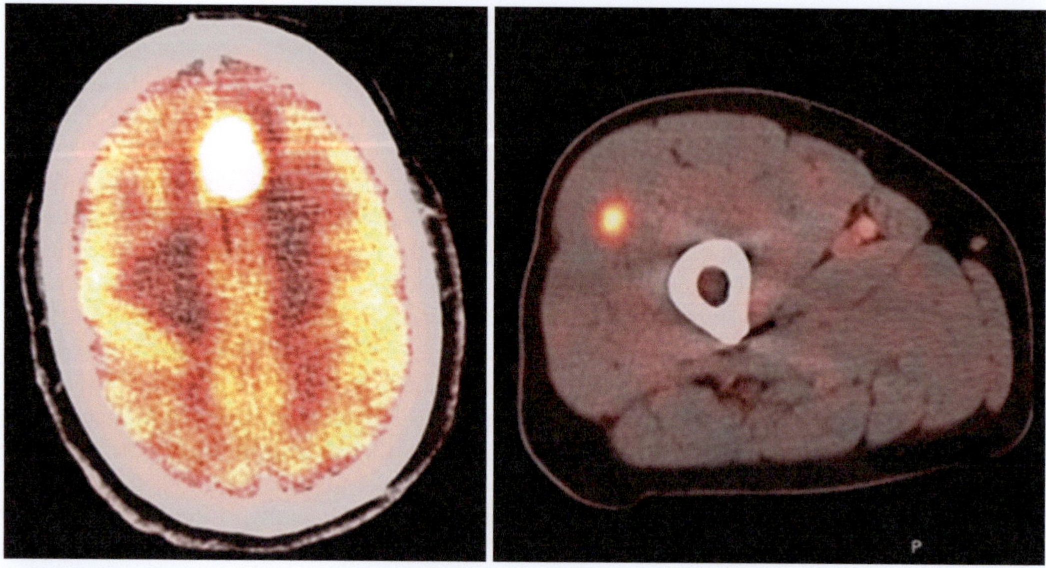

Fig. 4.3 Brain metastasis needs to be windowed with a high upper limit to be visible (note relative low uptake of normal brain), whereas muscle metastasis needs to be windowed with a lower upper limit (note relative intensity of muscle around it)

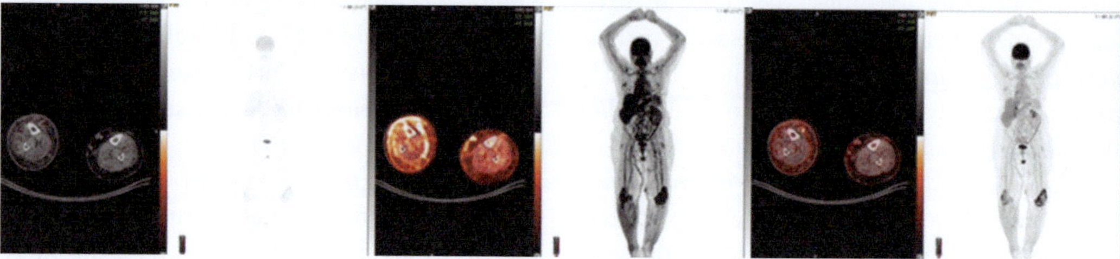

Fig. 4.4 Windowed too high (upper limit 50), too low (upper limit 2), and adequately (upper limit 6). Notice that the lesion in the right leg is difficult to see in the first case and benign variations in the tissue appear significant in the second

metastases (and melanoma is often very avid) may be visible on PET with proper windowing. Occasionally a tumor in the bladder may be seen as well.

Also visible on the MIP immediately are large extravasations and contaminations, appearing as large FDG-avid blotches. They will often be intensely avid (far more than any actual tumor, with SUVs in the hundreds) and will be recognizable as such, but should be identified to remove any confusion. In addition, extravasated FDG is eventually consumed by macrophages and brought to lymph nodes, possibly producing false positives in the nodal drainage pattern of the extravasation, so one should be aware of extrava-sations when they occur. The site of injection should also be noted—a mildly avid right axillary node becomes much more worrisome than a left axillary node if the original injection site was the left antecubital fossa.

If there are no obvious metastases, it then is useful to look at the usual drainage patterns of the tumor. Melanoma tends to spread to lymph nodes before going to other organs. In general, melanomas of the upper extremities drain to the axillae (Fig. 4.5) and melanomas of the upper extremities to the inguinal region (Fig. 4.6). Occasionally, epitrochlear nodes near the elbow or popliteal nodes behind the knee may also be seen to have metastases. Melanomas of the trunk may drain to

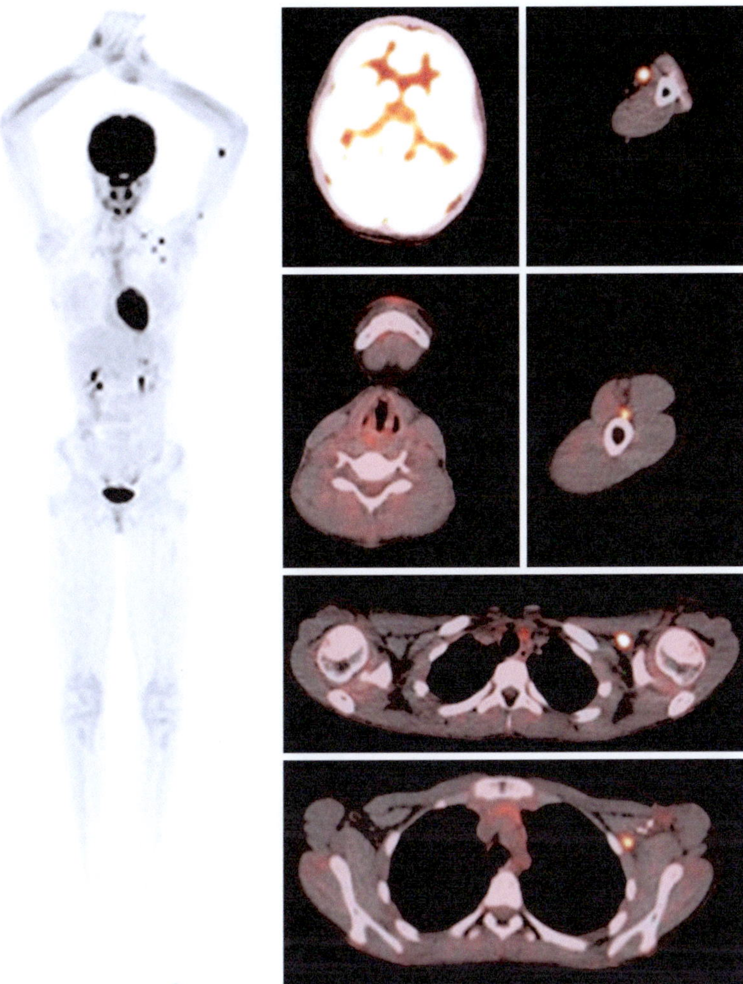

Fig. 4.5 Arm melanoma with axillary and subpectoral metastases

either or both axillary or inguinal sites—they tend to drain to the closest one, but nothing is certain and all four sites should be examined.

Sarcoma, conversely, tends to invade locally or spread to the lung (Fig. 4.7), so particular attention should be paid to the lung, although lymph nodes should also be examined.

Systematic Approach: Part by Part

Once the whole-body images have been examined, the patient should be examined body segment by body segment. In general, we move head to toe, as with the physical exam, using the usual quasi-radiology division into head and neck, chest, abdomen and pelvis, and lower extremities

and musculoskeletal system. Some readers prefer to view using fused images, while others prefer having separate CT and PET images and looking at both. One caution with the use of fused images is that registration may be imperfect, with the head and neck (usually the last part of the scan), lower chest (Fig. 4.8) and upper abdomen (due to diaphragmatic motion), and extremities being common trouble areas. It is usually fairly obvious when misregistration has occurred; if it has, separate viewing of CT and PET images and often a look at non-attenuation-corrected images is in order [1]. We will briefly discuss important CT findings to beware of at the end of each section.

It is also worth warning of "satisfaction of search." A patient may have more than one disease, and discovery of one large, prominent find-

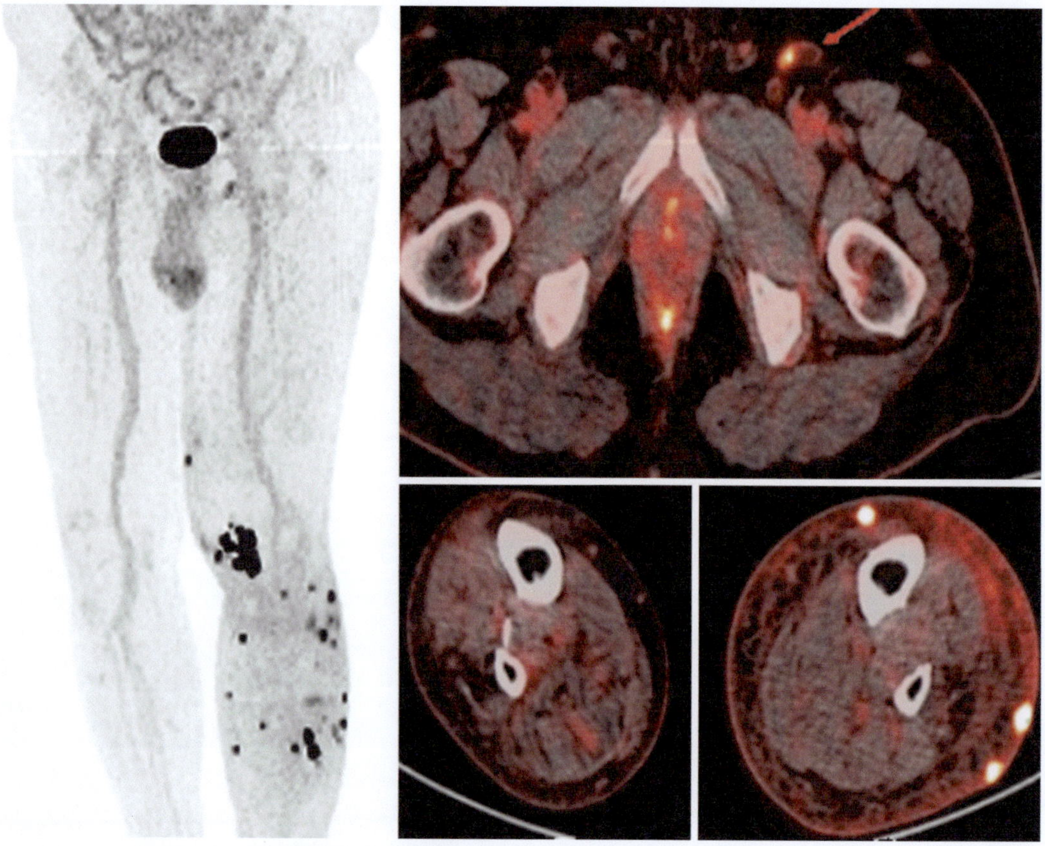

Fig. 4.6 Leg melanomas with metastasis to inguinal lymph node (arrow)

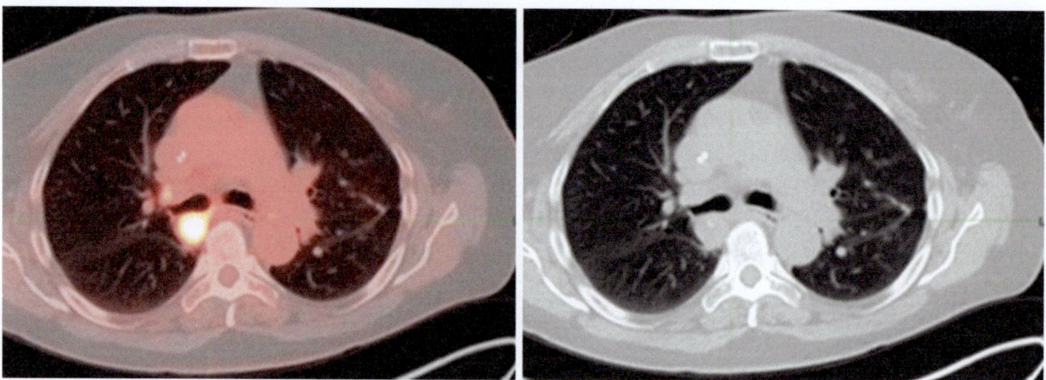

Fig. 4.7 Lung metastasis from recurrent sarcoma

ing may encourage a reader to stop looking and ignore other findings that may be just as important. Finding a pulmonary nodule, for example, does not mean a subtle periaortic node may not be present as well. The "big four" target sites of the brain, lungs, liver, and bone, as well as the relevant lymph nodes, should be specifically examined in each patient.

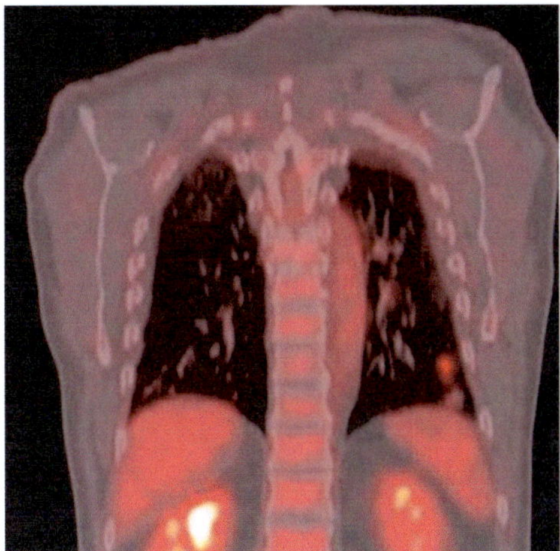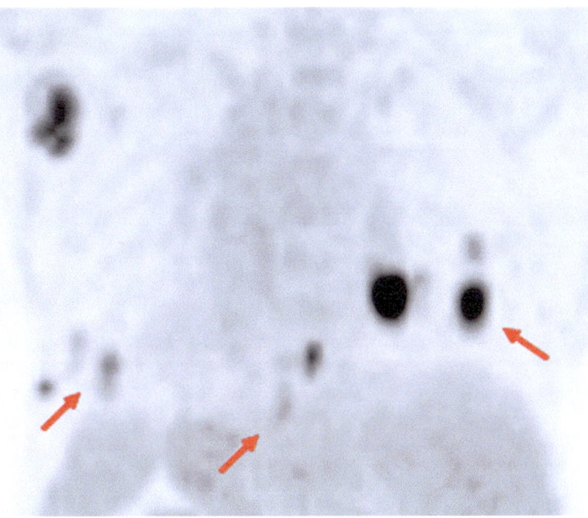

Fig. 4.8 Misregistered clear cell sarcoma lung metastasis. The lesion as depicted on PET is substantially superior to that on CT, likely due to the patient having taken a deeper inspiration on CT than on PET. On MIP images, streaks from motion (arrows) during acquisition are visible

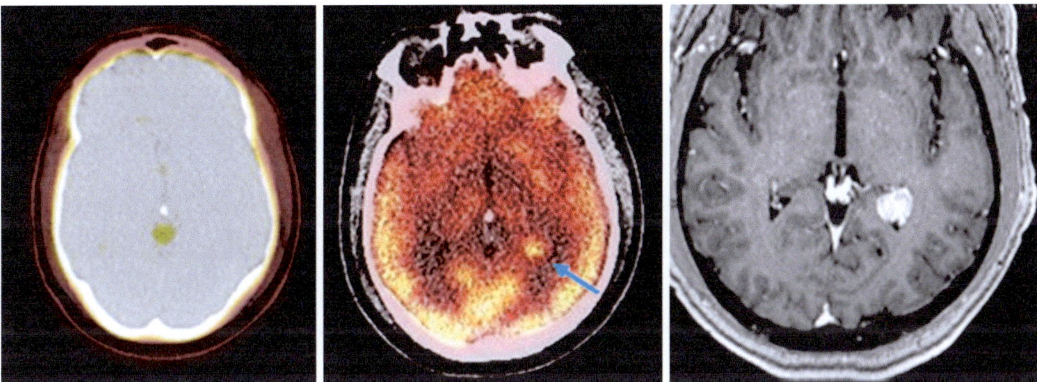

Fig. 4.9 Choroid plexus metastasis is invisible with standard windowing with max SUV 6, but windowed to max SUV 20 a hot spot is visible (arrow). MRI clearly confirms metastasis at this location

Head and Neck

As with the MIP, it is generally worth examining the brain. While sensitivity of PET for brain metastases is low [2] (and brain MRI is much more effective), if a brain MR is not ordered due to what is felt to be a low chance of metastatic disease, the PET gives at least some chance to detect one (Fig. 4.9). In general, the brain should be viewed using a typical brain window for CT and windowed to a higher upper limit for PET, in order to bring out brain lesions that would otherwise be obscured by the intense physiologic brain activity.

Moving on to the head and neck, there are many sites of interest. Normal structures which may display intense avidity (generally not to be confused with melanoma metastases) include Waldeyer's ring, including the adenoids, palatine tonsil, and lingual tonsil (Fig. 4.10), as well as the tongue and vocal folds (Fig. 4.11), which will light up if the patient has talked during the uptake period. (It is difficult to get some people not to speak for an hour.) In general, physiologic processes are symmetric—systemic activation of lymphatic tissue will tend to light up both sides at once—and relatively diffuse, such that diffuse

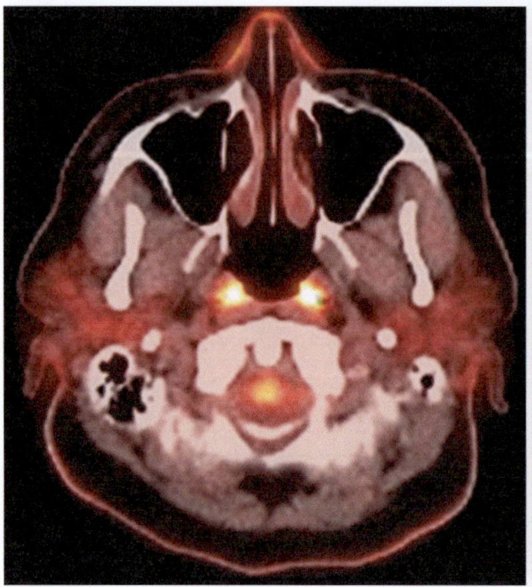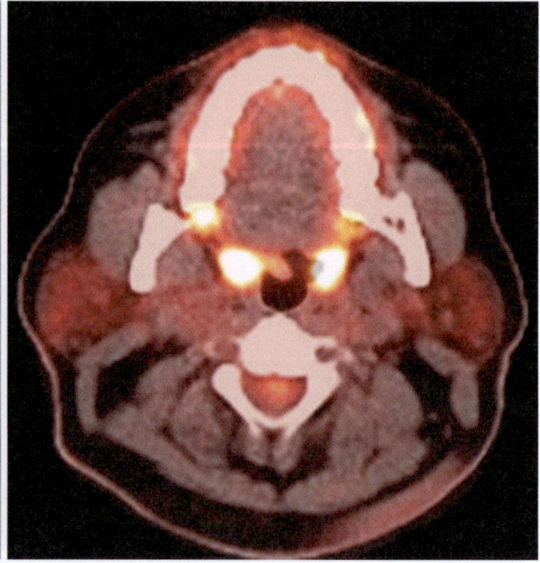

Fig. 4.10 Uptake in Waldeyer's ring. Given its symmetry, this is most likely benign physiologic uptake; more asymmetric uptake might suggest a focal malignancy (possibly a second primary) or metastasis, although local inflammation might also be involved

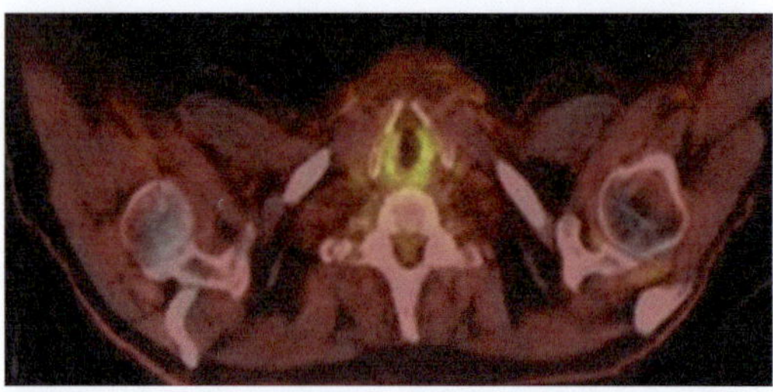

Fig. 4.11 Symmetric vocal cord uptake is usually physiologic. If the left side is less avid, however, it can reflect a tumor in the AP window in the chest or elsewhere along the course of the left recurrent laryngeal nerve

uptake in a structure is less worrying than a focal "hot spot."

The head is also a common site of melanoma due to its relatively high degree of sun exposure. The head and neck contains many lymph nodes in close proximity to each other. While the seven-level otolaryngology classification can be useful in describing the location of lymph nodes, it is designed for squamous cell carcinomas of the aerodigestive tract and does not include many nodes, such as mastoidal and occipital, which may be important sites of drainage for a scalp melanoma, for example. If one is not certain of the precise nomenclature of a node, describing local landmarks may be useful.

As inflammation lights up on PET just as cancer does, deciding whether a node is hot enough to call malignant is a difficult process. Some considerations include history (has the patient recently had an infection or surgery in the area, which may cause inflammation and hence a false positive?), the original site of disease (the same mildly avid jugular node is much more likely to be a malignant metastasis if a primary melanoma is on the cheek than if it is on the leg), symmetry (bilaterally symmetric metastases exist but are relatively rare), and CT appearance of the node (round, larger nodes with effacement of the hilum and in particular cystic or necrotic components are more likely to be malignant than oval, smaller nodes with a preserved hilum and without such components) [1]. Even so, judging a node benign or malignant is often a difficult judgment call.

It is also important to look at the subcutaneous tissues for nodules that may not be in typical nodal beds, but nonetheless represent sites of metastasis (Fig. 4.12). Uptake within fat with absolutely no CT correlate, if diffuse, symmetric and seen in a younger person, more likely repre-

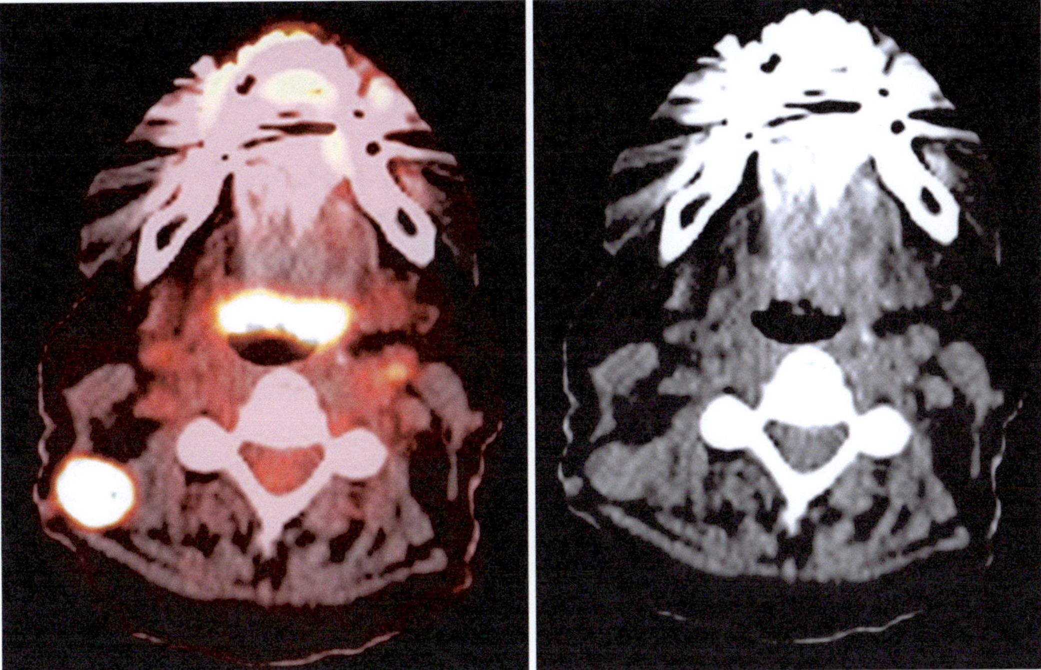

Fig. 4.12 Subcutaneous neck nodule. This is roughly in the location of a level 5 cervical node, but melanoma metastases can also be found in locations not corresponding to standard lymph node locations

sents brown fat, a normal variant commonly seen in colder weather. However, focal uptake with no CT correlate presents something of a conundrum. In this case we would advise to look carefully for a small nodule that may be misregistered; if none is found, directing careful attention on follow-up may be the best strategy. The thyroid may have metabolically active nodules, and these have a reasonable risk of malignancy ranging from 15% to 36% depending on the meta-analysis [3, 4]; if a hot spot is found in the thyroid, this should be brought to the clinician's attention in the impression and a thyroid ultrasound recommended if this has not already been done.

Small muscles may light up with muscular activity and become confusing. If purely due to anxiety, they will usually be symmetric, but in the case of asymmetric activation due to muscle strain, often after surgery, they can be hard to tell from small metastases, particularly if the patient moved their head during the scan. In this case a look at the maximum intensity projection images can be useful [2].

A look at the calvarium and later face and spine is also worthwhile; many tumors send metastases to the bone, and melanoma and sarcoma are definitely no exception.

Important CT findings to be on the lookout for in the head and neck include hemorrhagic or ischemic strokes (Fig. 4.13) or large brain tumors. If an acute stroke or hemorrhage is detected, the referring physician should be called immediately and the patient held and directed to the emergency room if they are still present.

Chest

As one moves into the chest, it is normal to look first at the lungs, which occupy most of the cross-sectional area and, receiving close to 100% of the body's blood supply, are common sites of metastasis from both melanoma and sarcoma (as well as many, many other tumors). There are different schools of thought on this, some holding that the lungs should be left for last to avoid ignoring

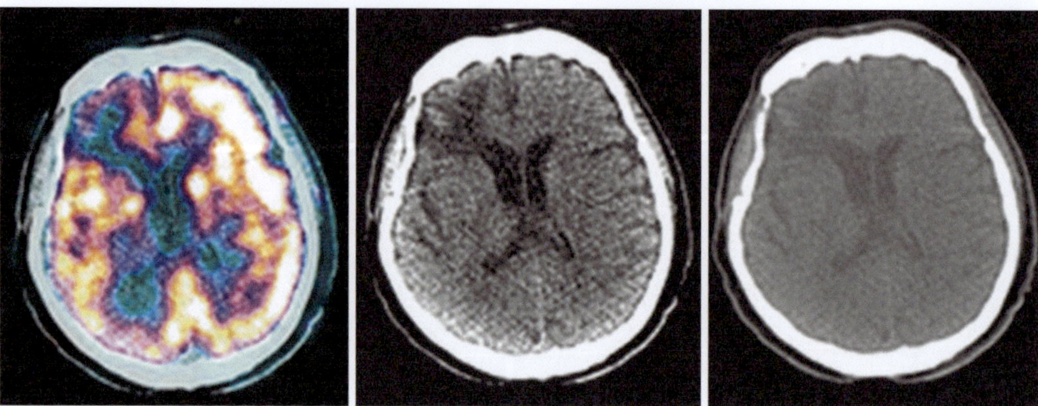

Fig. 4.13 This is an old stroke, visible in the right frontal lobe by the lack of uptake. Unfused CT shows the low attenuation characteristic of an old stroke—new strokes will show a more subtle blurring of the gray-white matter differentiation. Note that this is much more visible on the brain window images (center) than on the general soft = tissue window images (right). In most cases, strokes are old and well-known, but correlation with old imaging is recommended

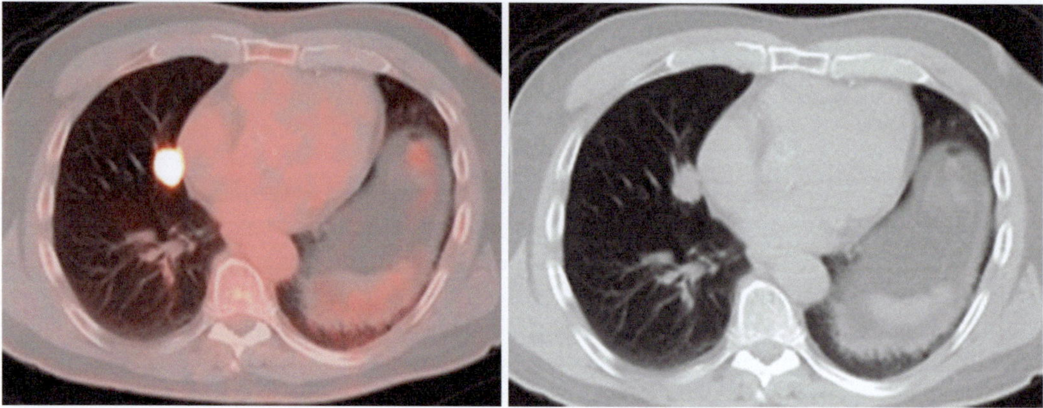

Fig. 4.14 Typical metastatic lung lesion—round and intense. Note that some primary lung lesions can have this appearance as well. Metastases to lungs are quite common

other thoracic structures, others holding that as a high-yield structure they should be examined first to quickly identify patients who are not candidates for surgical resection.

Whatever one's order of operation, the lungs are a major target of metastasis (Figs. 4.14 and 4.15) as well as one of the more common sources of primary cancers, and one should pay close attention to them. Generally, one scrolls up and down through the lungs, looking for nodules or masses. The normal branching of the bronchial and arterial trees produces vessels that are round in cross-section, and this is one of the most tech-nically challenging parts of the body to read. However, normal structures have a tree-like fractal branching pattern that moves from larger to smaller as one moves peripherally, and focal swellings are suspicious. Metastases, of course, may not connect to the bronchial or arterial trees at all, at least at CT resolution.

Telling whether a nodule or mass (a mass is over 3 cm) is primary or metastatic can be diffi-cult. Metastases tend to be round in shape, whereas primary cancers are more likely spicu-lated (Fig. 4.16), but these rules are not absolute, and some primary tumors such as carcinoids are

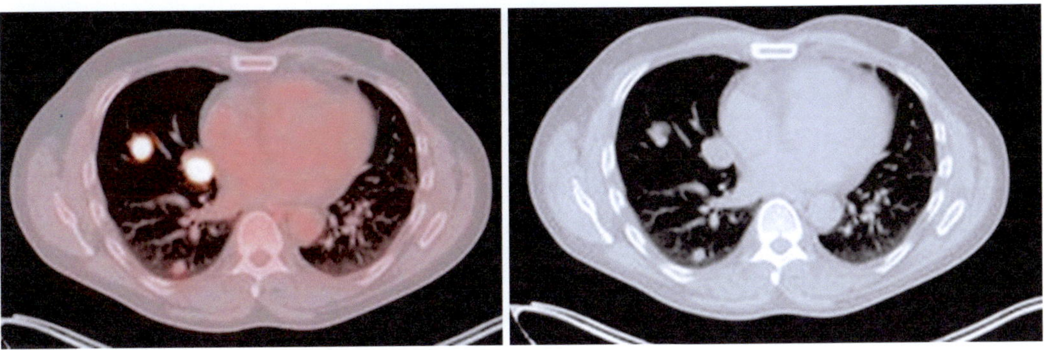

Fig. 4.15 Clear cell sarcoma with multiple lung metastases. Despite the different histology, these metastases have a roughly spherical appearance, similar to melanoma metastases in the previous image

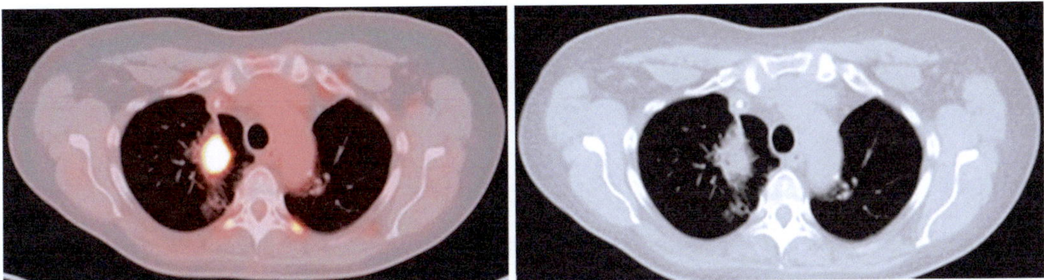

Fig. 4.16 Primary lung cancer, spiculated in appearance. It can sometimes be difficult to tell a second primary from a pulmonary metastasis, although primary lung cancers will tend to have a more irregular appearance

often round in shape. A biopsy may be required. Whatever the case, a "hot" or even "warm" nodule or mass is suspicious for malignancy. Exactly how "hot" is "hot" enough to be called malignant again requires judgment. Previous work on telling whether nodules were benign or malignant focused on SUVmax [5], but the many variations due to size, motion artifact, etc., as well as the problem of "hot" granulomas and "cold" adenocarcinomas and carcinoids, have made SUV an unreliable guide. In particular, due to issues involving volume recovery and partial volume effects [6], uptake will appear higher in larger tumors up to about 3 cm, so a lesion that grows larger without any changes in metabolism per cubic centimeter will appear to grow brighter as well.

Presently, we consider any activity in a nodule under 1 cm or any activity above mediastinal blood pool in a nodule over 1 cm suspicious. In general, PET is not sensitive for detecting lesions below about 8 mm, so lesions with visible avidity that are much smaller than this are likely to be very avid indeed and hence suspicious. Similarly, larger nodules with no avidity are felt more likely to be benign, or at least a low-grade tumor [7].

It is also worth mentioning that, since infection is a common source of false positives, and the lungs are a common source of infection, pneumonia as well as inflammatory diseases like pulmonary fibrosis (Fig. 4.17) will be "hot" on PET and may be confused with malignancy if one is not careful. They will tend to have different appearances on CT, however. Scarring from radiation may be avid and has a linear appearance not seen in natural processes (Fig. 4.18). CT images for PET-CT are taken in shallow inspiration, and the appearance may be somewhat different from stand-alone chest CTs taken in deep inspiration, particularly near the bases.

While there is an entire chapter on artifacts and pitfalls, one worth mentioning here is the breathing artifact at the bases [2]. The diaphragm is one of the largest muscles and one in near-

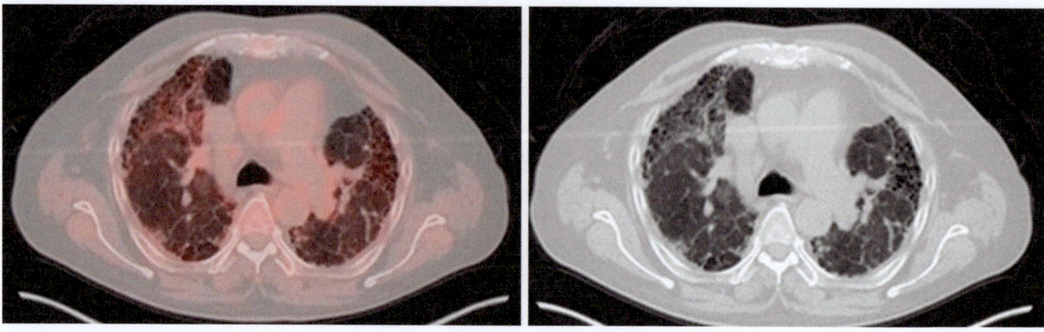

Fig. 4.17 Pulmonary fibrosis. Inflammation, like cancer, is hot on PET, and the area of uptake can often be seen to correspond to the area of fibrosis where inflammation is occurring. It can occasionally be confused with cancer

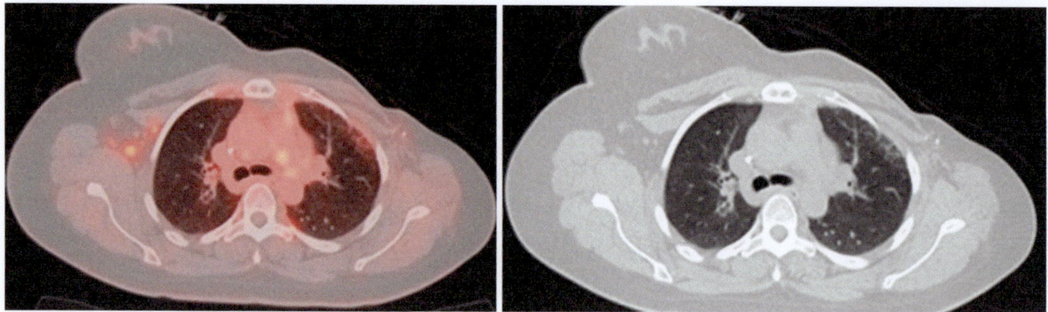

Fig. 4.18 Radiation fibrosis from radiation to breast (note mastectomy) with impact on surrounding lung—notice the linear contour

constant motion throughout normal physiologic functioning, and while we attempt to coach patients on shallow breathing to allow it to be in a similar position on the CT and PET, this is often difficult, especially with sick patients who may have poor breath control. As a result, misregistration is often greatest near the diaphragm, with the position of lung nodules on CT often quite different from their position on PET. This can lead to false negatives where the nodule appears cold because its PET position is registered a few slices up or down from its CT position. One countermeasure is to view the CT and PET separately in this region. Non-attenuation-corrected images may also be useful, as attenuation correction will be thrown off by misregistration.

While examining the lungs, it is also worthwhile to examine the pleura. Pleural metastases are much more common from primary lung cancers than from melanoma or sarcoma, but the well-known tendency of melanoma to send metastases to odd places means the pleura are at least worth investigating. Unfortunately, one generally cannot tell by avidity whether a pleural effusion is benign or malignant, as plenty of effusions with inflammatory causes may be "hot." A rind of soft tissue, generally with an irregular appearance, is much more suspicious for spread to the pleura (Fig. 4.19).

Once the lungs have been evaluated, one can turn one's attention to the mediastinum, usually defined simply enough as everything between the lungs (or to be exact the visceral pleural surfaces). The mediastinum contains the heart, great vessels and pulmonary vessels, esophagus, trachea, and many lymph nodes. Among these, the heart, great vessels, and pulmonary vessels are rare sites of metastasis radiologically (though some pathologic studies suggest cardiac metastases may be more common than often thought), and the heart in particular has variable and sometimes very intense uptake, so PET findings here

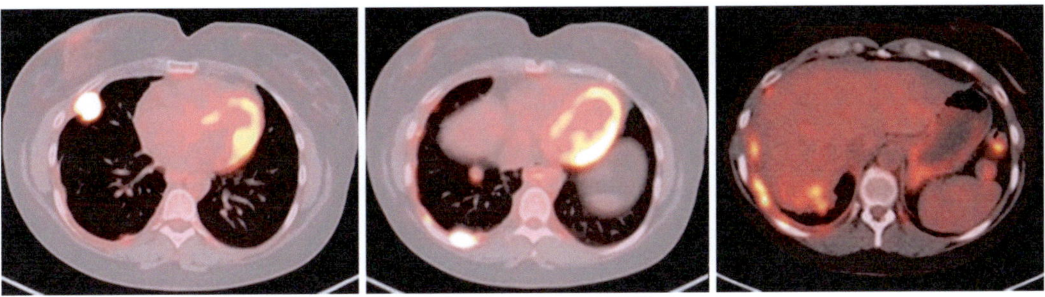

Fig. 4.19 Metabolically active pleural disease in this patient with melanoma

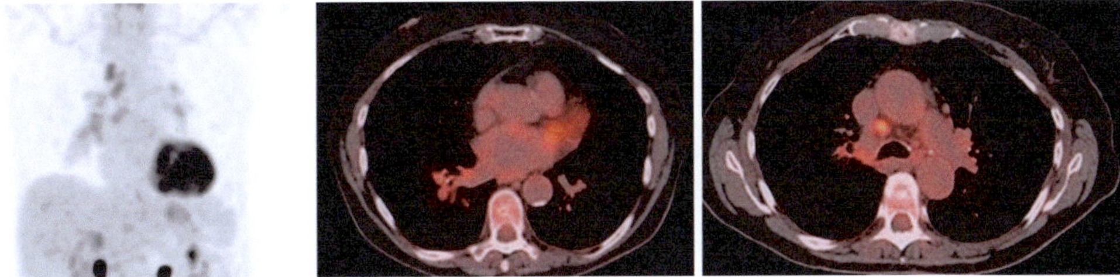

Fig. 4.20 Low-grade mediastinal and hilar uptake, bilaterally symmetric and possibly due to a small right lower lobe bronchopneumonia. The mild uptake and relative symmetry suggest a benign etiology

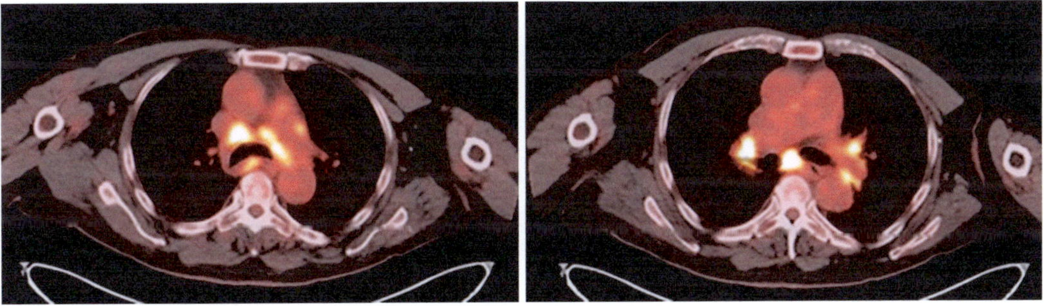

Fig. 4.21 Intense, symmetric mediastinal and bilateral hilar uptake characteristic of sarcoid

are relatively rare [2]. The esophagus and trachea are not commonly targets of metastasis either, although esophageal inflammation from chemotherapy in patients who have already been treated should at least be commented on to avoid clinicians reading the study on their own coming to the wrong conclusion. Inflammation from gastroesophageal reflux can also be seen.

Often a metastatic target, however, are lymph nodes. Mediastinal and hilar nodes are more commonly targets of metastasis from primary lung lesions, but can sometimes be targets of melanoma spreading down lymph node chains.

One possible false positive to beware of is that low-level mediastinal and hilar uptake is fairly common and easily confused with spread of disease (Fig. 4.20). The distinction here is that it is bilaterally symmetric or close to it, and mediastinal and hilar uptake should be similar in level [2]. In cases where there is a granulomatous disease such as sarcoid, it can be quite florid (Fig. 4.21). Metastases, conversely, tend to be sharply focal in a few areas. While diffuse mediastinal and hilar metastasis *may* exist, it is usually accompanied by widespread disease elsewhere in the body (in melanoma and sarcoma).

When looking at the chest, one should not forget the superficial soft tissues. Axillary (and adjacent subpectoral) nodes are the preferred site of drainage for upper extremity malignancies and frequent sites of drainage for trunk melanomas. As a result, one should always make sure to check the axillary nodes on both sides. Similar to the case with the mediastinum and hila, low-grade bilaterally symmetric axillary nodes can be seen in viral infections. HIV is a particularly notorious cause of this, and one should check the medical record for a systemic disease that could cause diffuse inflammation; occasionally, this can even be the cause for diagnosing a systemic illness even if the scan is negative for melanoma!

The breasts can also have additional primary malignancies, especially but not exclusively in women (Fig. 4.22). Additionally, melanoma in particular can send metastases to subcutaneous tissues and muscles, so one should look carefully for hot lesions here as well. Cutaneous "hot" spots may indeed be additional melanomas or may be local infections, so this is a place to draw attention to the site and refer the clinician to correlate with physical examination.

Finally, a glance at the ribs is wise, as the bone is a common target for metastasis from many tumors. As there are many ribs (usually twelve), it is difficult to follow each one individually, but a look at the ribcage as a whole can allow one to see many metastases. The sternum, scapulae, and clavicles should be examined too, as should the proximal humeri.

One important CT finding is the presence of a pneumothorax (Fig. 4.23). This may be a medical emergency depending on size and pressure and should prompt an immediate call to the referring clinician on detection. Other important findings to report include pleural effusions (Fig. 4.24), pericardial effusions (Fig. 4.25), pulmonary consoli-

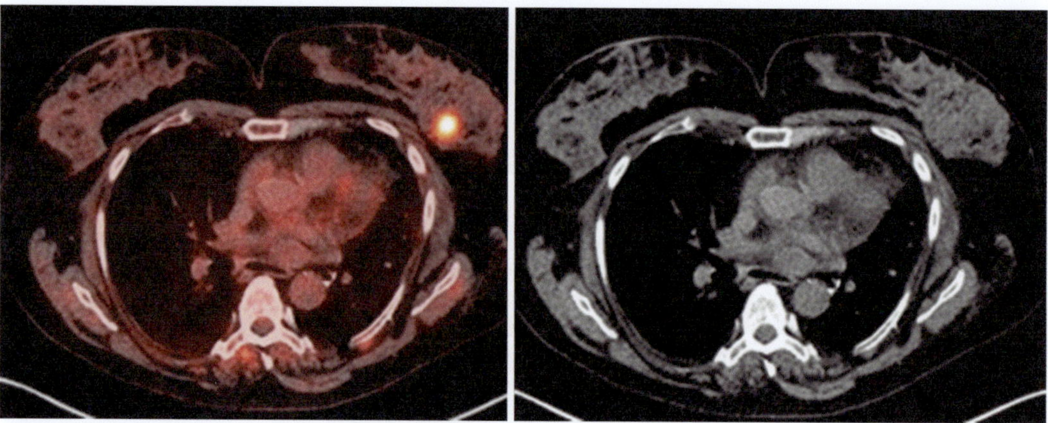

Fig. 4.22 Intense breast lesion, incidentally discovered, not visible on CT

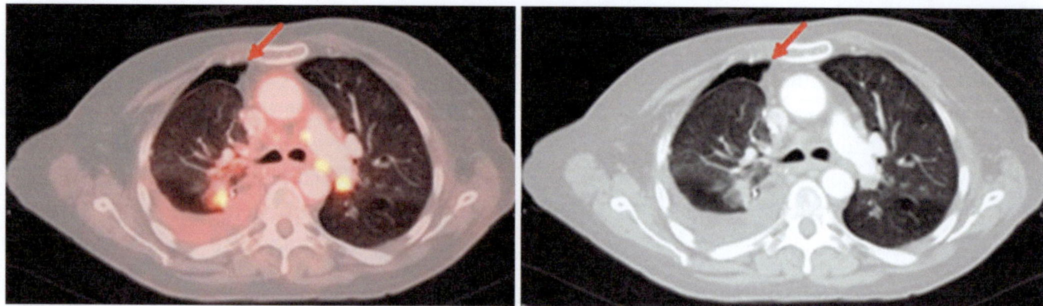

Fig. 4.23 Small pneumothorax (red arrow) incidentally found on chest CT

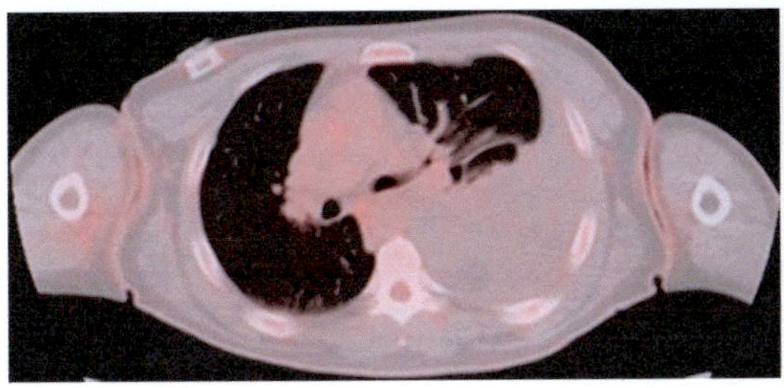
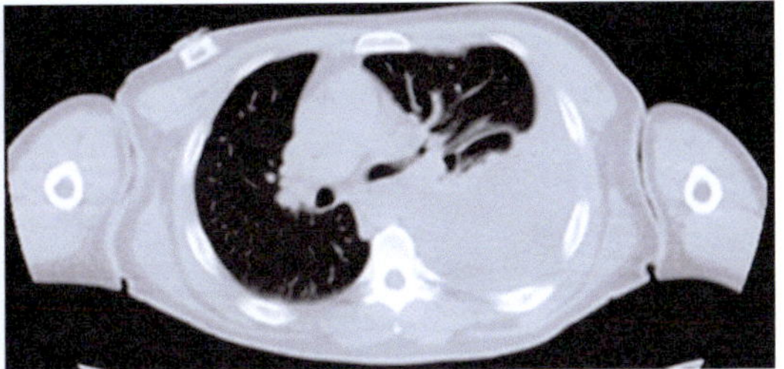

Fig. 4.24 This large non-avid pleural effusion in a patient with a non-avid desmoplastic round cell tumor may be benign or malignant; the lack of avidity suggests a benign etiology, but this is not certain

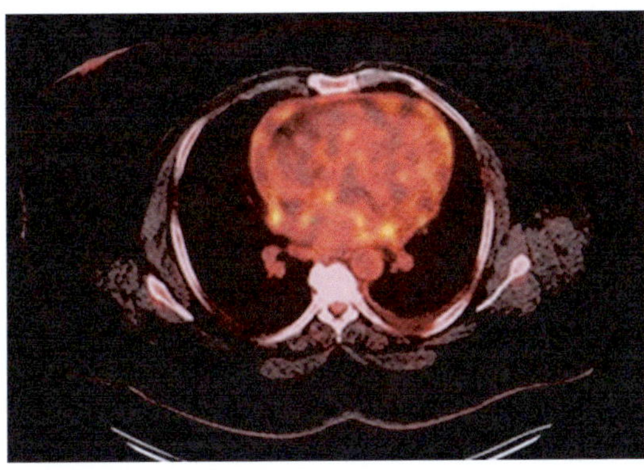
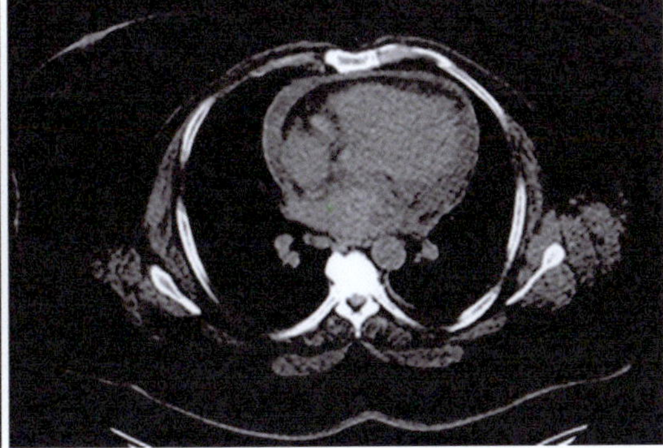

Fig. 4.25 This pericardial effusion is metabolically active, as could result from either benign inflammation or tumoral infiltration

dations such as pneumonia, and coronary calcifications (Fig. 4.26), which suggest coronary artery disease. Signs of a median sternotomy and coronary artery bypass grafts may be seen as well. Occasionally, one may see an aneurysm here.

Abdomen and Pelvis

The wide variety of organs here makes interpretation of the abdomen and pelvis relatively complex. While, as in most cancers, the liver and lymph nodes are common sites of metastasis, the viscera may become targets as well in melanoma.

The liver is a common target for metastasis in melanoma, with its dual blood supply meaning cancers have two methods of ingress. The liver has moderate FDG uptake, enough that it is used for benchmarking uptake in various applications. However, the somewhat grainy uptake means that metastases can be more difficult to detect, and while PET may find some metastases CT or MR

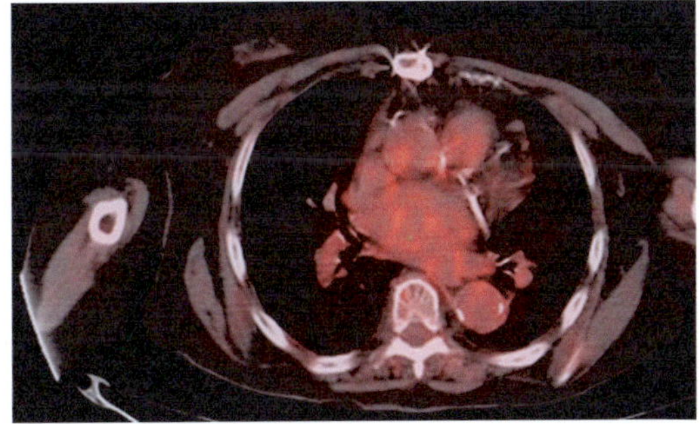

Fig. 4.26 Coronary artery calcification. This can suggest coronary artery disease, though specificity is rather low. It is usually worth calling attention to in the findings section at least

do not, the reverse is also true. As a result it is often useful to look at the CT separately, possibly using a liver window to see liver lesions better (Fig. 4.27). If there is continued clinical concern for liver metastasis despite a negative PET/CT, MRI can be useful in the liver [2].

Lymph nodes are also common sites of metastasis. While axillary nodes drain relatively quickly

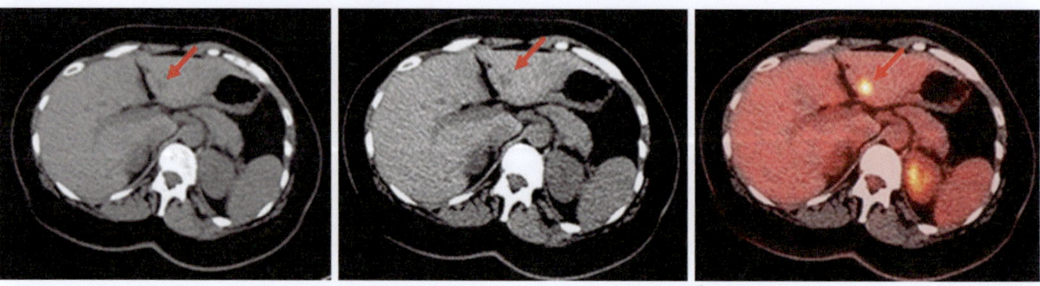

Fig. 4.27 Liver metastasis (arrows) is better seen on liver window (middle) than on soft tissue window (left) on CT. On PET (right), lesion clearly is quite avid and malignant

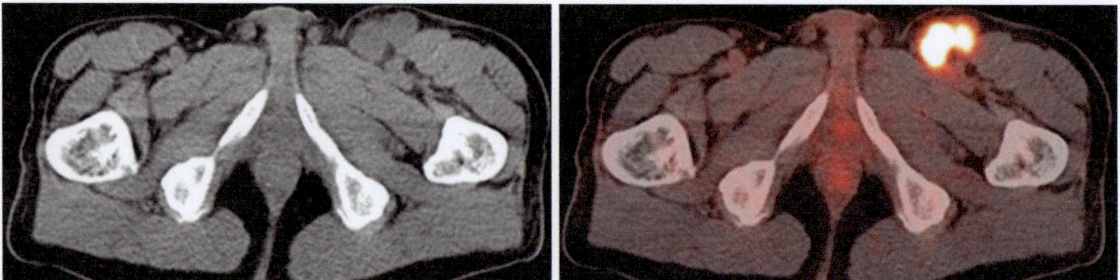

Fig. 4.28 Round, large, asymmetric inguinal node lacking fatty hilum, known melanoma. The heterogeneous uptake suggests necrosis

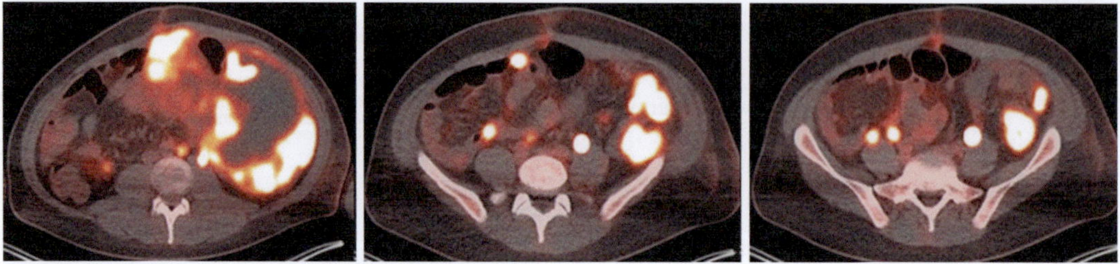

Fig. 4.29 This large desmoplastic round cell tumor (the same as previous patient with this tumor) has periaortic, right common iliac, and bilateral external iliac metastases

into subclavian trunks and reach the mediastinum, disease entering the inguinal nodes draining the lower extremities passes to external iliac and common iliac nodes along lumbar trunks and finally periaortic nodes before entering the thorax. Similarly, lymph leaving the bowel (and malignancies with it) drains into mesenteric nodes. As a result, there is a wider range of areas that must be checked for metastasis in the abdomen.

Inguinal nodes, draining the legs, often show mild, symmetric uptake and indeed have the largest acceptable dimensions for short axis apart from the subcarinal and lower aortic nodes [1]. Inguinal nodes are seen as suspicious if uptake is particularly intense (much more than liver) or asymmetric, particularly if there is a lower extremity melanoma ipsilateral to the node or the node has a malignant appearance by CT (round, lacking fatty hilum, large) (Fig. 4.28).

Mesenteric nodes may also be sites of metastasis, particularly if the disease has spread to the bowel. It is worthwhile in the case of a melanoma (assuming it is of the usual cutaneous source) to exclude a visceral source of inflammation which might be another cause.

Retroperitoneal nodes (Fig. 4.29), along the major vessels, are common sites of spread once disease has passed the inguinal nodes; in sarcoma cases they may be earlier sites of spread. In general, metastases will pass to the external iliac, then common iliac, and then perioortic/aortocaval nodes, but few malignancies are this regular in their behavior. All of these areas should be examined for enlarged or avid nodes.

The viscera are less common sites for metastasis, but melanoma in particular is notorious for sending metastases to uncommon locations. The bowel is a reasonably common target (Fig. 4.30), but evaluation of the bowel is complicated by the variable and sometimes intense uptake that can be seen in the bowel and particularly the colon [2]. Hot spots in the colon, if solitary, may reflect primary colon cancers or polyps with malignant potential, and a solitary area of focally increased uptake should prompt a colonoscopy (Fig. 4.31). An exception would be if the patient already has widespread metastatic disease and detecting a colon cancer early would have little effect on quality or duration of life. Metformin, a common

oral hypoglycemic, causes the entire bowel to become avid and may complicate diagnosis of bowel disease.

Other viscera are usually less important as far as evaluation goes, though it is wise to check them systematically, as melanoma in particular sends metastases to odd places. The gallbladder is rarely a target but can be easily checked along with the liver. The spleen does accumulate metastases and should be checked, although solitary splenic metastases are rare. The adrenal glands are much more commonly the site of spread from lung cancers, although adrenal metastases are well-known. Adrenal adenomas are also quite common, and generally adrenal nodules more avid than liver are considered suspicious (Fig. 4.32; as benign adenomas and bilateral adrenal hyperplasia can produce abnormal uptake, an MRI or contrast-enhanced CT using an adrenal protocol may be useful if uncertainty persists [2]. Evaluation of the kidneys and ureters

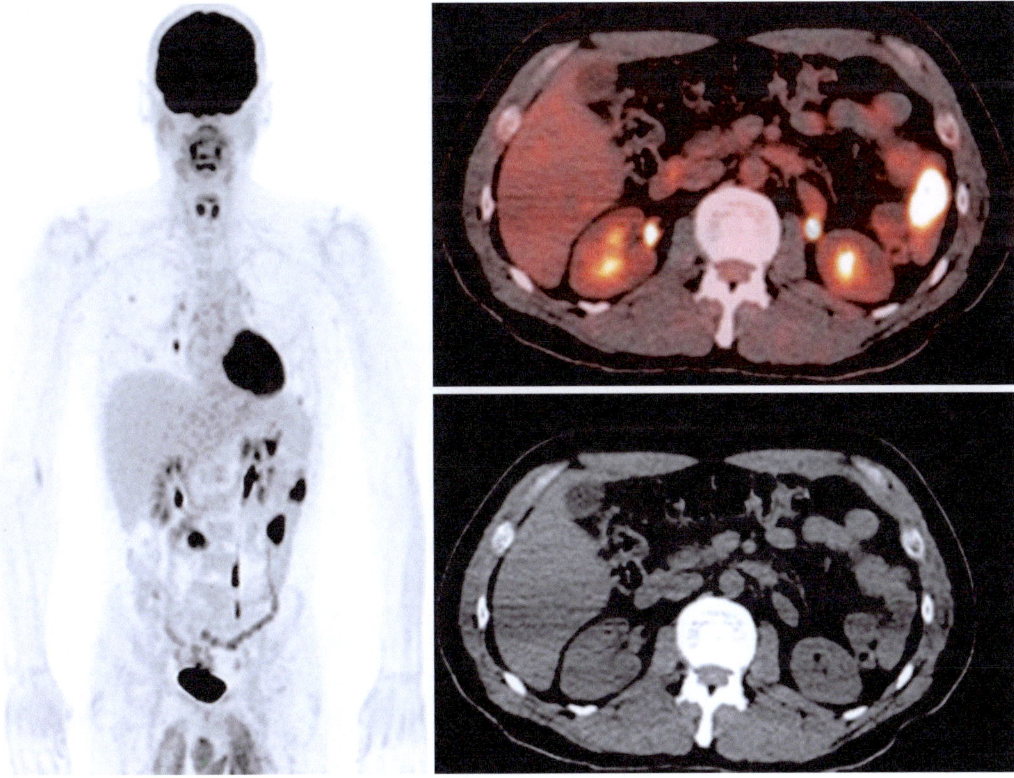

Fig. 4.30 Bowel metastasis from melanoma. Bowel metastases are often difficult to see on CT, even with oral contrast; if solitary bowel metastasis is suspected, colonoscopy may be in order to investigate it

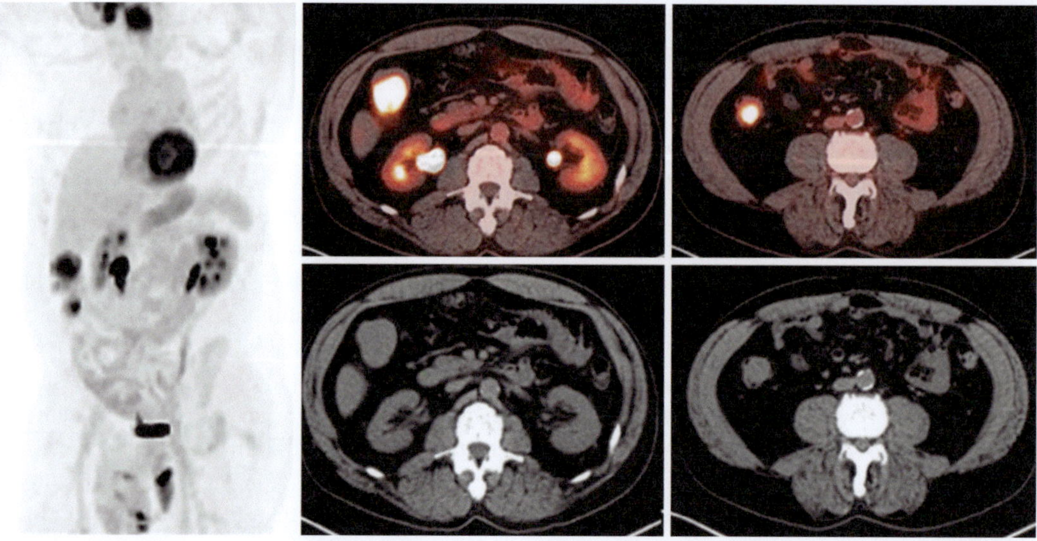

Fig. 4.31 Two focal areas of increased uptake in the colon, corresponding to masses on CT (poorly visualized without oral contrast); one proved malignant and the other a premalignant polyp on colonoscopy. Bowel metastases, primary colon cancer, and polyps are hard to tell apart, so focal areas of uptake in the colon should prompt a colonoscopy, unless the patient's chance of survival are otherwise poor and this is unlikely to be of any benefit

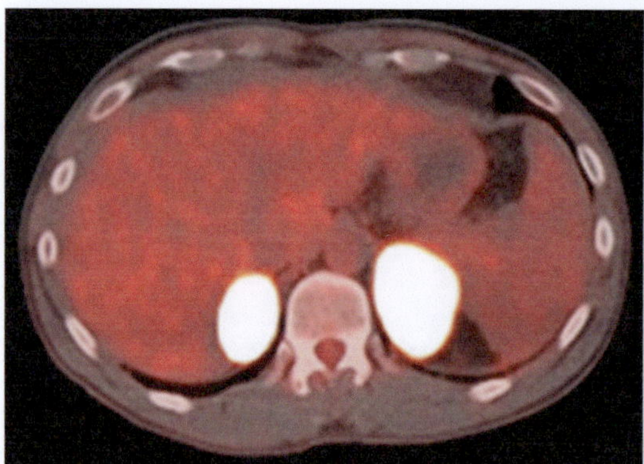
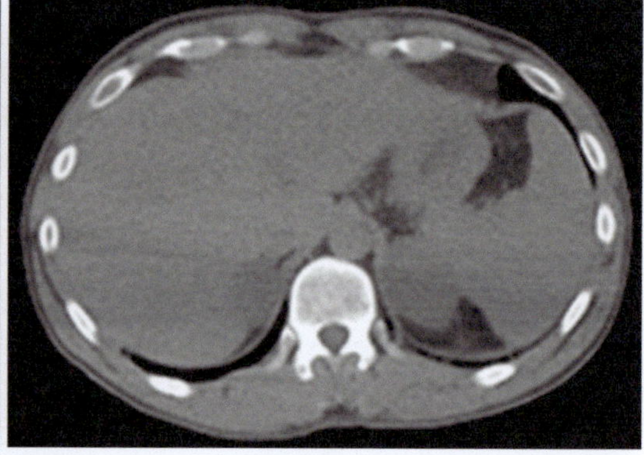

Fig. 4.32 Bilateral adrenal metastases. The liver is often used as a cutoff for determining "how hot is too hot" for adrenal nodules. Avid adrenal nodules can be further investigated by contrast-enhanced CT or MRI using special adrenal nodule protocols

is difficult given the normal physiologic excretion of tracer into the collecting system, but metastases are sometimes visible, and primary renal cell carcinomas are occasionally found (and may not be avid). A focus that localizes to the ureter is much more likely to be urine in the ureter than an actual metastasis to this organ (Fig. 4.33). Renal cysts, if large enough, are usually visibly non-avid. The bladder is generally difficult to evaluate given that large amounts of radioactive urine collect in the bladder, although windowing may allow the detection of masses—note that these may be seen as cold spots.

Reproductive organs such as the prostate (in men) and uterus and ovaries (in women) are uncommon targets of spread of disease. Avid foci in the ovaries in a woman of childbearing age may be entirely physiologic. Foci in the prostate along the course of the urethra may be similarly physiologic, but correlation with PSA is at least useful given the high background rate of prostate cancer in older men.

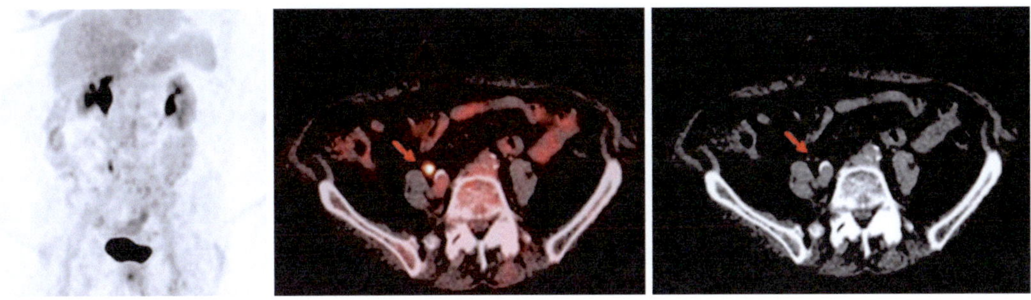

Fig. 4.33 Uptake localizing to ureter (arrows). Uptake has a linear, vertical, superolateral-inferomedial orientation and localizes to the ureter on CT. It can be easily confused with a retroperitoneal node

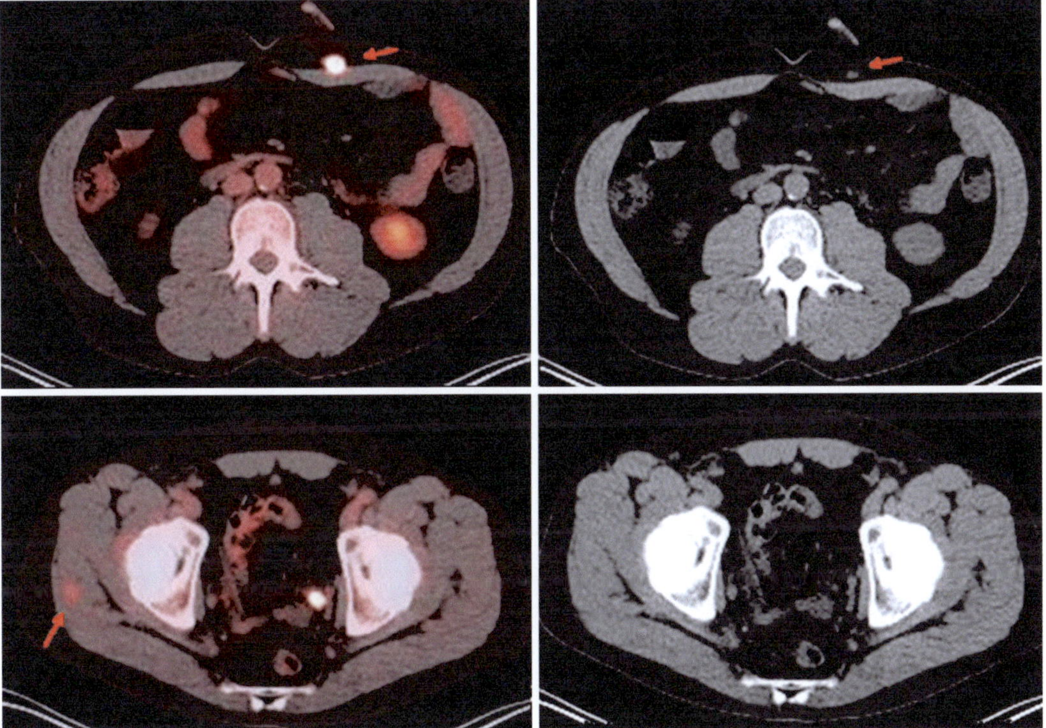

Fig. 4.34 Subcutaneous and muscular melanoma metastases (arrows). Note that muscular metastases in particular may be unimpressive and even invisible on CT without PET; the relatively high contrast of subcutaneous fat makes the metastases easier to see

Soft tissues and bones are important in the abdomen and pelvis. Injection granulomas from subcutaneous injections of insulin or other drugs may be avid and appear as false-positive sites; these are usually sorted out with a check of the patient's history and, if necessary, a note to the clinician about a physical examination. As in the head, neck, and chest, melanoma may send metastases to the subcutaneous tissues and muscles of the abdominal wall (Fig. 4.34).

Checking the skeleton in the abdomen and pelvis is important as much of the skeletal mass is here. The pelvis should generally be checked in multiple planes, both axial and coronal at the least, whereas a single sagittal view can see most of the spine unless the patient is very scoliotic. In

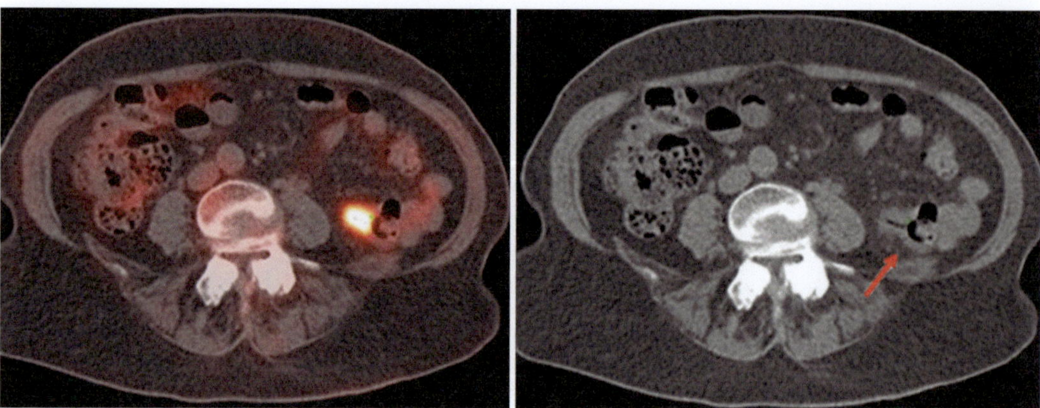

Fig. 4.35 Focus of uptake localized to a diverticulum in the colon (arrow), with mild soft tissue stranding surrounding the diverticulum, is suspicious for diverticulitis. Free air from perforation may also be seen

the skeleton, it is also important to look at the scan CT only using bone windows, as subtle sclerotic metastases may be present.

The abdomen and pelvis are notorious for the variety of CT findings that may exist, and of course CT of the abdomen and pelvis is the preferred method of diagnosing abdominal pain in many areas due to the wide variety of pathologies that may exist. Fortunately, most of these produce inflammation and are FDG-avid. Diverticulitis (Fig. 4.35), appendicitis, cholecystitis, and pancreatitis are all FDG-avid stranding, so the inflamed organ will be FDG-avid in addition to the CT findings such as edema and fat stranding. Pyelonephritis may be somewhat more difficult to diagnose as the kidney may have increased or decreased uptake. Bowel obstruction may not produce increased uptake, but the dilated loops of bowel are easy enough to recognize. Kidney stones may not produce visible FDG changes as they occur in a system with high background uptake, but are easy enough to detect on CT, and can be seen with the fused images turned off.

Musculoskeletal System and Extremities

The musculoskeletal system, practically speaking the bones and muscles for the purpose of searching for malignancy, is present throughout each part of the body and hence can be searched

when previously searching the head and neck, chest, and abdomen and pelvis. An additional search at the end is nonetheless prudent, as one is frequently focused on the viscera on an initial run-through.

If the scan is a whole-body scan (head to toe), as is commonly done for melanoma, a final look at the legs is at least prudent. One can scroll down using the soft tissue window and then scroll back up using the bone window and then go up and look at the skeleton as one moves upward toward the head. Non-axial plane reformats are often useful for the skeleton, given its craniocaudal extent relative to other organs and the importance of a whole-skeleton evaluation given the problems with diffuse versus patchy disease, as described below. A sagittal reconstruction allows one to view the entire spine at once unless significant scoliosis is present, and coronal reconstructions allow one to see much of the pelvis in one view. A major complication in interpretation of the skeleton is the low-grade bone marrow activity [8] (Fig. 4.36) which is normal and increases after the growth factors frequently given with chemotherapy (Fig. 4.37) [2]. Metastases generally produce a lumpy, multifocal appearance (Fig. 4.38). The MIP and sagittal and coronal sections can be useful in telling these apart. It is worth mentioning that metastases may be hidden by the intense bone marrow uptake.

Muscles can be targets of metastasis in melanoma (something much less common in other

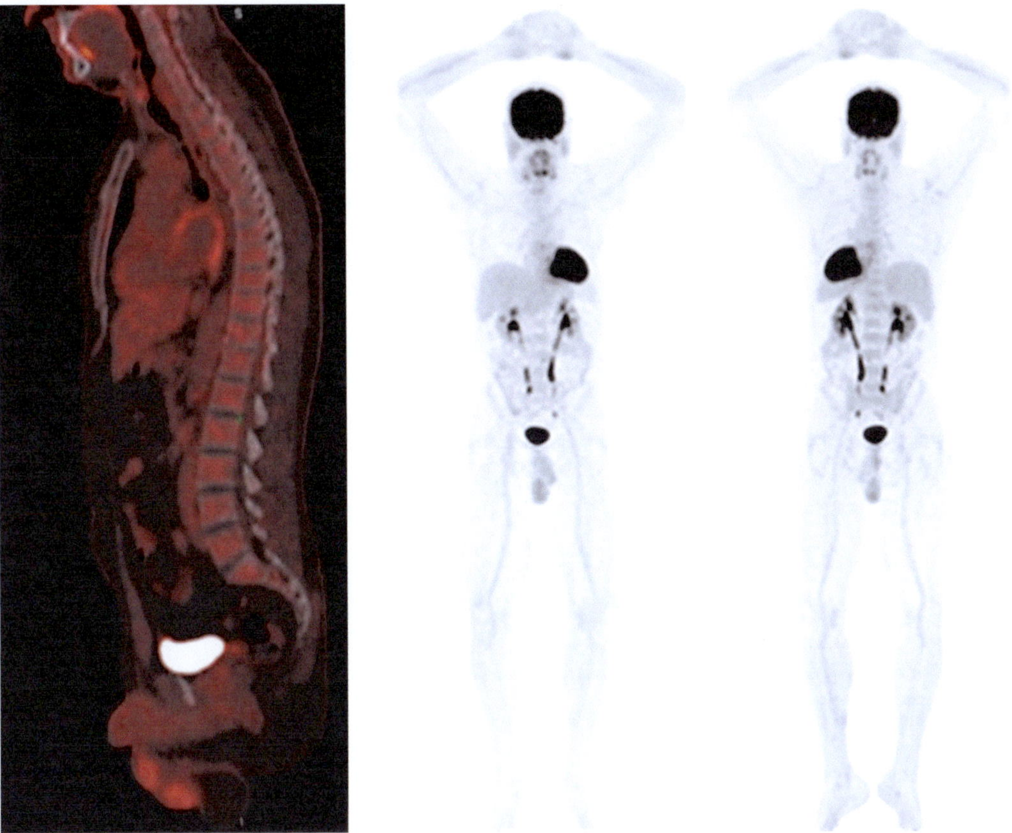

Fig. 4.36 Relatively normal bone marrow uptake. There is uptake in the axial and proximal appendicular skeleton, but it is not immediately obvious on the MIP unless rotated posteriorly

cancers). As such focal areas of uptake within muscle are much more concerning. This must be differentiated from physiologic activity due to the patient using the muscle during the uptake period [8] (Fig. 4.39). Usually this is simple enough as physiologic muscle uptake lights up the whole muscle in linear or triangular, muscle-shaped patterns, but smaller, short muscles in the neck may occasionally cause confusion.

Issues Specific to Melanoma

Surgical Field

Important in evaluation of melanoma is knowledge of prior surgical fields. Melanomas may recur multiple times in the same area, and it is important to know where the patient has been resected in order to pay special attention to those areas (Fig. 4.40). Postsurgical changes may be seen as well, but are usually more low grade and diffuse [2]. In addition, the duration of time from the last surgery should be known, as the area may continue to display uptake for a few weeks or even months after surgery. The reader should also be aware of any nodal dissections performed to stage the melanoma, not only as a possible site of metastasis, but because removal of a nodal basin may mean that recurrence occurs in other nodes nearby instead. Surgical clips can help show the site of axillary or inguinal (or epitrochlear, popliteal, or jugular) nodal dissection.

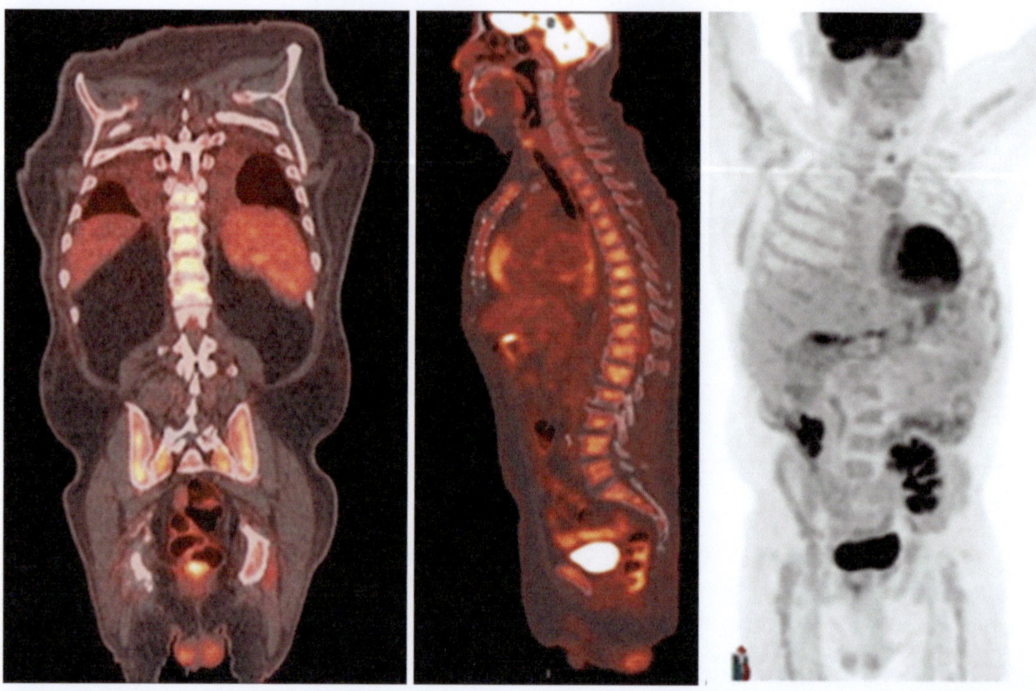

Fig. 4.37 Relatively homogeneous bone marrow and splenic uptake from growth factors. Note the uniform uptake throughout the spine (the sagittal view is usually good for this unless there is substantial scoliosis) and the slightly increased intensity of the spleen vis-à-vis the liver

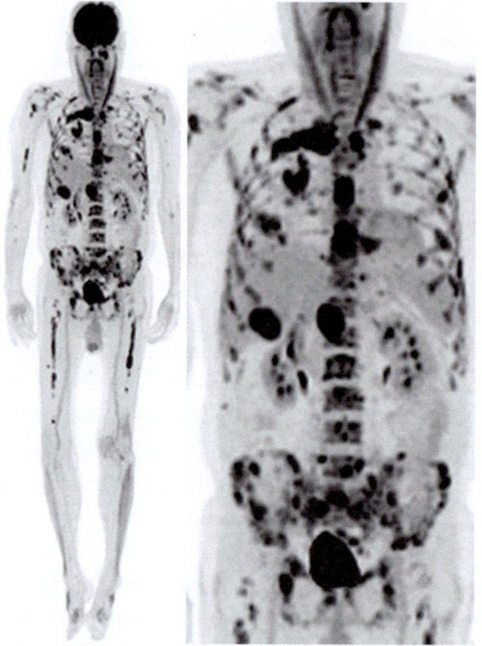

Fig. 4.38 Heterogeneous skeletal uptake from metastases—note the lumpy and heterogeneous uptake pattern, particularly in the spine, as opposed to the smoother uptake in the axial and proximal appendicular skeleton usually seen with bone marrow activation. Liver and bowel metastases are also present

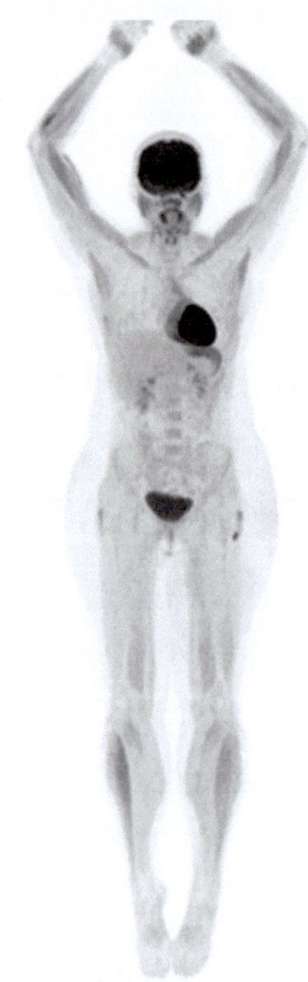

Fig. 4.39 Muscle uptake reflecting motion during the uptake period

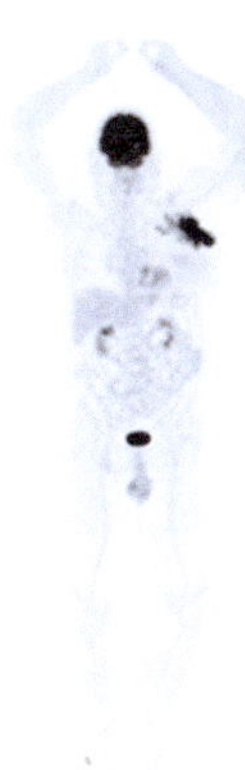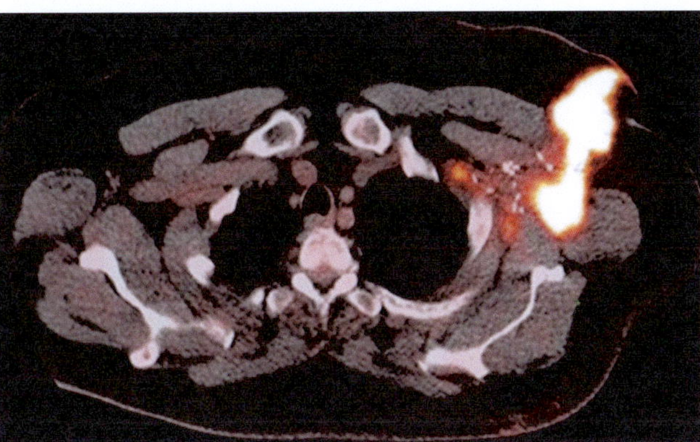

Fig. 4.40 Recurrence in surgical bed. Arm melanomas frequently drain to the axilla, and in this case, after an axillary nodal dissection, this arm melanoma presented with a recurrence in the axilla. PET-CT clearly demonstrates the large, confluent axillary mass

Whole-Body Imaging

Most cancers are imaged from skull base to mid-thigh, the idea being that the low sensitivity of PET for brain metastases makes including the brain useless, and metastases to the lower extremities are rare in the absence of numerous other metastases. Melanoma is imaged from vertex to toes (literally whole-body imaging), the idea being that given its tendency to spread all over the body, scanning the scalp and legs becomes useful. This is somewhat controversial, as isolated leg metastases are relatively rare even in melanoma [9, 10]. Melanoma is somewhat unique in this regard (the only other tumor we scan this way at our institution is multiple myeloma), and there is an argument for scanning skull base to mid-thigh for melanoma as well. The exception, of course, is melanomas of the lower extremities, where the lower extremities should be scanned in their entirety to detect the primary and any in-transit disease, and melanomas of the scalp, in which the whole skull should be included for the same reason.

NAC Image Use

Scans for melanoma often make use of non-attenuation-corrected (NAC) images, which have greatly decreased uptake in the inside of the body (Fig. 4.41), but increased uptake in the skin and lungs, which have counts suppressed by attenuation correction algorithms as part of their normal function. This remains somewhat controversial, but in the case of melanoma, may be relevant due to the possibility of skin lesions undetected on attenuation corrected images [2]. As with boosting the gain on any imaging system, noise rises as well as signal, but given the ease of correlating with physical examination on the skin, this may be worth doing.

Unusual Metastasis Locations (but Not in Melanoma)

The most common sites are lung, liver, bone, and brain, but significant numbers of metastases are also seen to bowel, adrenal, pancreas, heart, kidney, and spleen, as well as all the other viscera [11]. As a result, every organ should be checked, as described in the section-by-section lists above, and even relatively poorly perfused sites such as the subcutaneous tissues may become targets.

Immunotherapy

Immunotherapy has been a powerful new addition to the armamentarium of medical oncologists, with many previously untreatable cases of metastatic melanoma showing response to therapy. However, new side effects related to immunotherapy are being discovered, many of which are visible on PET/CT. In particular, the immune system may attack normal organs, which in addition to the obvious organ damage and consequent

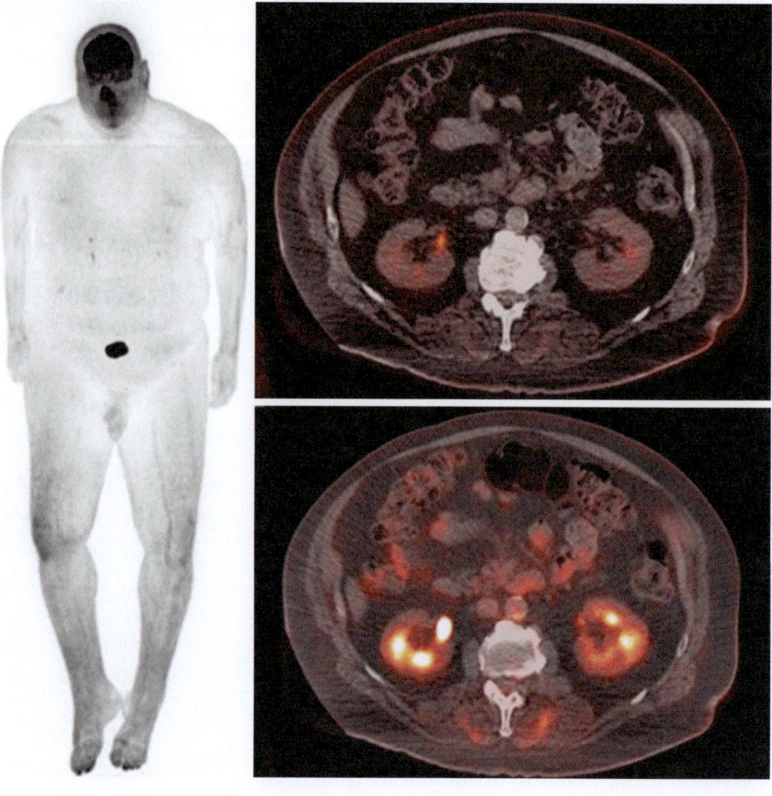

Fig. 4.41 NAC IMAGES, MIP, and FUSED (with AC image for comparison). Notice the higher uptake in the skin and significantly decreased uptake in the viscera

pathology appears as inflammation—and hence a false positive—on FDG-PET.

Current immunotherapies for melanoma include treatments targeted at mutations of the BRAF gene which result in constitutive activity of the MAPK or MEK cell proliferation and growth pathways and immunotherapies aimed at activating cytotoxic T cells to attack the melanoma. BRAF-targeted medications include oral BRAF inhibitors (vemurafenib, dabrafenib, or encorafenib) and MEK inhibitors (cobimetinib, trametinib, or binimetinib) [12].

With BRAF inhibitors, there may be increase in keratoacanthomas or squamous cell carcinomas, which may appear as metabolically active skin lesions and be seen on PET; as these are difficult to distinguish from cutaneous metastases, the reader should simply call attention to them, as being cutaneous lesions they will be easy to detect by physical exam. Lesions may fail to decrease in size despite therapy being effective, but FDG uptake usually occurs more rapidly (the terminal gene of the MAPK pathway, ERK,

decreases glycolysis when downregulated). These inhibitors may also cause activation of the immune system, and one may see activation of lymph nodes in the lymphatic drainage basin of metastatic sites and increased splenic uptake, reflecting an immune flare, particularly if tumor shrinkage also occurs [12].

Immunotherapies aimed at stimulating the immune system currently consist of antibodies that inhibit physiological inhibition of the immune system (thus making the immune system more active). These include antibodies to the CTLA4 receptor (ipilimumab) and to the PD1 receptor on activated T cells (pembrolizumab, nivolumab). Anti-CTLA4 agents cause infiltration of lymphocytes into sites of disease and germinal center activity in draining lymph nodes. Anti-PD1 agents increase cytotoxic killing by T cells. These can also produce a variety of toxicities (usually presenting at about 6–8 weeks) in various organs, most commonly the thyroid but also the pituitary, adrenals, lungs, liver, pancreas, and bowel; often the inflammation can be seen on

PET as increased activity. As with BRAF inhibitors, one may see reactive nodal uptake in the drainage basin of metastases and diffuse splenic uptake, as well as a sarcoid-like symmetric hilar and mediastinal nodal pattern, more common with pulmonary metastases [12].

Accompanying CT findings include colonic wall thickening, pericolonic fat stranding, and possible perforation and free fluid for colitis, mild hepatomegaly, periportal lymphadenopathy, and periportal edema for hepatitis, and diffuse groundglass and reticular opacities, consolidation, and traction bronchiectasis for pneumonitis [12].

CTLA-4 agents in particular have been known to produce false-positives for progression due to the infiltration of lesions (which can cause an apparent increase in size) or the appearance of new ones due to immune infiltrate (which are not actually new cancers). While baseline lesions may shrink or durable stable disease may occur as with other agents, other patterns including response after initial "worsening" (pseudoprogression) and simultaneous response in baseline lesions and presence of new lesions which also result in partial or complete response have also been described [13].

Due to the possible problems with new areas of uptake representing either new tumor (progression) or areas of immune response (response), separate immunotherapy guidelines have been produced for assessing immune response to therapy (immune-related response criteria, irRC). Generally, new measurable lesions on CT are incorporated into total tumor burden (rather than representing progressive disease and hence treatment failure), and progressive disease is defined as more than a 25% increase in total tumor burden compared with nadir, in two consecutive observations at least 4 weeks apart. Formal criteria for PET do not yet exist, but new lesions in common sites of toxicity such as the adrenals, bowel, or pituitary should not necessarily be assumed to be new sites of metastasis [13]. A follow-up examination in 1–2 months with new lesions that are felt to be possibly due to immune reaction (whether due to new lymph nodes in a relatively diffuse distribution more typical of inflammation than tumor, presence of increased splenic uptake, or localization in a typical target organ for adverse reactions such as bowel or pituitary) may be useful [14].

Issues Specific to Sarcoma

Heterogeneity of Uptake and Grade

Sarcomas are often heterogeneous in degree of aggressiveness, and the grade of the sarcoma may be underestimated if the wrong area within it is selected for biopsy. As dedifferentiated sarcomas tend to be both more aggressive and more FDG-avid, areas of high SUV more likely represent areas of high histologic grade, which can then be targeted for biopsy (Fig. 4.42) [15]. Attempts to grade tumors solely by SUV have been made, but generally find a high degree of overlap between benign and malignant tumors [15].

Metastases

Unlike the extremely wide range of metastases produced by melanoma, bone and soft tissue sarcomas often metastasize to the lungs. Retroperitoneal sarcomas often spread to the liver, and myxoid liposarcomas often spread to the retroperitoneum, spine, and paraspinous soft

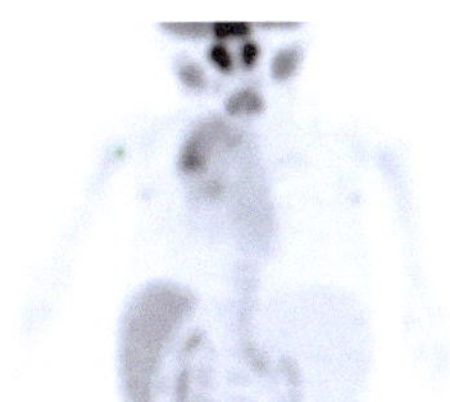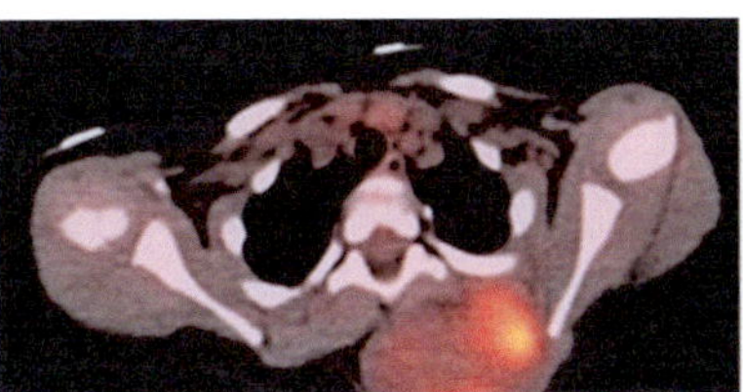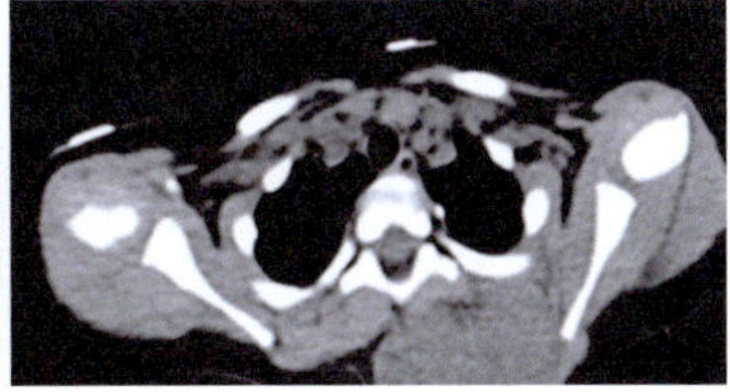

Fig. 4.42 Largely poorly avid fibrosarcoma with smaller area of more intense uptake. This area was targeted for biopsy

tissues. Synovial sarcoma, rhabdomyosarcoma, angiosarcoma, clear cell sarcoma, and epithelioid sarcoma often spread to locoregional lymph nodes, like other cancers [15] (Fig. 4.43).

Sarcomas are generally not as avid as melanomas (Fig. 4.44), and while not in the category of tumors unable to be staged by FDG-PET (like carcinoid or prostate cancer), careful attention to both PET and CT is useful.

CT, which is most sensitive for small lung lesions, is thus necessary for full staging of a sarcoma. As most modern scanners now include a CT, this is generally not an issue, but older PET-only scanners may require addition of a separate CT scan. The reader should also inspect the lungs carefully for smaller lung metastases [15].

Response to Therapy

Lacking the extensive use of immunotherapy, a decrease in uptake after chemotherapy usually predicts tumor response. GIST tumors in particular often display a decrease in response after treatment with imatinib before decreasing in size [15].

Joint Replacements

One problem with extremity osteosarcoma in particular is that limb-salvage therapy with endoprosthetic replacement produces metallic artifacts from prosthetics on both CT and MR. PET is generally less affected by these artifacts intrinsically, but errors in attenuation correction may also hamper PET interpretation. A look at the non-attenuation-corrected images can be helpful, particularly as attenuation is less important in most extremity lesions. Also, chronic periprosthetic inflammation will take up FDG and may produce false positives. The reader should be aware of this and look specifically for focal areas of increased uptake [15].

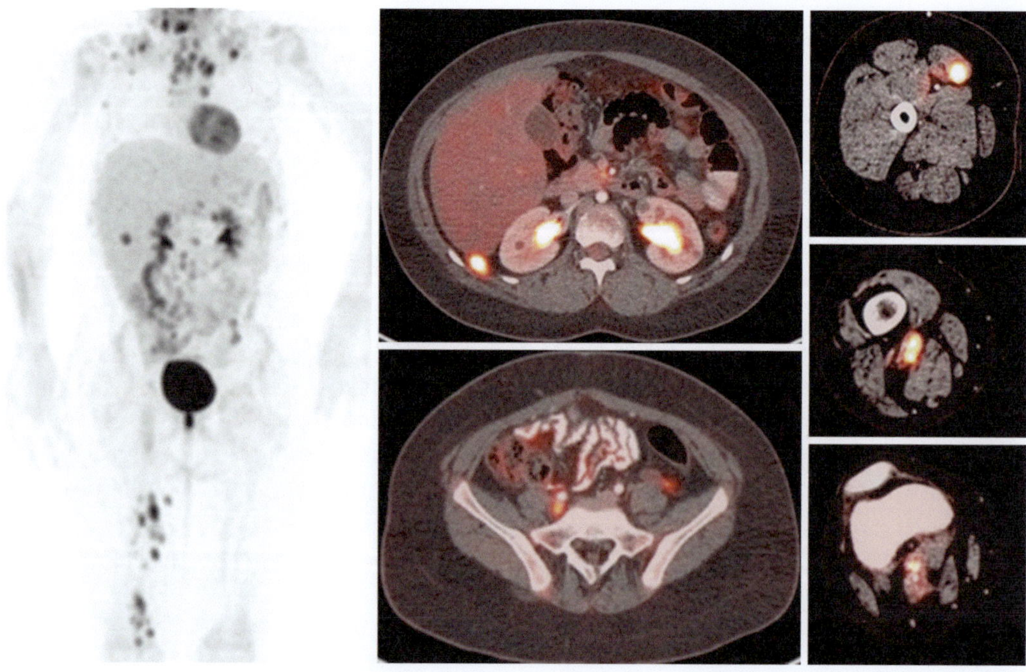

Fig. 4.43 This thigh rhabdomyosarcoma spread to local nodes, as well as a variety of more proximal and distant locations. Note that retroperitoneal nodes, while not that avid overall, are nonetheless visibly avid

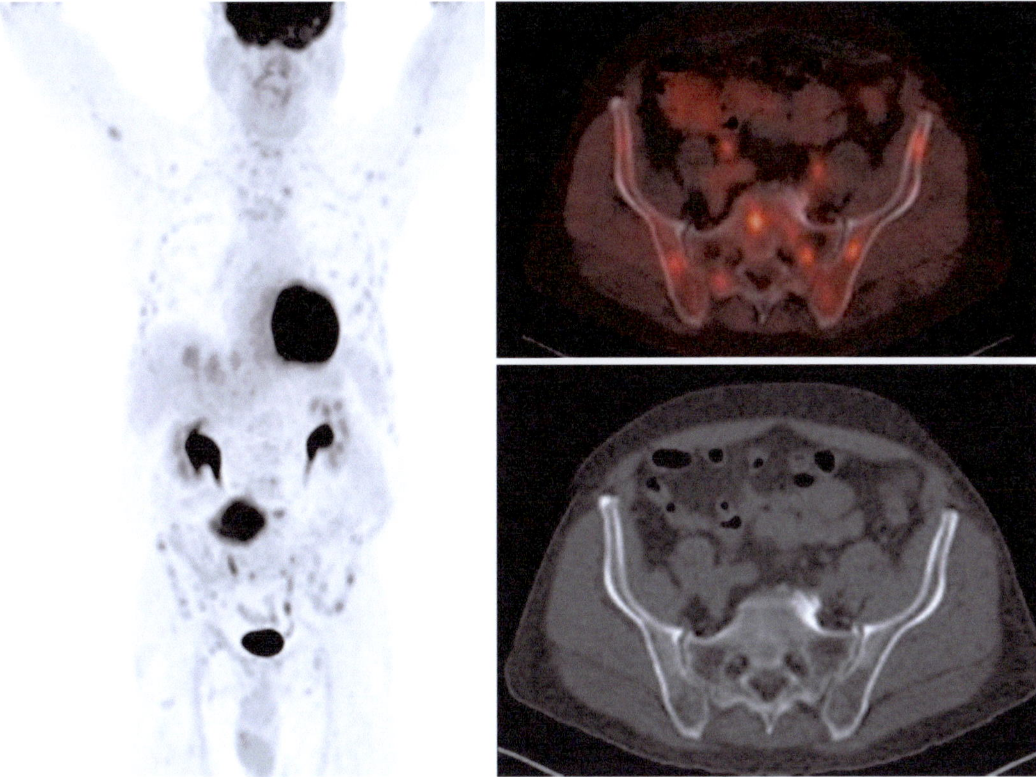

Fig. 4.44 Metastases to the bone. This retroperitoneal sarcoma has diffuse but relatively poorly avid bony metastases, which are even more subtle on CT

References

1. Wallitt K, Yusuf S, Soneji N, Khan SR, Win Z, Barwick TD. PET/CT in oncologic imaging of nodal disease: pearls and pitfalls: RadioGraphics fundamentals | online presentation. Radiographics. 2018;38(2):564–5.
2. Bourgeois AC, Chang TT, Fish LM, Bradley YC. Positron emission tomography/computed tomography in melanoma. Radiol Clin N Am. 2013;51(5):865–79.
3. Nayan S, Ramakrishna J, Gupta MK. The proportion of malignancy in incidental thyroid lesions on 18-FDG PET study: a systematic review and meta-analysis. Otolaryngol Head Neck Surg. 2014;151(2):190–200.
4. Treglia G, Bertagna F, Sadeghi R, Verburg FA, Ceriani L, Giovanella L. Focal thyroid incidental uptake detected by (1)(8)F-fluorodeoxyglucose positron emission tomography. Meta-analysis on prevalence and malignancy risk. Nuklearmedizin. 2013;52(4):130–6.
5. Patz EF Jr, Lowe VJ, Hoffman JM, Paine SS, Burrowes P, Coleman RE, et al. Focal pulmonary abnormalities: evaluation with F-18 fluorodeoxyglucose PET scanning. Radiology. 1993;188(2):487–90.
6. Adams MC, Turkington TG, Wilson JM, Wong TZ. A systematic review of the factors affecting accuracy of SUV measurements. AJR Am J Roentgenol. 2010;195(2):310–20.
7. Groheux D, Quere G, Blanc E, Lemarignier C, Vercellino L, de Margerie-Mellon C, et al. FDG PET-CT for solitary pulmonary nodule and lung cancer: literature review. Diagn Interv Imaging. 2016;97(10):1003–17.
8. Basu S, Kwee TC, Surti S, Akin EA, Yoo D, Alavi A. Fundamentals of PET and PET/CT imaging. Ann N Y Acad Sci. 2011;1228:1–18.
9. Loffler M, Weckesser M, Franzius C, Nashan D, Schober O. Malignant melanoma and (18)F-FDG-PET: should the whole body scan include the legs? Nuklearmedizin. 2003;42(4):167–72.
10. Webb HR, Latifi HR, Griffeth LK. Utility of whole-body (head-to-toe) PET/CT in the evaluation of melanoma and sarcoma patients. Nucl Med Commun. 2018;39(1):68–73.
11. Dasgupta T, Brasfield R. Metastatic melanoma. A clinicopathological study. Cancer. 1964;17:1323–39.

12. Wong ANM, McArthur GA, Hofman MS, Hicks RJ. The advantages and challenges of using FDG PET/CT for response assessment in melanoma in the era of targeted agents and immunotherapy. Eur J Nucl Med Mol Imaging. 2017;44(Suppl 1):67–77.

13. Guldbrandsen KF, Hendel HW, Langer SW, Fischer BM. Nuclear molecular imaging strategies in immune checkpoint inhibitor therapy. Diagnostics (Basel). 2017;7(2):23.

14. Perng P, Marcus C, Subramaniam RM. (18)F-FDG PET/CT and melanoma: staging, immune modulation and mutation-targeted therapy assessment, and prognosis. AJR Am J Roentgenol. 2015;205(2):259–70.

15. Kandathil A, Subramaniam RM. PET/computed tomography and precision medicine: musculoskeletal sarcoma. PET Clin. 2017;12(4):475–88.

Review of PET/CT Images in Melanoma and Sarcoma: False Positives, False Negatives, and Pitfalls

5

Jorge Daniel Oldan

While FDG-PET is a powerful modality for staging, restaging, response assessment, and surveillance of both melanoma and sarcoma, it is prone to a few pitfalls that the reader must be aware of. Both false positives and false negatives have been known to occur.

False Positives

The most common cause of false-positive FDG-PET is inflammation [1]. White blood cells, in particular macrophages, accumulate glucose and thus its analog FDG, resulting in increased uptake in the local region which can be confused with presence of tumor [2]. This is known to be a problem with a variety of tumors, and melanoma is no different. This is somewhat different from the case with MR and CT where increased vascularity leads to increased contrast enhancement, though both cases may sometimes be seen. The effect is well-known enough FDG-PET has been used to look for foci of occult infection in fever of unknown origin.

As benign inflammation tends to decrease in uptake over time whereas malignancy tends to continue to accumulate glucose, some have advocated dual time-point imaging to distinguish between inflammation and malignancy. The effect is not reliable enough to be useful, however [3], and dual time-point imaging has generally not proved sensitive or specific enough to be useful, however.

In general, benign inflammation can be due to iatrogenic causes or to actual inflammation or infection (Figs. 5.1 and 5.2).

Recent Therapy

One of the most difficult causes to disentangle from malignancy is recent local therapy. Surgery or radiation will produce inflammation and hence uptake. It is for this reason that an inspection of the recent history of surgery, radiation, and chemotherapy the patient has had is important when interpreting examinations.

Surgery in particular can produce local inflammation persisting for months afterward (Fig. 5.3) [4]. The degree and duration are heavily dependent on the type of surgery, with larger procedures producing more uptake and larger amounts of uptake. Linear uptake is usually recognizable as surgical, and changes in local anatomy (e.g., from a cystectomy with neobladder—Fig. 5.4) may provide evidence of a recent procedure. In addition, the presence of surgical clips should be noted. (This is one reason to inspect a site using

J. D. Oldan (✉)
Department of Radiology, Division of Molecular Imaging and Therapeutics, University of North Carolina, Chapel Hill School of Medicine, Chapel Hill, NC, USA
e-mail: jorge_oldan@med.unc.edu

© Springer Nature Switzerland AG 2021
A. H. Khandani (ed.), *PET/CT and PET/MR in Melanoma and Sarcoma*,
https://doi.org/10.1007/978-3-030-60429-5_5

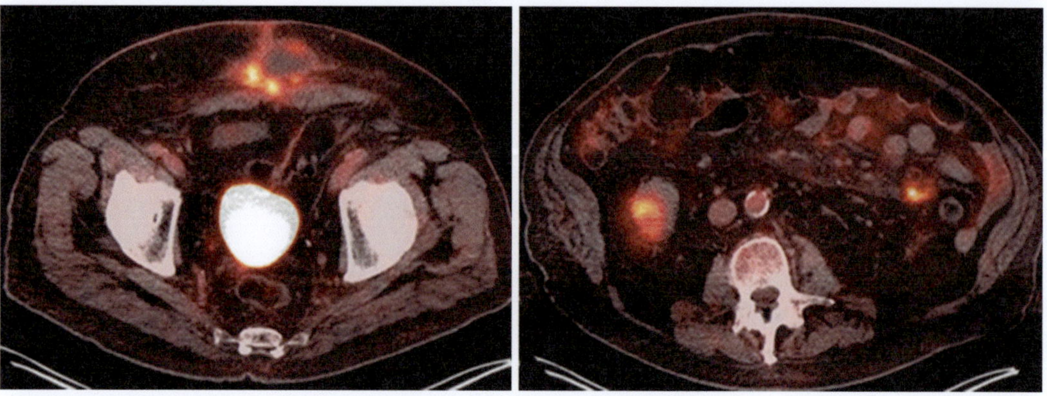

Fig. 5.1 Peripheral uptake and uptake in draining lymph nodes from large abdominal wall abscess

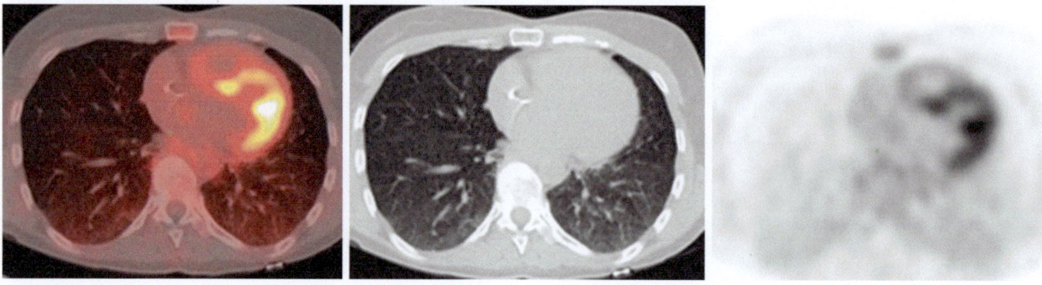

Fig. 5.2 Diffuse lung inflammation, with mild ground-glass opacities on CT and uptake on PET

at least one sequence other than fused images, as surgical clips may be obscured by intense uptake on fused images—Fig. 5.5.) In some cases, there may be no recourse other than to simply say "recommend attention on follow-up," but usually the localization and specific pattern of surgical uptake can give the answer.

Radiation can produce a great deal of uptake, and radiation fibrosis can make reading the scan challenging. Fibrosis in the lungs can appear as a secondary mass, whereas radiation changes in the soft tissue, while generally not confused with malignancy, can make mass lesions hard to see. One useful property of radiation changes is their limitation to the area of the radiation port—they will have sharp geometric borders unlike any physiologic or other pathologic process [4].

The bone marrow (and often the spleen) will often show increased uptake after either chemotherapy or the growth factors such as Neulasta given with it. This can decrease sensitivity for metastases to these areas. Conversely, an inciden-

tal finding that can sometimes indicate the presence of prior radiation if missing from the provided history is decreased uptake in multiple contiguous vertebral bodies (from local myelofibrosis) (Fig. 5.6).

In general, the precise duration to wait after any sort of therapy is unclear. Chemotherapy usually cannot be stopped, so the scan is done before the initiation of the next cycle. Postsurgical uptake is quite variable, but a few weeks are usually sufficient to at least figure out what is actually recurrence. Uptake from radiation can last a long time. Unlike the timing of the wait from other types of treatment, this has been heavily studied, with the head and neck squamous cell carcinoma literature finding a good negative predictive value for radiation done 3 months after (whereas 1 month after is generally not sufficient). While the American Society of Nuclear Medicine and Molecular Imaging does not have specific guidelines for how long to wait, the European Association of Nuclear Medicine's

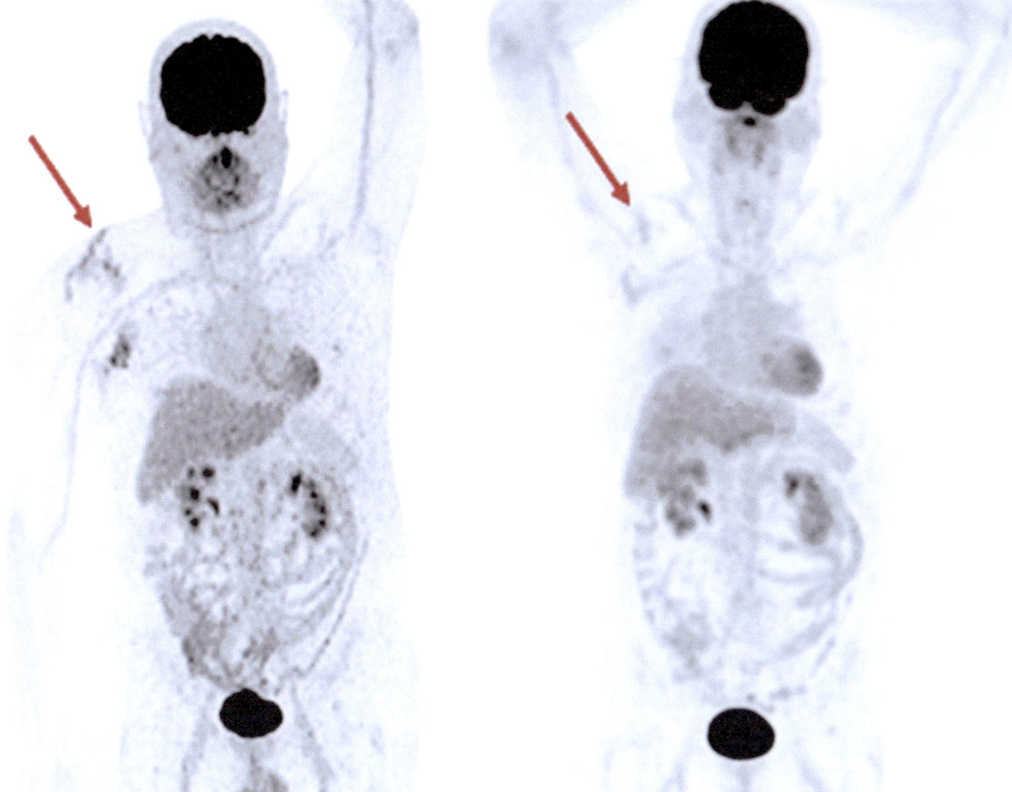

Fig. 5.3 Right shoulder melanoma surgical site shortly after resection and approximately 1 year later (arrows). Most of the immediate uptake has died down, but vague postsurgical changes have still died down

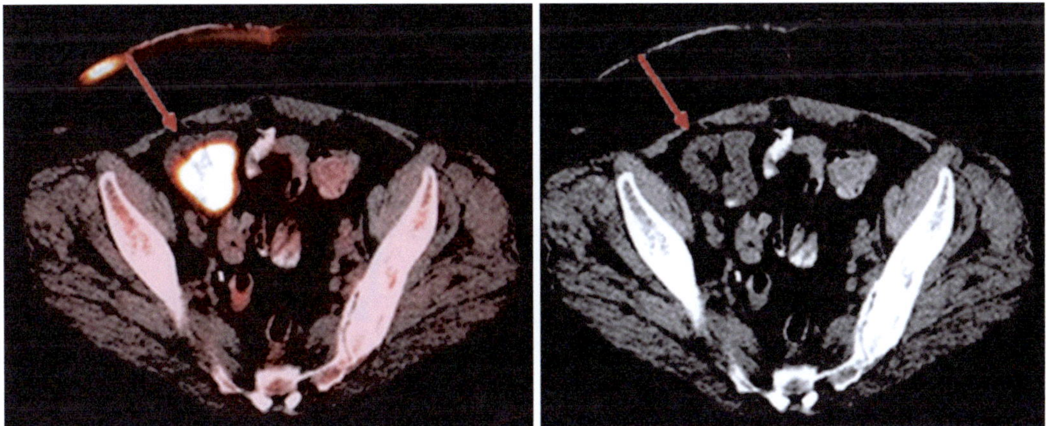

Fig. 5.4 Intense uptake in neobladder after cystectomy (arrows); the CT appearance is of loops of bowel filled with low-attenuation fluid (urine), which is extremely FDG-avid (as the tracer is excreted in the urine)

guidelines does suggest 10 days for chemotherapy, 2 weeks for growth factors such as G-CSF and GM-CSF, 6 weeks for surgery, and 2–3 months for radiation [5].

Many of the newer immunotherapy drugs such as ipilimumab and pembrolizumab may produce false positives due to inflammation from immune-related adverse events, such as arthritis

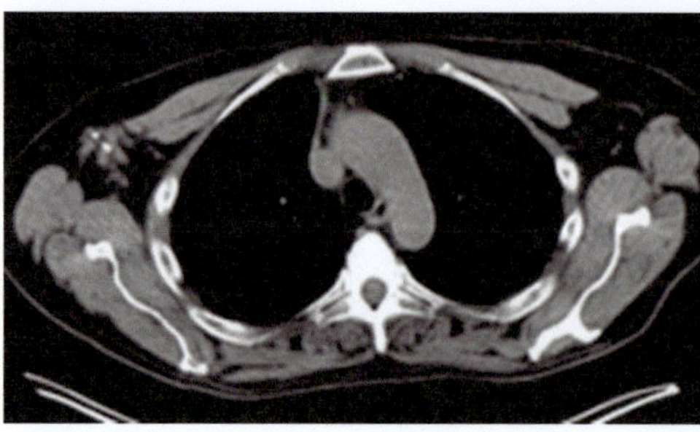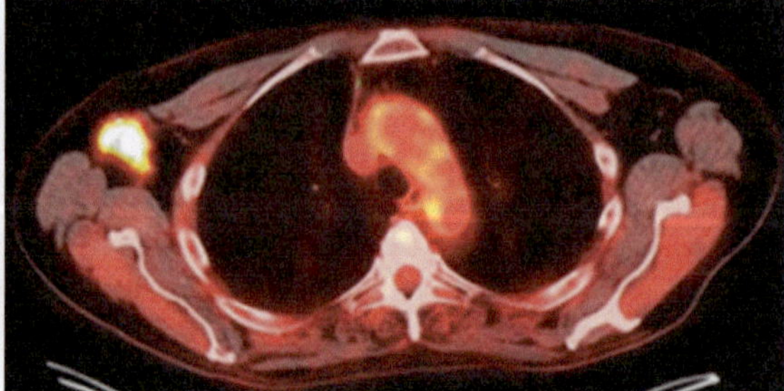

Fig. 5.5 Axillary surgical clips are obscured by intense uptake from recurrence; suppression of PET from fused image reveals them

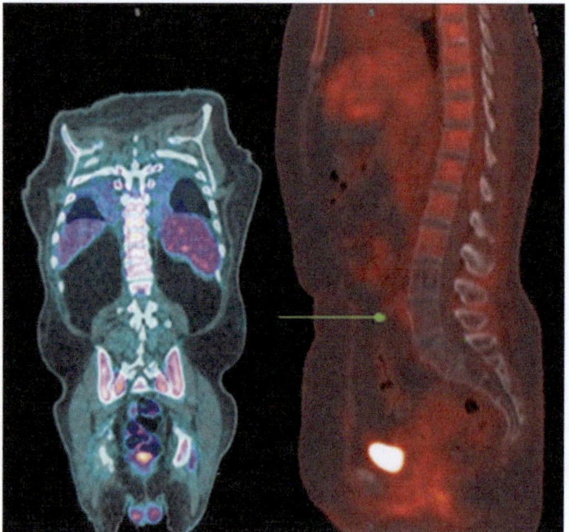

Fig. 5.6 Diffuse spine uptake and spleen greater than bone marrow liver uptake typical of Neulasta. A lack of uptake in the lower L-spine (arrow) suggests prior radiation therapy to this area

and colitis [6] and a sarcoid-like mediastinal and hilar lymphadenopathy [7] or thyroiditis [8]; this has been described in a variety of cancers, but melanoma is no exception. While the false positives may be confusing, the presence of these findings may actually correlate positively with progression-free survival [6, 7] or early response [8], although the relationship of colitis has been questioned [9]. A few different response criteria such as IPERCIST [10] and IMPERCIST5 [11] have been formulated, but presently the most widely used is presently iRECIST [12], which has a category of "immune unconfirmed progressive disease" where progression must be confirmed on a follow-up scan. Given the wide variety of protocols, it can be difficult to determine what exactly the benchmark in a research trial is unless this is communicated directly from the referring clinician, so the safest approach is to refrain from definitively calling "progression" in the presence of new lesions on immunotherapy and to simply note the presence of new lesions in patients on these drugs.

Inflammation/Infection

Inflammation and infection will also show increased uptake—thus bacterial infections will show locally increased uptake, whereas viral infections, being more systemic normally, will tend to show increased uptake in multiple nodes around the body. HIV quite notably can cause low-grade uptake in axillary and inguinal nodes (Fig. 5.7). This tends to be bilaterally symmetric, unlike a local infection or local spread of disease.

Granulomatous inflammation such as that in tuberculosis, mycobacteria, or fungi, as well as inflammatory diseases such as sarcoid, is a well-known cause of false positives on FDG-PET for a variety of tumors (Fig. 5.8) [2]. The nodular nature of granulomatous inflammation is particularly confusing as it can look like a spherical metastasis. Granulomatous inflammation tends to be in a more symmetric or systemic pattern, but this is often difficult to tell. A history of exposure to TB or fungi may be of use.

A related pattern is the often-seen low-grade mediastinal and bilateral hilar nodal uptake seen in many patients on FDG-PET (Fig. 5.9). This may be related to granulomatous inflammation (as described above) or may have to do with other low-grade inflammatory processes. Nonetheless, it tends to be rather diffuse, low-grade, and sym-

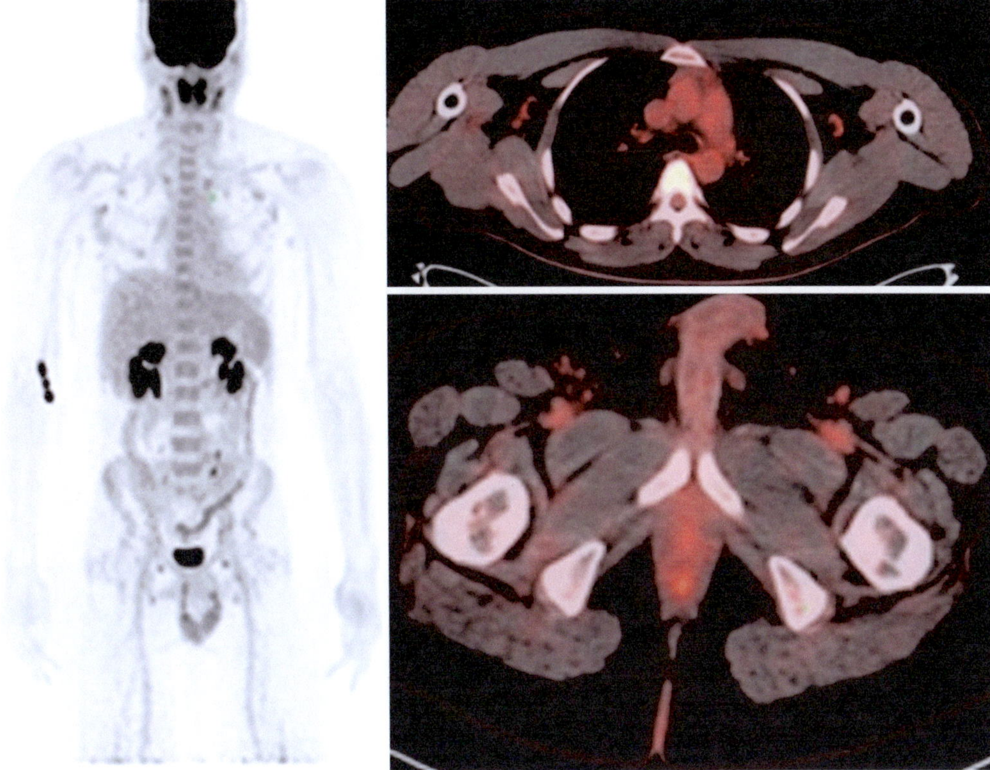

Fig. 5.7 Low-grade uptake in axillary and inguinal nodes from HIV

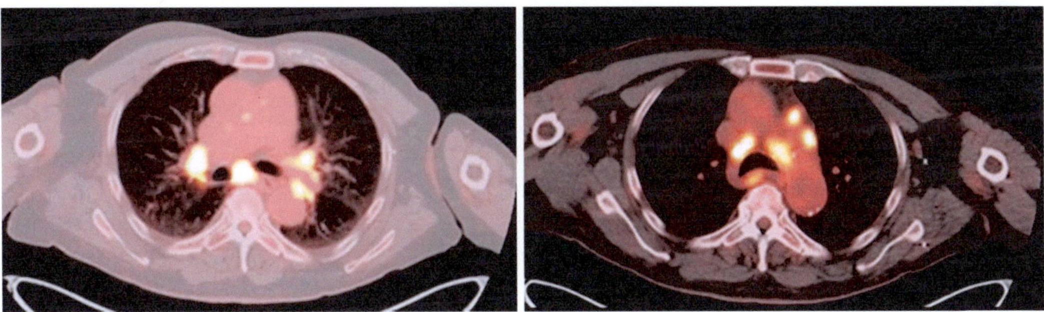

Fig. 5.8 Bilateral mediastinal and hilar nodal uptake typical of sarcoid or other inflammatory reactions

metric, and melanoma, as a cutaneous tumor, will tend to spread to axillary and inguinal nodes before reaching the mediastinum. Of course, if there are many focal nodes on one hilum, a primary lung tumor may be responsible.

Degenerative change is another common source of abnormal uptake. While this is more of a common problem with bone scintigraphy, mildly increased activity can be seen at the site of degenerative changes in many cases (possibly as a result of accompanying inflammation).

Generally localization is sufficient to identify change as degenerative (metastases to osteophytes do occur but are rare). Once in a while an insufficiency fracture in a site affected by radiation may occur.

With all the questions about inflammation, one can wonder if simply waiting for the resolution of the infection (or treatment of the autoimmune disease) may help in imaging. In fact we do recommend not imaging patients, particularly in non-urgent setting such as surveillance, until any

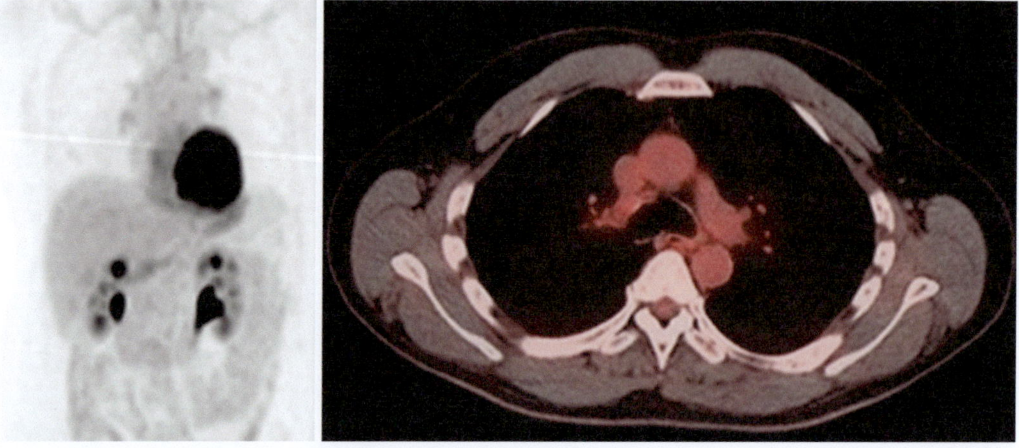

Fig. 5.9 Low-grade mediastinal and bilateral hilar uptake. Sometimes a visible site of infection is visible, more often not. If the uptake is mild and symmetric enough, this is often ruled benign

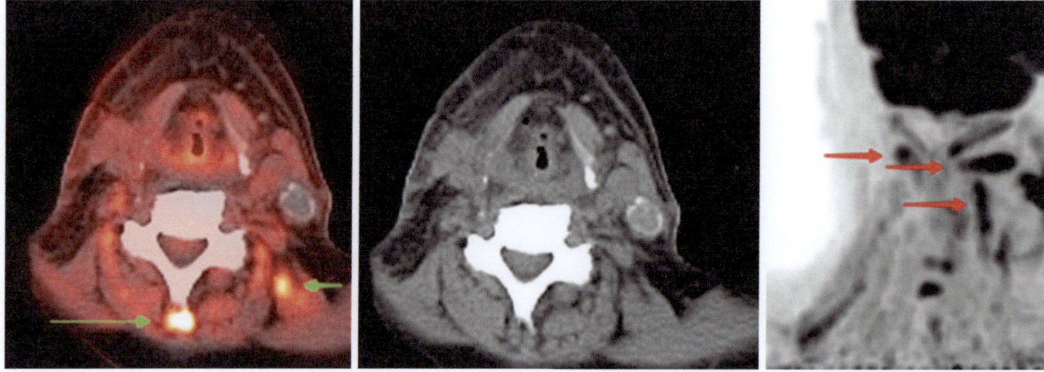

Fig. 5.10 Intense uptake in numerous small muscles of the head and neck (arrows) can be confused for nodal metastatic disease. (A non-avid calcified node is, in fact, visible anteriorly)

known existing inflammatory diseases have resolved. However, this may not always be an option if imminent treatment is necessary or the patient has a chronic inflammatory disease that is unlikely resolve completely.

Another cause of abnormal uptake apart from inflammation is extravasation [4]. In addition to reflecting sites of actual physiologic uptake by glucose-using processes, FDG is a physical substance that has to be injected. In cases of extravasation, it will be picked up by macrophages and brought to the draining lymph node. As the patient is imaged at 1 hour, the initial extravasation may not be visible if small (though it often is). The relevance is that uptake may be seen in a draining axillary node on the side of the injection and mistaken for the spread of tumor. The node will, of course, appear normal. Noting that the abnormal uptake is on the same side as the site of injection is usually sufficient to exclude metastasis. It is for this reason that one notes the side and site of injection and injects opposite to the side of any lesion. Right axillary uptake in a patient with a right upper extremity melanoma injected in the right antecubital fossa could represent either extravasation or spread of tumor, but if the same patient were injected on the left, one could be fairly sure the uptake was related to spread of malignancy.

Physiologic uptake in muscles is usually distinguishable by its diffuse intensity and linear, rather than nodular, contour. However, the small muscles of the neck may occasionally be confusing, particularly if activated unilaterally due to prior surgery in this region (Fig. 5.10).

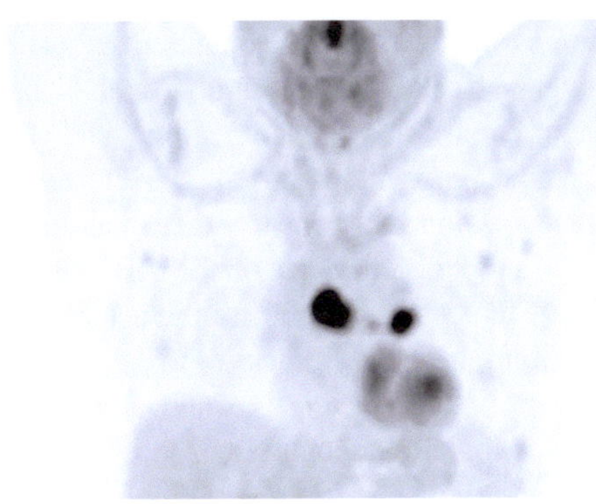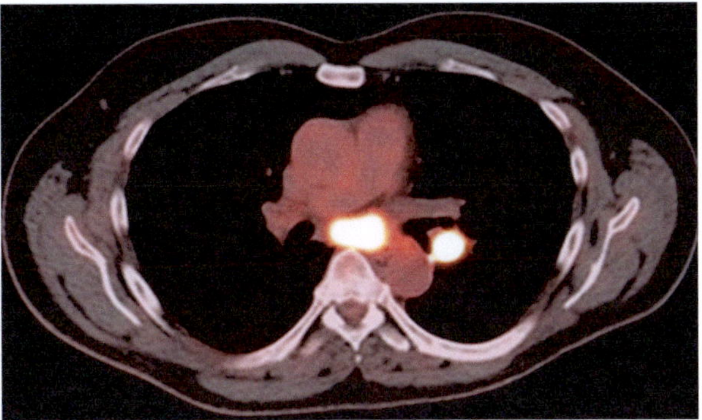

Fig. 5.11 Unilateral hilar and mediastinal nodes, more typical of a primary lung tumor (resected) than metastases

Finally, other tumors will of course take up FDG, and one may find a tumor one was not expecting. The various incidental hot spots that may be either benign or malignant are discussed below, but malignant-appearing lesions (classically a spiculated lesion in the lung, but other common sites of malignancy such as the breast or kidney are also possible) may be seen in a variety of places (Fig. 5.11). Whether this truly represents a *false* positive is a matter of semantic debate, but they are nonetheless serious health problems to be dealt with like any other tumor.

False Negatives

High Background Organs

The brain is famously high in background uptake on FDG scans, which greatly decreases sensitivity for metastases [4]. Even melanoma, which is quite FDG-avid, can be difficult to see over the high background brain uptake. In some cases, large metastases may be seen as cold spots. In general, while it is worth inspecting the brain for "hot" areas that may be metastatic, brain MRI is a much more sensitive test for brain metastases. (CT, even with contrast, is a poor substitute.)

Bone marrow usually displays at least some uptake, although this is increased (as described above) after the use of growth factors which stimulate blood cell formation [4]. The diffuse bone marrow uptake of active bone marrow is usually easy to distinguish from the multifocal, many-small-intense areas uptake of bone metastases. Even when the number of metastases is very large, it is usually easy to distinguish from diffuse bone marrow activation. The major concern is decreased sensitivity for metastases; for this reason the bone should be inspected on bone window at least once to look for non-avid lytic or blastic lesions.

Muscle metastases often have no CT correlate as the soft tissue density of metastases is similar to that of lung (contrast this with lung or bone). Muscle may also show physiologic uptake if the patient has moved during the uptake period (something difficult to completely prevent as people find it difficult to stay 1 hour without moving at all), but given the diffuse distribution in commonly used muscles this is usually easy to distinguish. Postsurgical changes may cause intense muscle uptake if muscles have to compensate for resected muscles on the other side (this is most commonly a problem in head and neck lesions where small muscles may be confused with nodal metastases) [4]. In this case it is often more obvious the uptake is muscular in nature on maximum intensity projection images.

The kidneys are a particularly perplexing case as cortical uptake is relatively mild but uptake in the collecting system (which holds urine full of excreted FDG) may be quite high. Renal metastases (a possibility with melanoma) may be confused with uptake in the collecting system. If the study can be done with intravenous contrast, renal metastases (or primary renal tumors) may be easier to detect.

In general, bladder metastases are impossible to detect on PET. A round lesion may be visible on CT, particularly if intravenous contrast has been administered, but any uptake will be drowned out by the intense, contiguous uptake of the urine in the bladder. Tumors contacting the bladder may occasionally be seen as a cold spot, but the PET is of no use in finding metastases to the bladder.

Brown fat is sometimes seen if the patient has been cold before the scan, particularly in younger patients and women [4]. This is one area where fused images are most useful as the intense uptake in the fat can be localized to the fat rather than a node (Figs. 5.12 and 5.13); of course, the neck is also a commonplace for nodes to be found [2].

Too Small to Characterize

PET is not reliable for *characterizing* lesions below about 1 cm (Fig. 5.14). Due to the relatively high distance gamma photons travel within the crystals that detect them, spatial resolution for nuclear modalities is relatively poor and par-

tial volume effects (where the uptake from a single voxel affects neighboring voxels) are prominent. Uptake in a single imaging voxel will also increase uptake in neighboring voxels, and a very intense lesion will appear larger than a less intense lesion of the same size on the PET. This is where the CT becomes useful, as the actual size of the lesion can often be determined from the CT. In addition, if a lesion is small enough, it may not accumulate enough tracer to be visible above background (which is usually nonzero) (this has been a problem in the use of SUVmax to characterize tumors as benign or malignant, as maximum voxel intensity will be affected by size up to a size of about 3 cm) [13].

However, it has been known to *detect* lesions below 1 cm (Fig. 5.15). The reason for this conundrum is that small metastases from very avid tumors (and melanoma is one such tumor) can successfully take up enough tracer to be significantly avid above background. A 4 mm, strongly avid, spherical lung nodule or axillary node is quite concerning for metastasis, particularly if multiple. This is particularly useful in low-background organs such as lung and fat

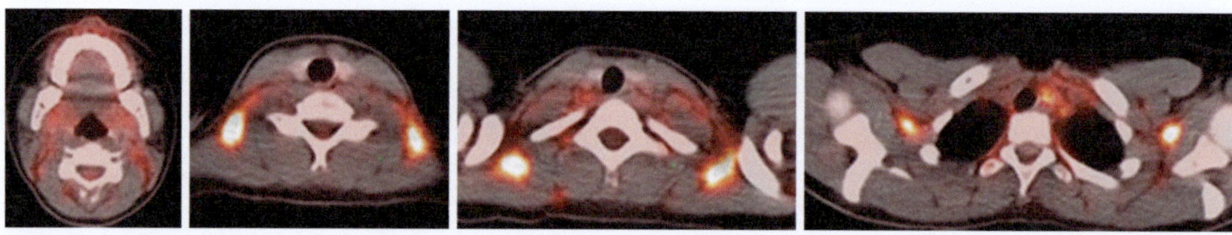

Fig. 5.12 Brown fat in standard locations—posterior neck fat and (less often) posterior mediastinal uptake

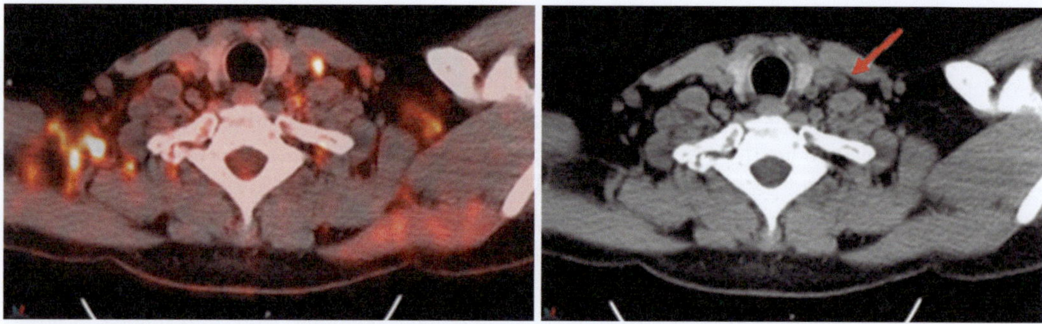

Fig. 5.13 Numerous foci of uptake localize to fat and likely represent brown fat. A single focus of uptake adjacent to the carotid on the left may represent an actual metastatic node

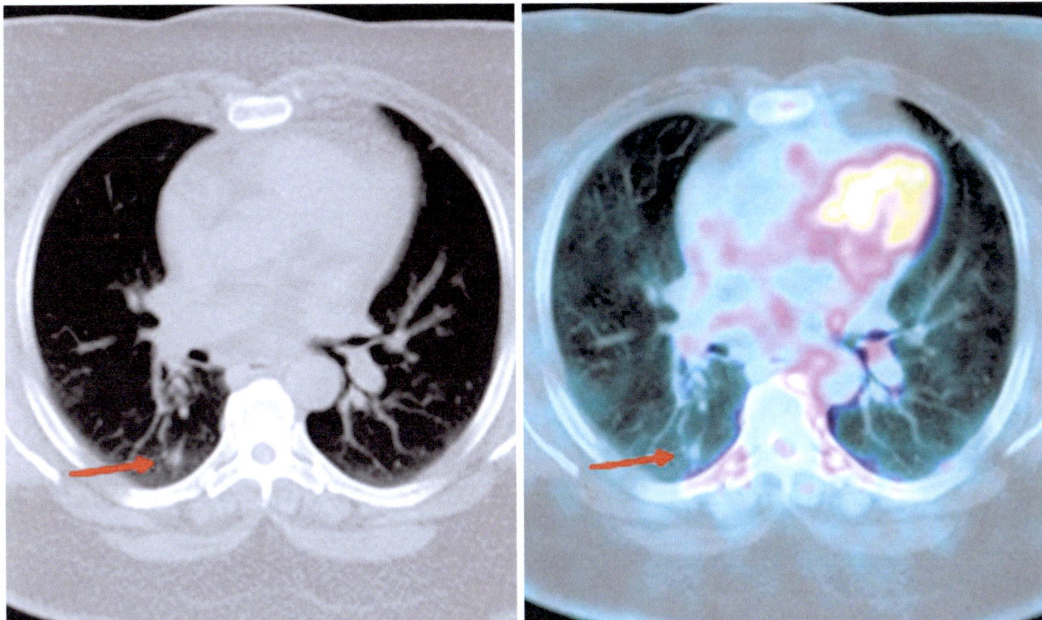

Fig. 5.14 Pulmonary nodules under about 1 cm (arrow) may be too small to characterize. As benign pulmonary nodules are common, they can usually be followed by CT as per Fleischner Society guidelines

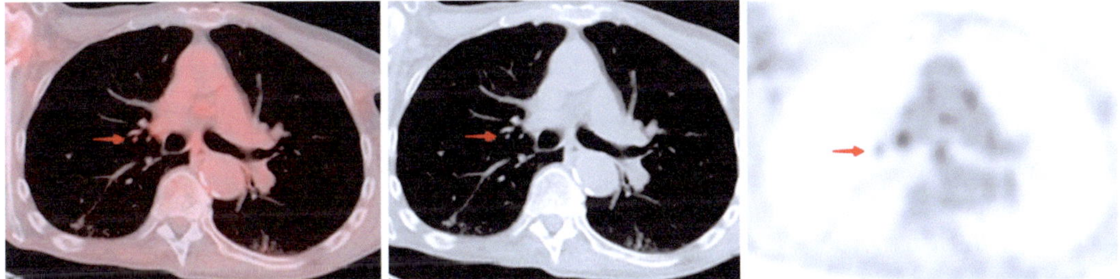

Fig. 5.15 Nodules as small as 2 mm may show visible uptake if intense enough, as in the case of this right perihilar nodule. While the negative predictive value at this size is poor, if there is reasonable suspicion for metastasis, the finding is at least concerning

(which nodes are usually surrounded by). Nonetheless, sensitivity decreases with smaller lesions, and in high-background areas such as the brain, a lesion must be a few centimeters in size to be visible at all on PET.

Too Superficial to Detect

A problem with superficial lesions is that, being spread out in two dimensions, they do not accumulate all their uptake in a single three-dimensional voxel the way a round metastasis does and hence have lower measured uptake. The attenuation correction algorithm also decreases counts from skin lesions (which being on the surface are not attenuated), and so at least a cursory look at non-attenuation-corrected (or NAC) images is in order. Usually superficial lesions are easy to detect, being right on the skin on the MIP. As non-malignant infections of the skin or minor injuries are avid and common, usually calling attention to the location and recommending correlation with physical examination is sufficient.

Involuntary (Breathing) and Voluntary Patient Motion

Patient motion has a number of problems. First of all, as the moving part of the body may occupy multiple positions in space during the imaging time, uptake will be decreased and "smeared" out over the multiple locations. This can decrease sensitivity and be quite confusing. Alternatively, the patient may be still during both PET and CT but move between the scans, causing the body part to be in different positions in the two different scans. In this case, the CT and PET should be viewed separately in the area of concern, and NAC images consulted as attenuation correction is often affected. Second, because modern attenuation correction algorithms use CT images to calculate attenuation, a part of the body may appear too hot or too cold on PET, possibly leading to either false negatives or false positives. NAC images may again be of use here. Third, there is the problem of misregistration. If fused images are used, the area of uptake may appear to be in a different location than it actually is.

This is most prominent with breathing. The diaphragm moves up and down during breathing and separates the lung from the liver on the right, both of which are common sites of metastasis. An added complication is that CT images take only a few seconds, whereas a PET bed position takes several minutes. The patient can hold their breath for CT, but not for PET; thus to have the two areas registered well requires the CT to be performed using shallow breathing, which is a change from usual CT protocol, where the images are acquired in deep inspiration to maximize lung expansion. Should the patient take a deep breath (if instructed by a technologist who usually does only CT) or breathe out of anxiety during CT acquisition, liver lesions may be projected over lung or vice versa. Usually lung lesions have a clear CT correlate, but liver lesions (particularly in a nonenhanced scan) may be difficult to confirm. In this case, the CT and PET should be viewed separately; lesions can often be seen to be clearly in the lung or in the liver on PET (Fig. 5.16). In addition, NAC images may be useful if attenuation correction is affected.

Physiologic bowel motion can often be problematic as well, placing bowel metastases in the mesentery or vice versa (Fig. 5.17), although this is difficult to prevent. (Some centers give glucagon before scans.) While looking at CT and PET image separately may still be of use, normal variation in physiologic bowel uptake decreases the utility of this somewhat. The CT images should be carefully inspected for presence of mesenteric nodules or nodules adjacent to or in bowel, but the relative low prominence of bowel metastases on CT (particularly without intravenous contrast) can lower the utility of this as well. If it affects management, a separate contrast-enhanced CT of the abdomen and pelvis may be necessary.

Finally, a patient may move their extremities. Given the relative lack of importance of extremity metastases (usually important only if the primary was an extremity lesion as by the time extremity metastases are present the trunk is usually affected), this may be less of an issue. However, if solitary metastases are suspected and will change management if present, the patient can be referred for physical examination, radiography, or MRI, depending on the precise location.

Adjacent to Nearby Uptake (Within the Surgical Bed)

Local metastases within the surgical bed may be confusing as they can be hard to distinguish from postsurgical changes. Careful reading of the history can be useful. If enough time has elapsed, an operative note may be available. However, in cases where scarring is genuinely difficult to distinguish from local recurrence, only reimaging in a few weeks may be useful.

Low-Grade Tumors

This is usually only a problem with sarcoma—melanoma is usually intensely FDG-avid and can be seen even at relatively small sizes. Low-grade tumors are usually better-differentiated and have less affinity for glucose and, as a result,

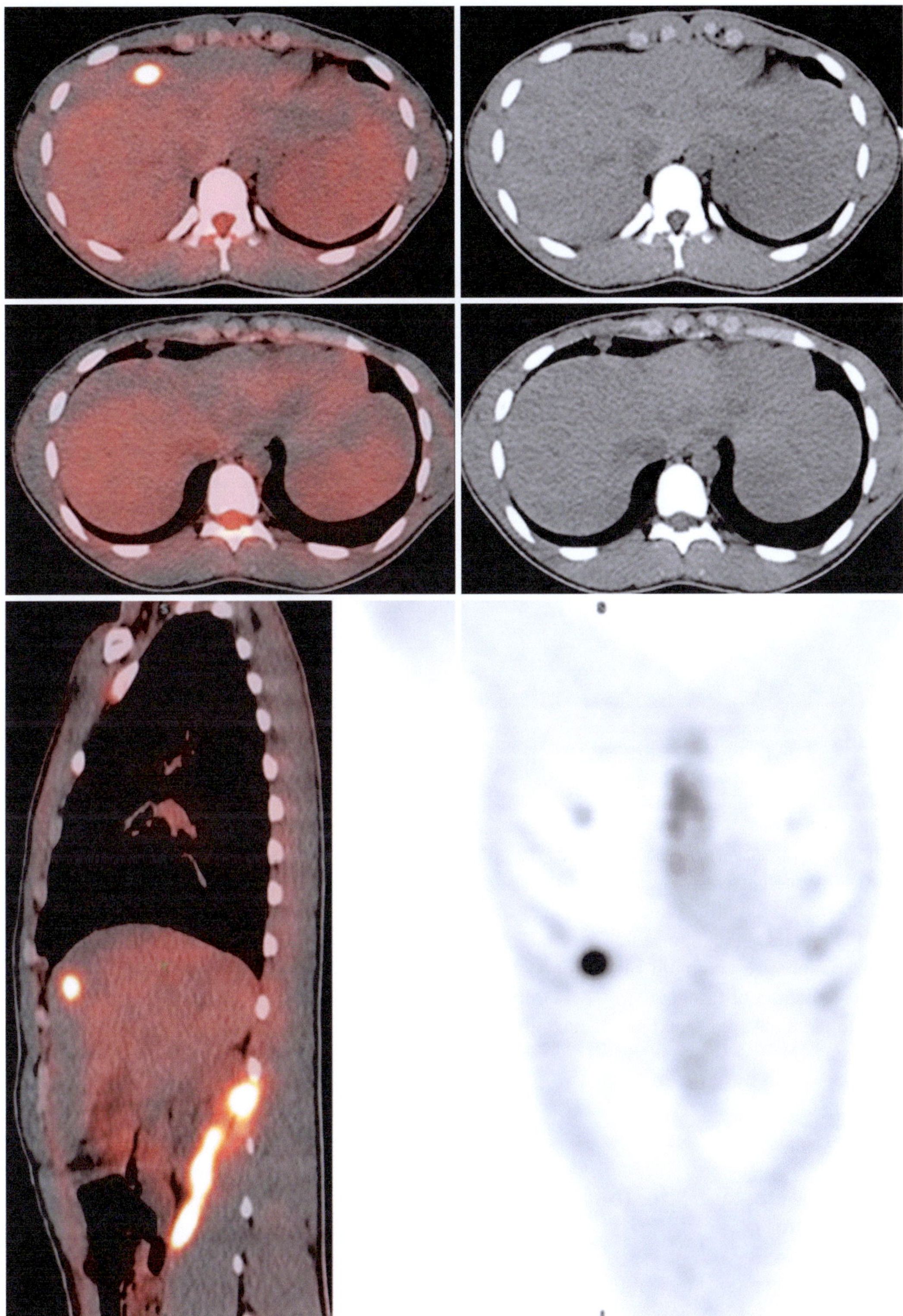

Fig. 5.16 At first glance, it would appear there is a liver metastasis and a non-avid lung metastasis, but cross-correlation with sagittal and coronal images makes clear there is in fact a single avid lung metastasis. Contrast-enhanced CT and/or MR of the liver might still be indicated

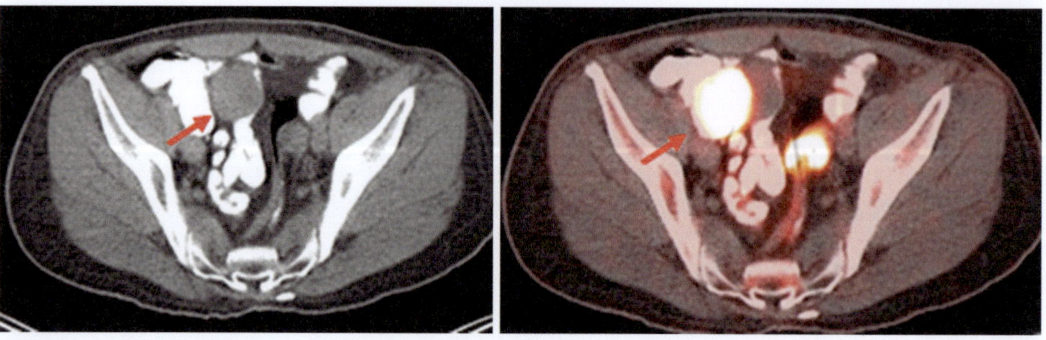

Fig. 5.17 While the metastases are localizable to the bowel, the CT and PET are clearly in different locations in front (arrow)

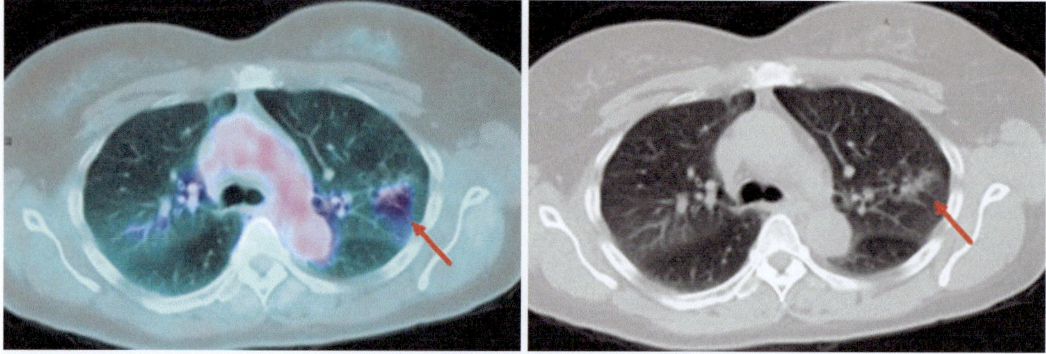

Fig. 5.18 Adenocarcinoma of the lung (arrows), well-known as an example of a malignancy often not (very) avid on PET

may take up relatively little FDG, decreasing the sensitivity of the test for metastatic disease. A variety of incidentally found tumors may have low FDG uptake, including renal, prostate, low-grade lymphoma, carcinoid or neuroendocrine, adenocarcinoma of the lung (Fig. 5.18), lobular carcinoma of the breast, and mucinous tumors of any organ [2].

Pitfalls

Unusual Metastasis Sites (but Not in Melanoma)

Melanoma is notorious for sending metastases to sites other tumors do not. While these are in many cases not particularly difficult to see if one is looking for them, sites that are usually benign in other tumors may not be so in melanoma.

Melanoma may send metastases to the viscera. While the liver and adrenal glands are common sites for metastases from various other tumors, other organs may become targets such as the spleen, pancreas, kidneys, heart, or even less common sites such as the gallbladder. In general, it is sufficient to simply remember to look closely at these organs as well. In some cases, such as the pancreas, it is not clear if there is a metastasis to a node near the organ or the organ itself. In many cases this is not important as systemic disease is present, but if it is crucial in any particular case, a contrast-enhanced CT (or MRI) can be used as follow-up.

A word on bowel metastases is warranted. The bowel moves involuntarily due to peristalsis, has

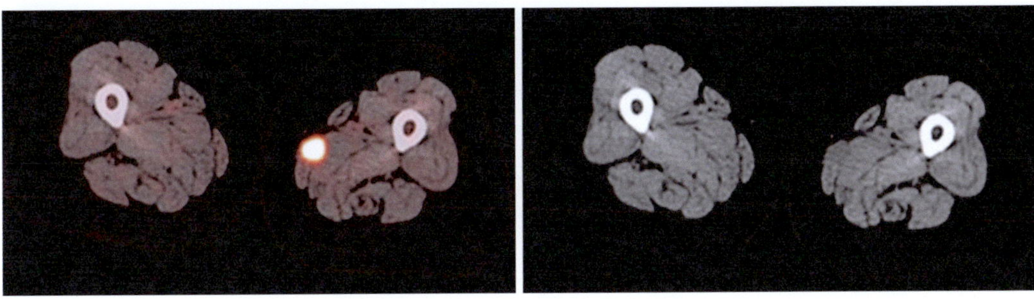

Fig. 5.19 Metastasis to thigh muscle from melanoma. The metastasis may be difficult to see on CT, which is where the typical high avidity of melanoma becomes useful

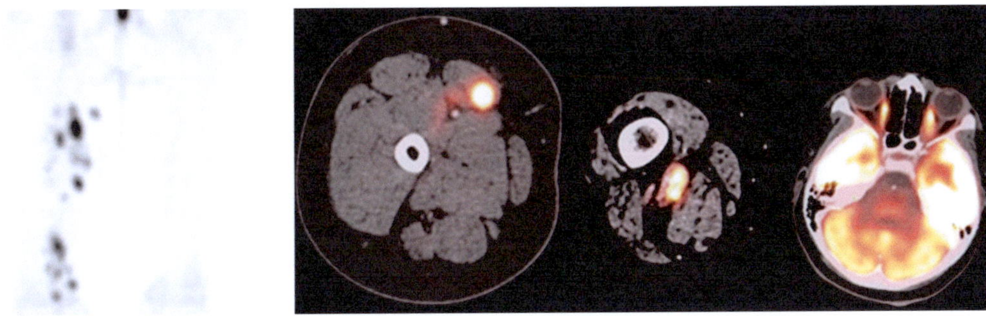

Fig. 5.20 This rhabdomyosarcoma sends multiple metastases to thigh muscles (and nodes). There is even a distant metastasis to a rectus muscle in the left orbit

variable uptake physiologically, and is prone to developing its own primary tumors which are FDG-avid. For this reason the bowel can be a very confusing site. For this reason careful attention to the bowel is warranted. Again, a contrast-enhanced CT may be useful. As described below, focal areas of uptake that appear roughly spherical in contour should be investigated by colonoscopy.

Muscle is a site of metastasis that is relatively specific to melanoma (Fig. 5.19). As such the muscles, including in the extremities, should be examined, particularly if the primary tumor is in the extremity itself. (A sarcoma may also spread locally from the extremities—Fig. 5.20.) If there is high physiologic uptake due to muscle activity, as described above, the CT should be examined carefully for abnormal lesions. In patients who have taken insulin or eaten shortly before the scan, there may be diffuse muscle uptake; this is why one should carefully interview patients and reschedule (if possible) if these things have occurred [2].

Cutaneous metastases are not unheard of, particularly with melanoma. As described previously, a careful look at the skin, particularly using MIP images and NAC images, should help to detect any lesions large enough to be visible on PET [4]. Physical examination correlation is advised as these lesions are usually fairly obvious.

Sites at Border of Image Field

Due to technical factors (fewer detectors are involved), noise rises as one approaches the border of the image field, and the last and first images are usually quite noisy. This can produce either false negatives or false positives. If a suspicious area is caught before the patient leaves, the area can be reimaged, this time in the center of the field of view. Additionally, it is important to pay close attention to protocolling in this situation; a skull base to mid-thigh protocol is particularly inappropriate for a scalp lesion (and some

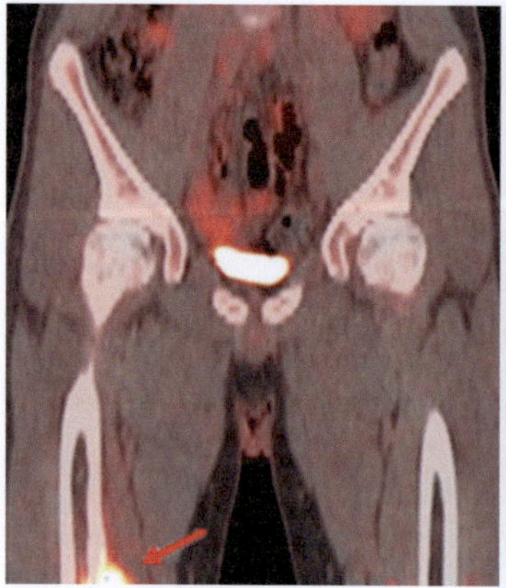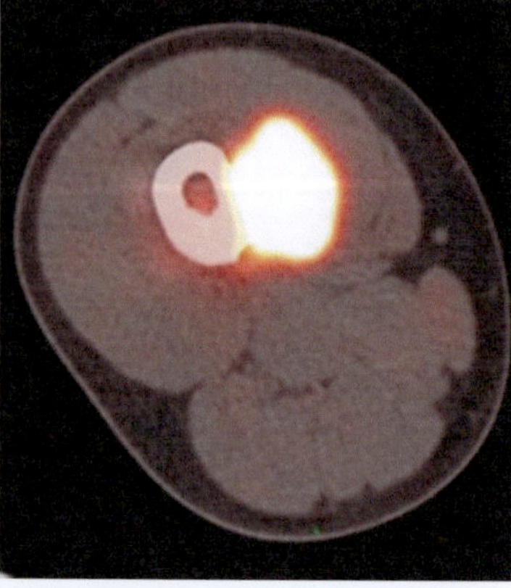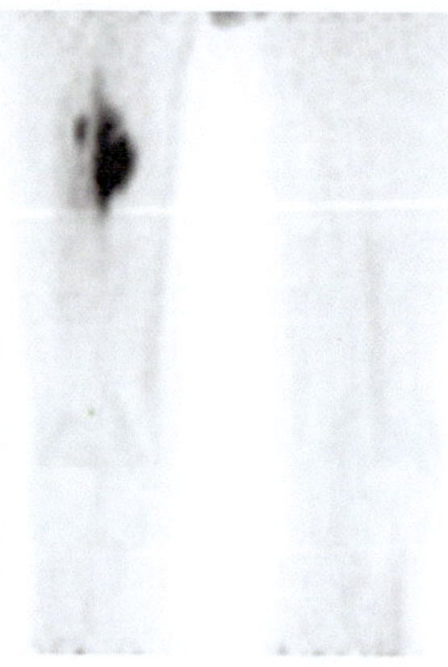

Fig. 5.21 This patient had a thigh sarcoma (arrow) that was nearly missed due to using a standard skull-base-to-mid-thigh protocol. The patient was brought back and the proximal lower extremities scanned to properly visualize the lesion itself

additional "air space" can be included even with a vertex to toe image) or thigh lesion (Fig. 5.21).

Obscured by Intense Nearby Uptake

In addition to high background uptake obscuring metastases to the brain itself, the high physiologic brain uptake obscures uptake in nearby areas such as the skull base due to partial volume effects. While difficult to work around, a careful look at the CT, particularly in often-missed areas of metastasis such as the clivus, can be of great use.

Uptake in the heart is quite variable, to the point where myocardial metastases, though described in many series, are difficult to detect by PET. In addition to the difficulty discovering metastases to the myocardium, uptake in cardiophrenic nodes may be obscured. Occasionally a nearby pulmonary metastasis may be missed as well; however, it is usually detectable on CT.

Uptake in the blood pool is not exceptionally high. However, a common problem is that retroperitoneal nodes (particularly in the aortocaval region) may be projected over the blood pool and mild uptake in retroperitoneal nodes may be difficult to distinguish from blood pool. Since it is only mild uptake that presents this problem (intense uptake in a retroperitoneal node will clearly be seen), an admonition to pay attention on follow-up exams may be sufficient. Alternatively, mild uptake in the retroperitoneal nodes may be confused with blood pool. In this case it is usually sufficient to be vigilant for enlarged nodes in this region. Viewing the CT and PET separately may be useful here.

Intense uptake in the bowel may be confused with mesenteric nodes (or vice versa), as described above. Another problem is that diffuse intense bowel uptake (Fig. 5.22), most commonly with use of metformin, a common oral hypoglycemic, may obscure the presence of nearby intense mesenteric nodes or omental metastases, producing a false negative. In this case, with intense bowel uptake, it is important to look carefully at the CT to see if there are any extra nodules within the abdominopelvic cavity. (One should also ensure the patient is actually *on* metformin, of course; if not the possibility of bowel inflammation should be investigated.)

New reconstruction algorithms have removed the prior problems with low-intensity areas surrounding the very intense bladder and obscuring nodes. Looking carefully for pelvic nodes nearby on CT can help deal with the problem of pelvic nodes becoming inconspicuous due to the proximity of the bladder. If these problems are still noted, repeating the reconstruction without scatter correction may be of use.

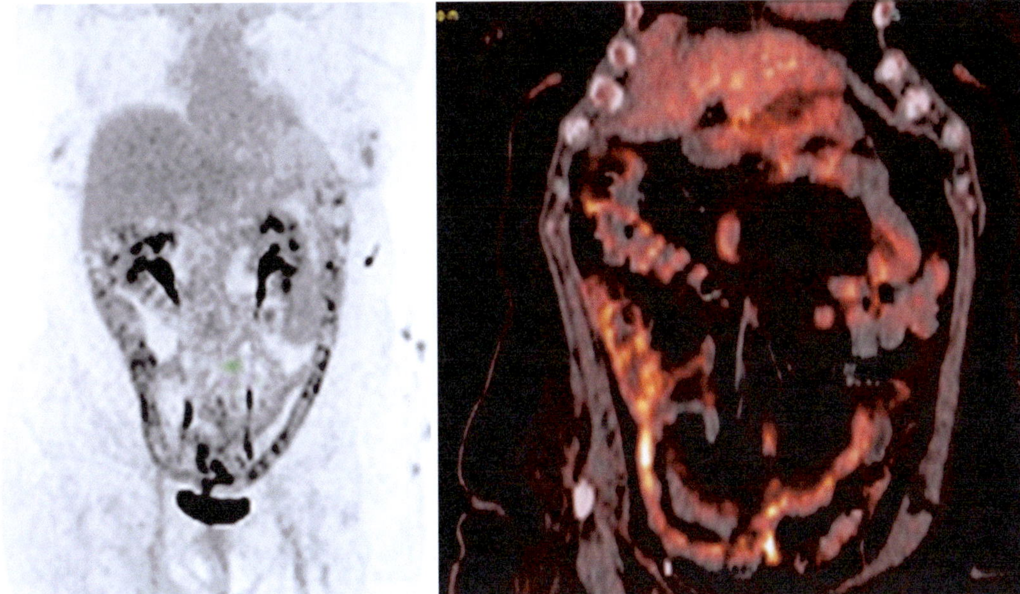

Fig. 5.22 Diffuse bowel uptake is seen with metformin use. The CT appears normal. It should be verified that the patient is actually on metformin

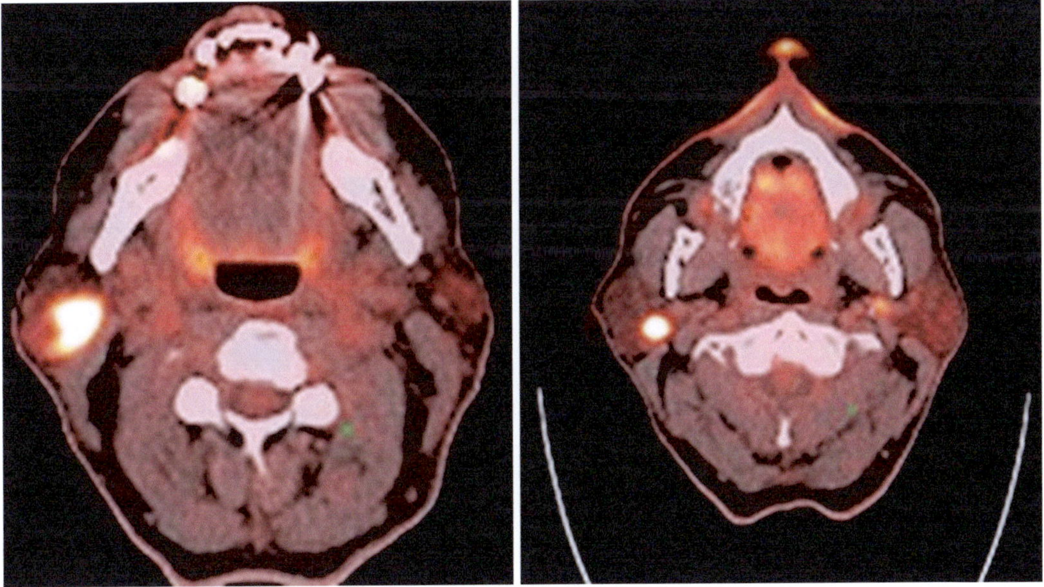

Fig. 5.23 Intense uptake from Warthin's tumors in the parotid gland

Incidental Findings on PET

A variety of areas of focal uptake can be noted on PET. In addition to metastases, some of these may be physiologic or even represent other primary tumors. In most cases these are usually benign but malignant frequently enough to require tissue diagnosis or other investigation.

Focal uptake in the parotid (Fig. 5.23) is seen in about 0.4% of cases and is malignant in about

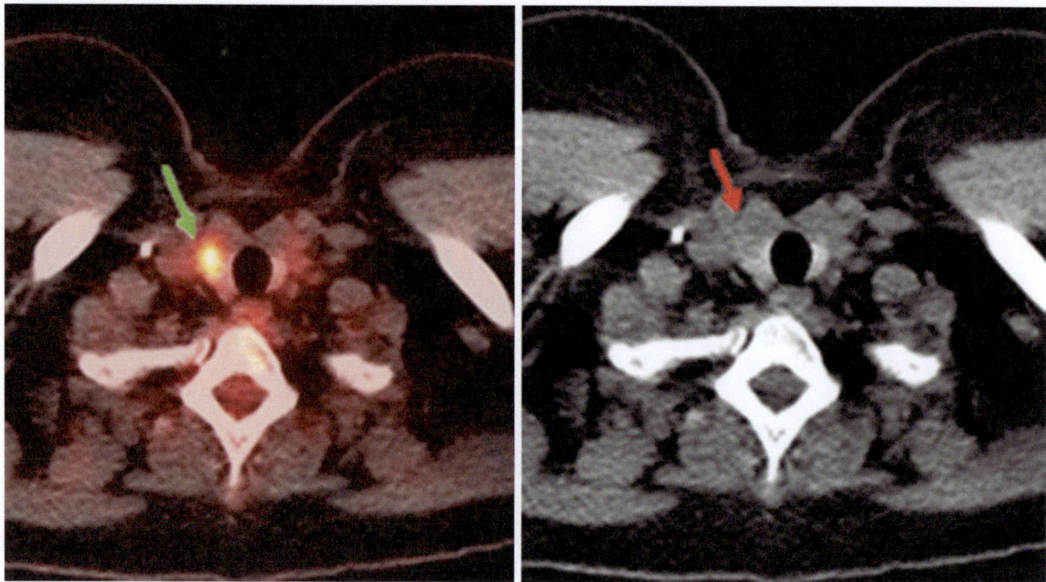

Fig. 5.24 Intensely avid thyroid nodule (arrow), corresponding to hypodense thyroid lesion. Metastases to thyroid exist, but primary nodules are much more common. Some are malignant

10% of those [14]. As such, it is more likely to represent a benign parotid tumor (Warthin's tumor is particularly notorious for being avid) than anything else. However, as some benign parotid tumors can become malignant, it is wise to at least refer these for further workup.

Focal uptake in the thyroid has been extensively studied and is the subject of three meta-analyses at the time of writing [15–17]. In summary, focal hot spots (Fig. 5.24) appear in about 2% of PETs [16], about 20–36% of incidentally discovered avid focal thyroid nodules are malignant [15–17], and only 1% of lesions are distant metastases [15]. As with many other tumors, while malignant lesions tend to have a higher SUVmax, there is enough overlap to prevent this from being useful [17]. Given the reasonably high frequency of thyroid malignancy, further workup of these lesions is useful.

Focal uptake in the breast occurs in 0.4% of cases (0.8% of women), but is malignant in 37–48% of these [18, 19], most commonly infiltrating ductal carcinoma. As such a mammogram and/or ultrasound should be obtained if focal uptake is visible.

Focal uptake in the colon is particularly concerning because even benign lesions (colonic adenomas) are often premalignant. Focal areas of colorectal uptake (Fig. 5.25) are seen in about 3.5% of cases, with 68% being premalignant or malignant, and SUVs not differing enough to tell apart benign, premalignant, or malignant lesions [20]. If it will affect clinical management, the patient should receive a colonoscopy to exclude a second malignancy; in the case of surveillance, the colon cancer may be more dangerous than the risk of recurrence from melanoma! However, in the case of patients with many other metastases, the presence of either a colonic metastasis or a second colon cancer may not make enough of a difference to justify an additional invasive procedure; our usual practice is thus to recommend colonoscopy "if clinically indicated." One should also look at the area on CT; if there is soft tissue stranding in the fat, free air, and many diverticuli, the patient may have diverticulitis instead (Fig. 5.26)!

It is worth paying attention to the uterus and ovaries, but the menstrual status of the patient should be kept in mind. Focal uptake in the ovaries may be physiologic if the woman is of childbearing age, as many focal uptake in the uterus (Fig. 5.27), although this should follow the uterine contour—a focal nodal area in the uterus is

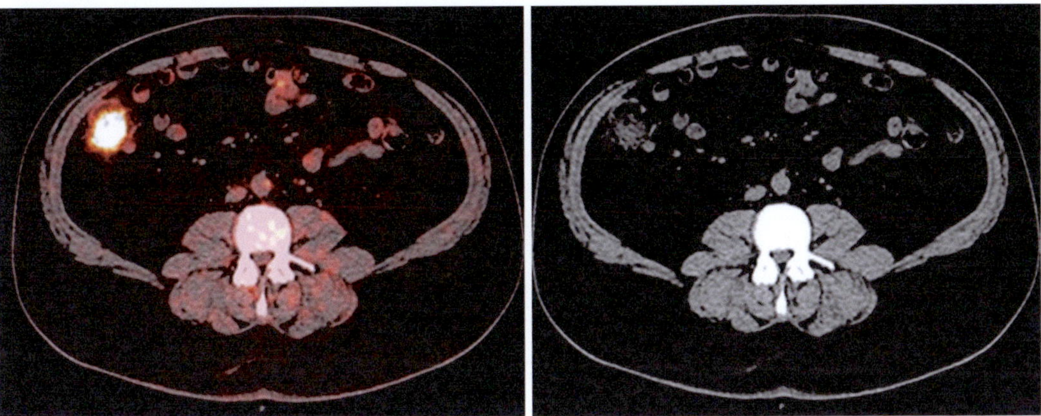

Fig. 5.25 Focal uptake in the colon may have a CT correlate or not, but either way if localized (rather than diffuse) should prompt a colonoscopy

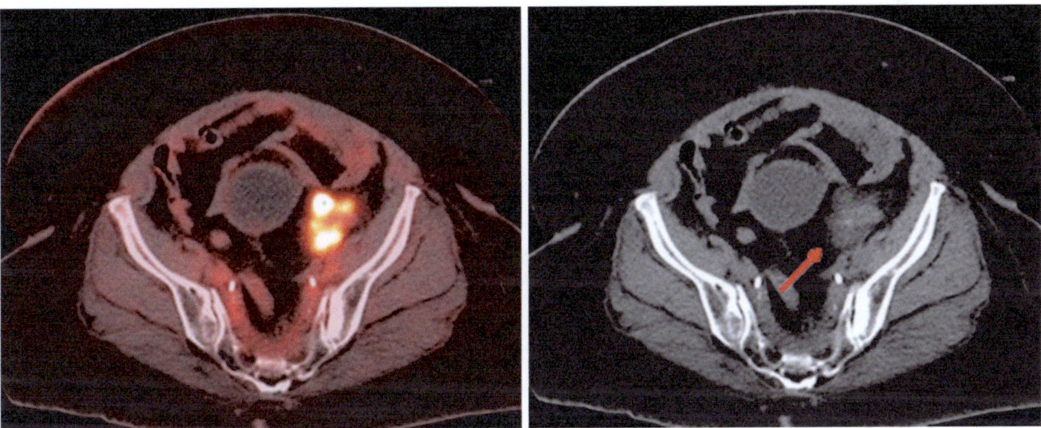

Fig. 5.26 Intense uptake corresponding to soft tissue stranding typical of diverticulitis. Unfortunately, this is often difficult to separate from metastasis

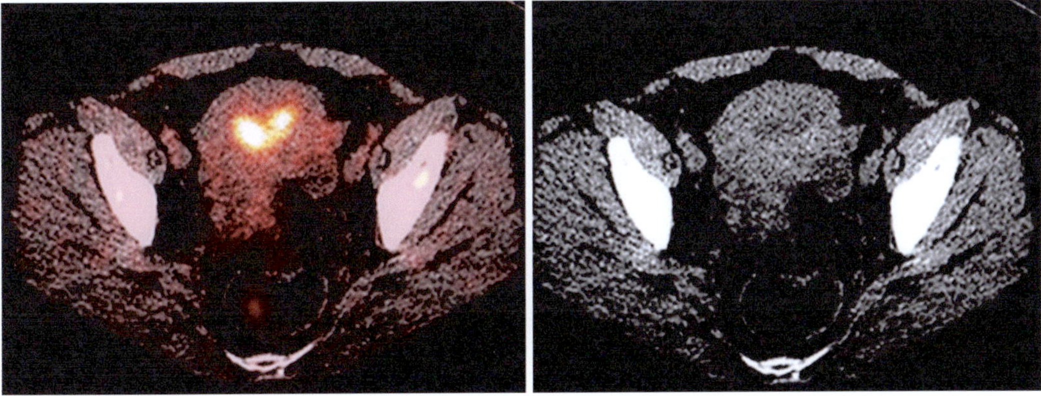

Fig. 5.27 Intense endometrial uptake reflects physiologically active endometrium in a woman of childbearing age. The uptake follows the contour of the endometrium on CT

suspicious. If the patient is not of childbearing age, or the lesion is otherwise suspicious on CT, an ultrasound is usually a good first step.

Prostate cancer is notorious for being non-FDG-avid, but this is not absolute. Very aggressive and unusual histopathologies of prostate cancer may be FDG-avid, and so incidental uptake does stand an increased chance of being malignant (Fig. 5.28). Incidental uptake is seen in the prostate in 2% of cases and is malignant in 17% of cases but 62% of those confirmed by biopsy [19]. As such further workup is wise and may begin with a PSA and digital rectal examination.

Naturally, an occult infection can also be responsible for focal FDG uptake. As such the CT should be examined to see if a clear explanation can be found; focally avid lung nodules in a typical peribronchial distribution may simply represent a lung infection (Fig. 5.29). If felt to be infectious, lung nodules may be followed up with CT alone; a PET is usually necessary as lesions visible on PET are usually visible on CT as well (the reverse is usually not true as many nodules may be too small to characterize).

Incidental Findings on CT

Incidental findings on CT are common; one study found them in 75% of cases [21]. Mercifully, most acute incidental findings on PET-CT, such as appendicitis, cholecystitis, and diverticulitis, are FDG-avid and have clear CT correlates. One that is cold on PET and must be dealt with immediately is the pneumothorax (Fig. 5.30); if not previously known, this should occasion a call to the clinician and on occasion a trip to the ED for the patient. In many cases it results from recent surgery and is known to the service, so a

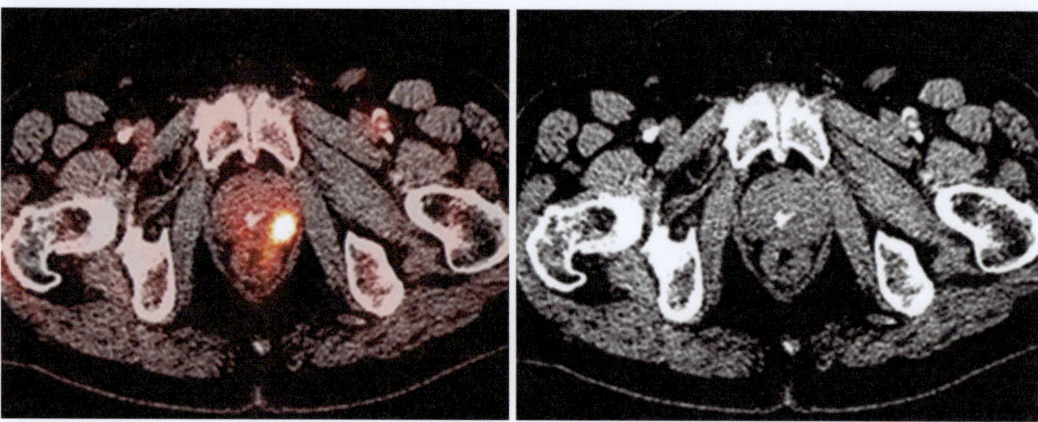

Fig. 5.28 Intense uptake in the prostate; these foci are malignant with a frequency high enough to justify workup. Often nothing is detectable on noncontrast CT

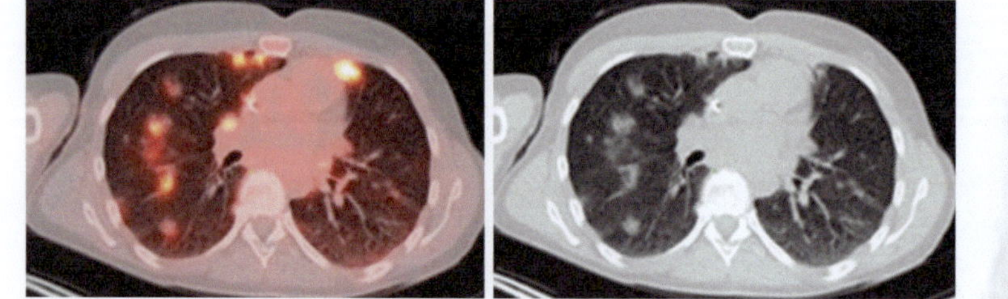
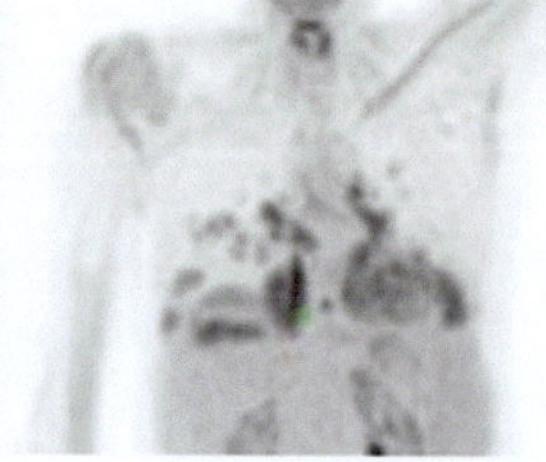

Fig. 5.29 Numerous metabolically active groundglass nodules. These do not have the solid appearance of lung metastases. While any one of these might be a primary lung carcinoma, the relatively diffuse, bilateral distribution is more consistent with infection

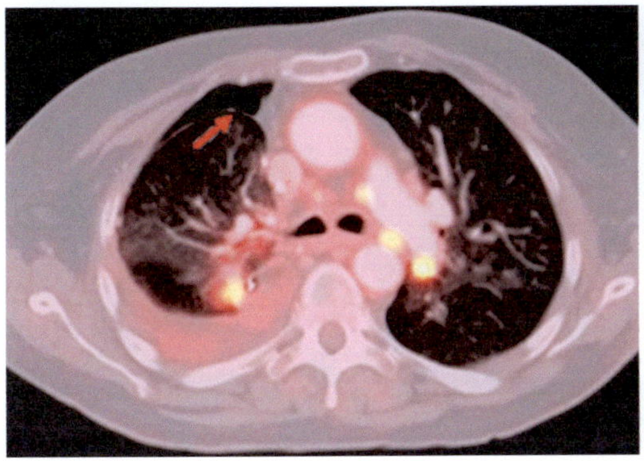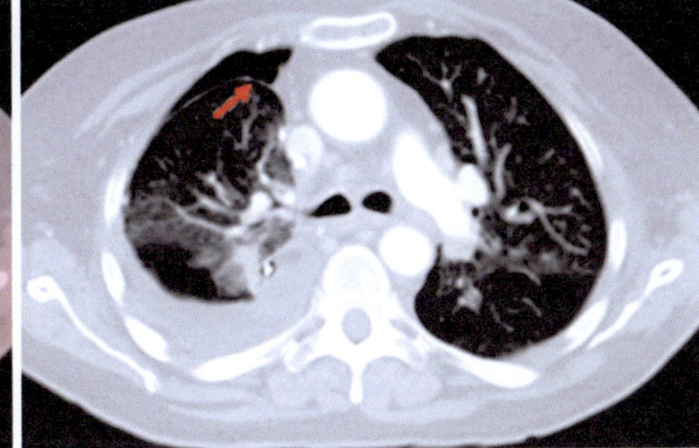

Fig. 5.30 Pneumothorax; note the area of absent lung markings located in the antidependent portion of the lung as air in the pleural space collects. This is slightly cold on PET as no FDG collects in the free air, but is better seen on CT (and all PET-CTs bear examination of the chest in the lung window to exclude this finding)

glance at the medical record is useful to avoid an embarrassing call.

Rarely, there may be an intracranial hemorrhage. While this can be difficult to see on PET, CT is fairly sensitive for this (particularly if acute), and hence examination of the head CT using brain windows is recommended to rule out this potentially lethal finding.

A variety of nonacute findings may be seen on CT, many non-avid on PET but nonetheless concerning or at least worthy of future follow-up. A lot of these are so frequent there are standardized protocols for handling them, which are updated every few years. The guidelines for handling lung nodules from the Fleischner Society were recently revised in 2017 [22] and are useful with incidentally discovered lung nodules.

The interpretation of abdominal lesions is its own, large field within medical imaging, but a few guidelines for incidental lesions may be given. Renal and liver cysts are usually visibly non-avid if large enough. If small enough, the usual guidelines for these lesions can be followed; generally, any lesion with CT attenuation under 20 Hounsfield units (HU) can be assumed to be a cyst. A renal (not hepatic) lesion with CT attenuation over 70 HU is assumed to be a hemorrhagic cyst and also benign. Adrenal nodules are similarly thought to be lipid-rich adenomas (and hence benign) with attenuation below 10 HU on a non-contrast examination; they are worrisome from the PET point of view with intensities greater than liver [23]. (Avid liver lesions are concerning given the frequency of metastasis to liver, and avid renal lesions are usually concerning as well given the high background uptake in the kidney.) Visceral lesions not meeting these criteria are not necessary malignant, but should be further worked up with a contrast-enhanced CT or MRI.

Apart from possible malignancies, one potentially dangerous finding that can be seen on abdominopelvic CT is an abdominal aortic aneurysm (Fig. 5.31). These are more common in patients with atherosclerosis; the diameter of the abdominal aorta should be no more than 3 cm. If higher, it is aneurysmal and should be followed at the very least; if over 5 cm surgery may be required.

A number of more minor incidental findings within the abdomen and pelvis are quite common. Kidney stones and gallstones may be seen and are usually nonemergent findings but bear mentioning. Diverticulosis without evidence of diverticulitis is quite common as well; one should mention it at least as a note to future clinicians. Avid areas within or near a colonic diverticulum may represent diverticulitis, and calling attention to this is useful for clinicians.

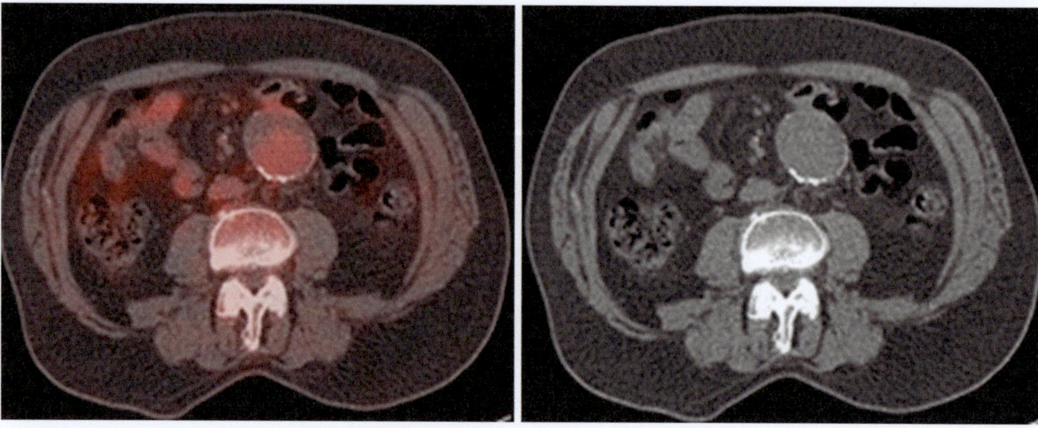

Fig. 5.31 Abdominal aortic aneurysm, viewed as a large abdominal aorta. This should be noted if seen

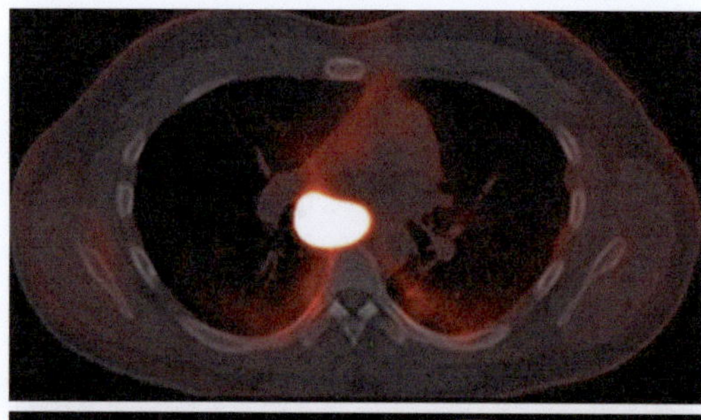

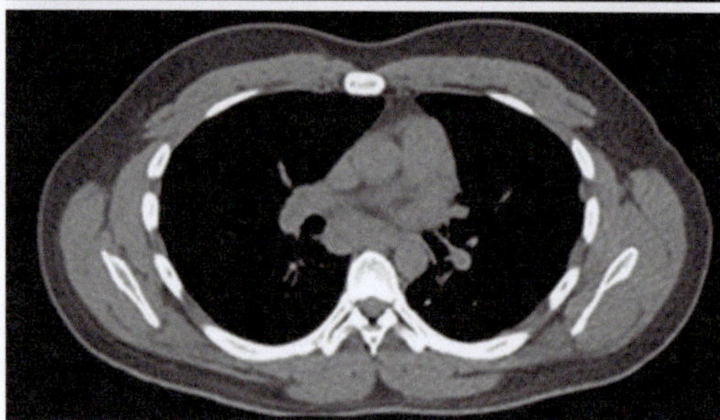

Fig. 5.32 This extremely hot node (SUVmax 55) appears to extend into the adjacent vertebral body on fused images, but is seen not to do so on unfused CT

Technical Artifacts (May Be False Positive or False Negative)

Volume Averaging Artifact

Very intense tumors will often appear larger on PET than on CT due to scatter and the relatively poor spatial resolution of the modality (Fig. 5.32), leading to the observation that assessing tumor size on PET is usually inaccurate. It is also well-known that calculations of SUVmax on tumors below about 3 cm are affected by the size of the tumor [13].

Attenuation Correction and Artifacts: Misregistration, Motion, Breathing

In most modern PET scanners, a CT scan is used for attenuation correction. While this is usually technically adequate, and allows the acquisition of a concurrent CT scan as well, in some cases (usually due to some variety of patient motion), attenuation correction artifacts can result. Even physiologic bowel motion can produce artifacts (Fig. 5.33), but musculoskeletal motion is more commonly the issue. Patients are advised to maintain shallow respiration (rather than taking a deep breath as with a conventional CT) and to hold still during the scan, but not everyone is able to comply, and even relatively mild motion during the scan can produce artifacts (Figs. 5.34 and 5.35). Even respiration can produce its own set of artifacts (Fig. 5.36), with lesions occasionally being projected from the liver into the lung (Fig. 5.37) or vice versa.

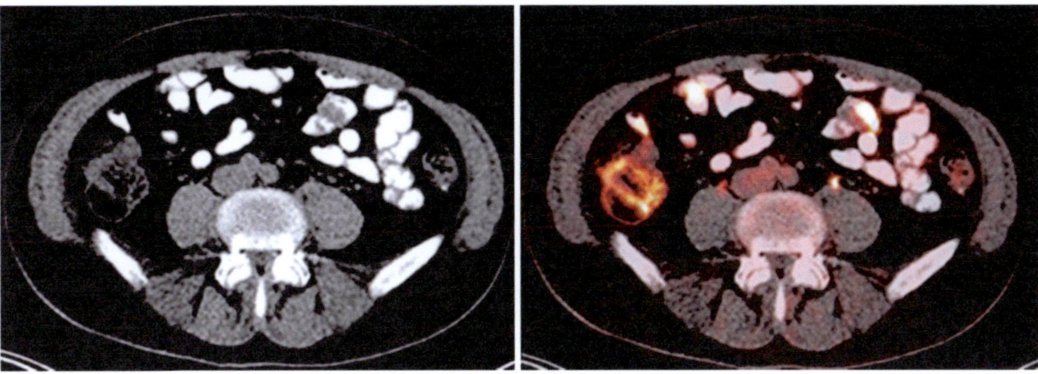

Fig. 5.33 Mass lesion in the bowel is imperfectly registered between PET and CT

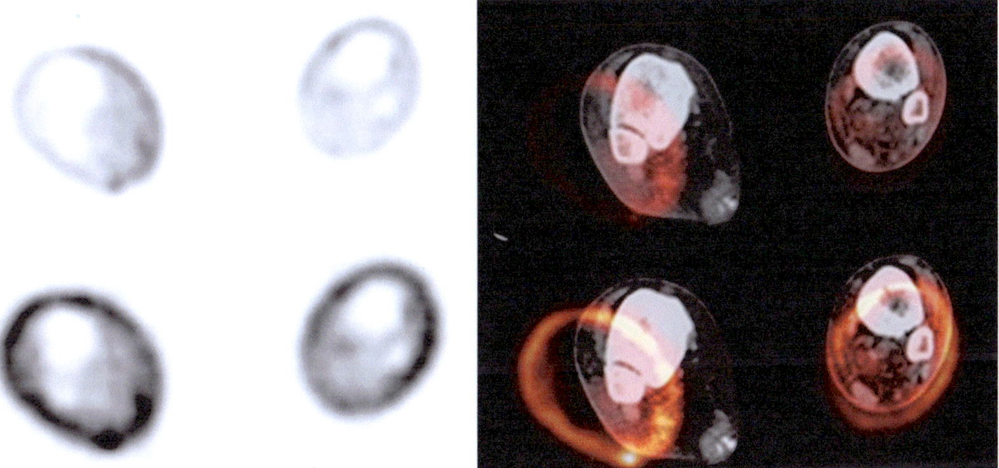

Fig. 5.34 AC (top row) and NAC (bottom row) PET and fused images. The (apparent) increased uptake in the medial right ankle is in fact an artifact of the lateral right ankle being projected over the air, with "corrected" atten-uation being falsely low. NAC images show this is not the case and, in fact, if anything the lateral ankle is more intense

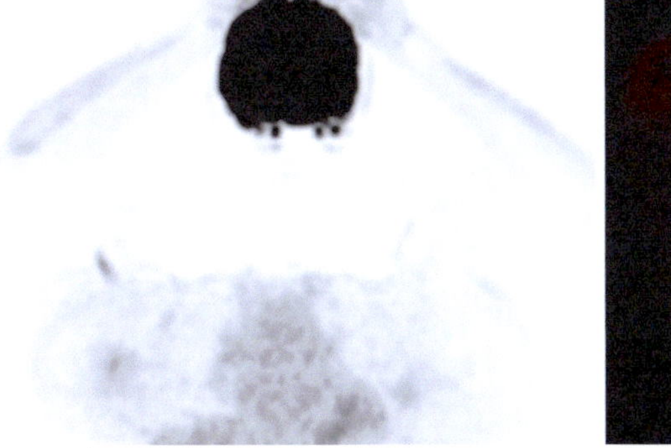

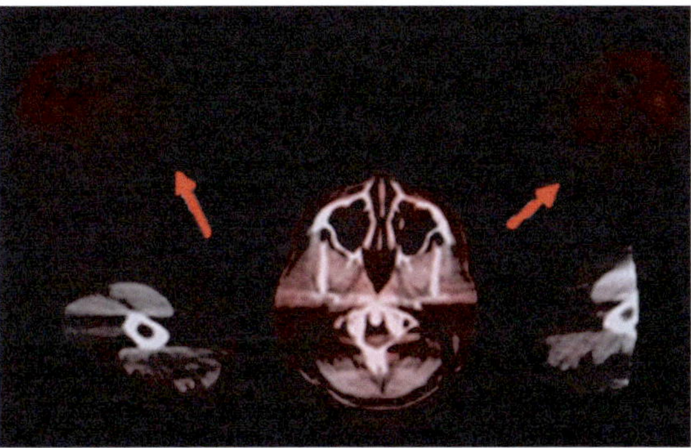

Fig. 5.35 The patient moved her arms downward during PET acquisition. Note the absent uptake in the neck region on MIP and the "gray" appearance of the proximal arms indicating no uptake, as well as the orange "ghosts" (arrows) anteriorly reflecting PET images registered to the empty air. This produces falsely low values for the PET as the PET scanner is attenuated but the CT does not reflect this. The PET scan was repeated in this area

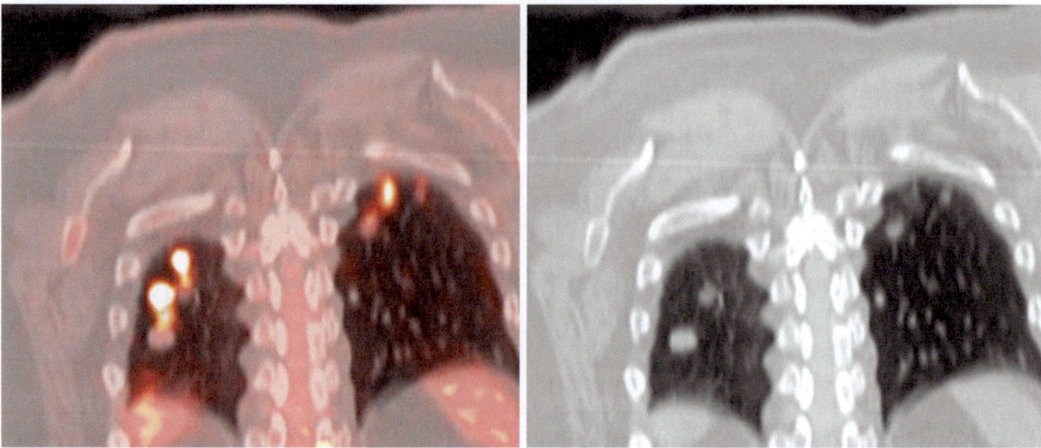

Fig. 5.36 Lung metastases from a clear cell sarcoma on PET are significantly displaced from their locations on CT

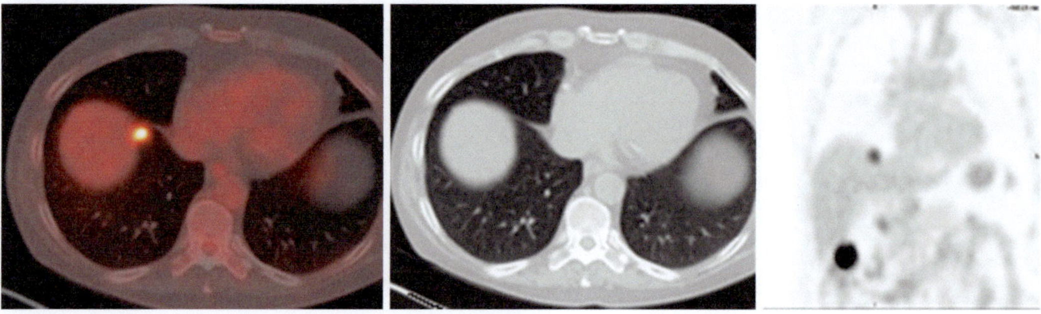

Fig. 5.37 Lesion apparently in the lung but not seen on CT is seen on coronal PET-only images to be localized in the liver

References

1. Kumar R, Mavi A, Bural G, Alavi A. Fluorodeoxyglucose-PET in the management of malignant melanoma. Radiol Clin N Am. 2005;43(1):23–33.
2. Wallitt K, Yusuf S, Soneji N, Khan SR, Win Z, Barwick TD. PET/CT in oncologic imaging of nodal disease: pearls and pitfalls: RadioGraphics fundamentals | online presentation. Radiographics. 2018;38(2):564–5.
3. Lococo F, Muoio B, Chiappetta M, Nachira D, Petracca Ciavarella L, Margaritora S, et al. Diagnostic performance of PET or PET/CT with different radiotracers in patients with suspicious lung cancer or pleural tumours according to published meta-analyses. Contrast Media Mol Imaging. 2020;5282698:2020.
4. Bourgeois AC, Chang TT, Fish LM, Bradley YC. Positron emission tomography/computed tomography in melanoma. Radiol Clin N Am. 2013;51(5):865–79.
5. Boellaard R, Delgado-Bolton R, Oyen WJ, Giammarile F, Tatsch K, Eschner W, et al. FDG PET/CT: EANM procedure guidelines for tumour imaging: version 2.0. Eur J Nucl Med Mol Imaging. 2015;42(2):328–54.
6. Sachpekidis C, Kopp-Schneider A, Hakim-Meibodi L, Dimitrakopoulou-Strauss A, Hassel JC. 18F-FDG PET/CT longitudinal studies in patients with advanced metastatic melanoma for response evaluation of combination treatment with vemurafenib and ipilimumab. Melanoma Res. 2019;29(2):178–86.
7. Sachpekidis C, Larribere L, Kopp-Schneider A, Hassel JC, Dimitrakopoulou-Strauss A. Can benign lymphoid tissue changes in (18)F-FDG PET/CT predict response to immunotherapy in metastatic melanoma? Cancer Immunol Immunother. 2019;68(2):297–303.
8. Nobashi T, Baratto L, Reddy SA, Srinivas S, Toriihara A, Hatami N, et al. Predicting response to immunotherapy by evaluating tumors, lymphoid cell-rich

organs, and immune-related adverse events using FDG-PET/CT. Clin Nucl Med. 2019;44(4):e272–9.

9. Lang N, Dick J, Slynko A, Schulz C, Dimitrakopoulou-Strauss A, Sachpekidis C, et al. Clinical significance of signs of autoimmune colitis in (18) F-fluorodeoxyglucose positron emission tomography-computed tomography of 100 stage-IV melanoma patients. Immunotherapy. 2019;11(8):667–76.

10. Goldfarb L, Duchemann B, Chouahnia K, Zelek L, Soussan M. Monitoring anti-PD-1-based immunotherapy in non-small cell lung cancer with FDG PET: introduction of iPERCIST. EJNMMI Res. 2019;9(1):8.

11. Ito K, Teng R, Schoder H, Humm JL, Ni A, Michaud L, et al. (18)F-FDG PET/CT for monitoring of ipilimumab therapy in patients with metastatic melanoma. J Nucl Med. 2019;60(3):335–41.

12. Seymour L, Bogaerts J, Perrone A, Ford R, Schwartz LH, Mandrekar S, et al. iRECIST: guidelines for response criteria for use in trials testing immunotherapeutics. Lancet Oncol. 2017;18(3):e143–52.

13. Adams MC, Turkington TG, Wilson JM, Wong TZ. A systematic review of the factors affecting accuracy of SUV measurements. AJR Am J Roentgenol. 2010;195(2):310–20.

14. Treglia G, Bertagna F, Sadeghi R, Muoio B, Giovanella L. Prevalence and risk of malignancy of focal incidental uptake detected by fluorine-18-fluorodeoxyglucose positron emission tomography in the parotid gland: a meta-analysis. Eur Arch Otorhinolaryngol. 2015;272(12):3617–26.

15. Nayan S, Ramakrishna J, Gupta MK. The proportion of malignancy in incidental thyroid lesions on 18-FDG PET study: a systematic review and meta-analysis. Otolaryngol Head Neck Surg. 2014;151(2):190–200.

16. Treglia G, Bertagna F, Sadeghi R, Verburg FA, Ceriani L, Giovanella L. Focal thyroid inciden-tal uptake detected by (1)(8)F-fluorodeoxyglucose positron emission tomography. Meta-analysis on prevalence and malignancy risk. Nuklearmedizin. 2013;52(4):130–6.

17. Shie P, Cardarelli R, Sprawls K, Fulda KG, Taur A. Systematic review: prevalence of malignant incidental thyroid nodules identified on fluorine-18 fluorodeoxyglucose positron emission tomography. Nucl Med Commun. 2009;30(9):742–8.

18. Bertagna F, Treglia G, Orlando E, Dognini L, Giovanella L, Sadeghi R, et al. Prevalence and clinical significance of incidental F18-FDG breast uptake: a systematic review and meta-analysis. Jpn J Radiol. 2014;32(2):59–68.

19. Benveniste AP, Marom EM, Benveniste MF, Mawlawi O, Fox PS, Yang W. Incidental primary breast cancer detected on PET-CT. Breast Cancer Res Treat. 2015;151(2):261–8.

20. Treglia G, Taralli S, Salsano M, Muoio B, Sadeghi R, Giovanella L. Prevalence and malignancy risk of focal colorectal incidental uptake detected by (18)F-FDG-PET or PET/CT: a meta-analysis. Radiol Oncol. 2014;48(2):99–104.

21. Adams SJ, Rakheja R, Bryce R, Babyn PS. Incidence and economic impact of incidental findings on (18) F-FDG PET/CT imaging. Can Assoc Radiol J. 2018;69(1):63–70.

22. MacMahon H, Naidich DP, Goo JM, Lee KS, Leung ANC, Mayo JR, et al. Guidelines for management of incidental pulmonary nodules detected on CT images: from the Fleischner Society 2017. Radiology. 2017;284(1):228–43.

23. Dong A, Cui Y, Wang Y, Zuo C, Bai Y. (18)F-FDG PET/CT of adrenal lesions. AJR Am J Roentgenol. 2014;203(2):245–52.

Eric Wolsztynski and Janet F. Eary

Conventional PET-Based Quantitation

Standardized Uptake Values

PET imaging data essentially consist of count and spatial information on photons emitted by positron decay of the PET radiotracer molecules within the body. The scanner output data represents the number of photons detected by the detectors at an imaging time point. This raw information is processed (or "reconstructed"), usually by the imaging device based hardware, to generate a final four-dimensional digital image of intensities that relate to these initial photon counts in the volumetric field of view, captured over a number of imaging time frames. We refer to a unit of this 3D image frame as a voxel (volume element). A higher intensity at a given voxel therefore indicates higher concentration of the administered radiotracer at that location.

In routine practice, the volumetric PET body tissue uptake information is converted into standardized uptake values (SUV) by adjusting the raw tissue radioactivity concentration measured within an image region of interest at time t, $C(t)$, for patient body weight W and injected dose D:

$$\mathrm{SUV}(t) = C(t)/(D/W)$$

Tissue SUV values are commonly expressed in g/mL, with concentration level $C(t)$ in MBq/mL, and injected radioactive imaging agent dose per unit weight D/W in MBq/g. SUV measures are considered unitless, on the basis that $C(t)$ can be defined as concentration in soft tissue, itself with a mass density of about 1 g/mL.

The above uptake value standardization convention remains the predominant choice for image analysis in the literature and in clinical practice, although alternative methods have been considered for generation of initial tracer concentration than that provided by body weight W, which is very sensitive to patient physiology [1]. The most widespread of these alternatives is the lean SUV (SUL), using lean body mass W-BF, where BF is body fat, in place of W.

E. Wolsztynski (✉)
Insight Centre for Data Analytics, School of Mathematical Sciences, University College Cork, Cork, Ireland
e-mail: eric.w@ucc.ie

J. F. Eary
National Institutes of Health/NCI/DCTD, Bethesda, MD, USA
e-mail: janet.eary@nih.gov

Volume of Interest Segmentation

PET-based quantitation consists of deriving statistical summaries of the image data-based volume of interest (VOI), many of which rely on accurate tumor size assessment. Delineation, or segmentation, of the VOI is therefore critical but

© Springer Nature Switzerland AG 2021
A. H. Khandani (ed.), *PET/CT and PET/MR in Melanoma and Sarcoma*,
https://doi.org/10.1007/978-3-030-60429-5_6

can vary significantly with the method chosen. The use of hand-drawn VOI segmentation masks determined by trained staff is most commonly performed, but this process is tedious and prone to human error and interoperator variability. A wide range of semi- and fully automated alternatives are also available. Some approaches consist of identifying VOI voxels that have values above a segmentation threshold defined as a fraction of the maximum SUV in the image or as a multiplier of the average background SUV level [2]. Such thresholding schemes tend to be sensitive to image contrast and noise characteristics [1, 3]. Other techniques consist of identifying contours of the VOI adaptively from the imaging data, by evaluating the likelihood that a given voxel belongs to the tumor according to its direct neighborhood voxel characteristics [1, 2]. Multimodality image analysis techniques also exploit the additional information provided at higher transverse spatial resolution by a coregistered CT or MRI scan when available. For example, FMISO-PET VOI masks of glioma volumes may be determined using image appearance in FLAIR sequence MRI data [4, 5]. Reproducible segmentation seems more likely to be achieved using a combination of automatic edge-detection techniques and expert assessment of its output [2].

Conventional Summaries and Their Use at Baseline and Follow-Up

Once a tissue VOI is obtained, PET tracer uptake distribution is traditionally analyzed in terms of SUV summaries, namely, its maximum value (SUV_{max}), average value (SUV_{mean}), average value within the SUV_{max} tissue neighborhood (SUV_{peak}), metabolically active tumor volume (MATV), and total lesion glycolysis (TLG = $SUV_{mean} \times$ MATV) [1]. Note that the term "glycolysis" here stems from the use of FDG as a tracer for tissue metabolism. Other PET imaging agents report on different tissue processes or status. For example, F-18 fluoromisonidazole is used to determine the level of tissue oxygenation. In analyzing FMISO-PET data, a value for total lesion hypoxia can be

determined. Several variations exist for the calculation of SUV_{peak} using a number of PET imaging agents. One common approach uses the average SUV within a 1 cubic centimeter tissue sphere centered at the voxel with intensity SUV_{max}, but the neighborhood could be, e.g., the 9-voxel cube centered at SUV_{max} instead of a sphere. As for MATV, the tissue volume analyzed could be roughly approximated by the product of the number of voxels within the VOI and the unit volume of a single voxel. Some refinements exist to account for fractional voxels at VOI boundaries.

The above summaries are used essentially for characterization of primary lesions. Metastases assessments can also be performed. In most instances, similar tissue uptake determinations are performed. Typically, the number of lesions and parameters such as their size and SUV_{peak} values are reported. Methodologies vary with the image specialist and the type and nature of the disease.

For PET-based therapeutic response assessment, it is common to compare the most active lesions before and after therapy. Several sets of guidelines have been created. The Positron Emission Tomography Response Criteria in Solid Tumors (PERCIST) was published in 2009 in an effort to adapt the former WHO and (more MR- and CT-appropriate) Response Evaluation Criteria In Solid Tumors (RECIST) guidelines to the specifics of FDG PET (tissue metabolism) imaging data [1]. PERCIST classification rules determine whether there is "complete metabolic response," "partial metabolic response," "stable metabolic disease," or "progressive metabolic disease" following therapy, taking into account the number of lesions and the proportional changes in size and SUV_{peak} in all measurable lesions.

Risk Characterization and Predictive Validation

The prognostic value of PET-derived biomarkers is traditionally assessed by means of survival analyses, which can be carried out in a number of ways and are interpreted with respect to the endpoint considered. Conventional endpoints used to describe patient risk, outcome, or therapeutic effectiveness are, most often, overall survival (OS) (duration of patient survival before they become lost to follow-up), progression-free survival (PFS), or disease-free survival (DFS). These endpoints are continuous in nature, in that all patients can be placed on a timeline that usually starts either on the day of diagnosis or baseline scan ($t = 0$), and allow for longitudinal survival analyses. Time to progression (TTP) is another commonly used reference, but OS and PFS are usually preferred. Other endpoints, such as fixed-term survival (e.g., 2-year survival: yes/no) or disease presence (yes/no), are discrete (binary or multilevel factors) and are used for patient classification into risk groups. The nature of the endpoint determines the type of statistical analysis that can be carried out for risk characterization.

Risk Characterization for Continuous Endpoints

For continuous endpoints, cohort information is longitudinal—it contains a record of duration along a timeline until the event of interest occurs or the patient becomes lost to follow-up (e.g., for OS or PFS). In this context, two complementary forms of statistical assessment are traditionally carried out, which evaluate (i) the predictive potential of risk variables of interest and (ii) the ability of predictive models based on these variables to segregate patients into risk groups. Hazard models (most often, Cox proportional hazard models [6]) are usually used for the former task; they provide a measure of the effect of an increase in a particular variable on patient risk (as defined by the endpoint considered). For the latter task, survival curve estimates (most often, Kaplan-Meier estimates [6]) are obtained and compared for subgroups of the cohort defined on the basis of a score determined from the risk variables.

Univariate hazard models focus on the individual effect of a variable on risk. For a given outcome type, they produce a hazard ratio (HR) that quantifies the change in risk for a unit increase of this variable, compared to a hypothet-

ical baseline population within which the variable has a value of zero. A HR equal to 1 indicates no effect; HRs less than or greater than 1, respectively, indicate reduction and increase in risk following a change in the variable. Table 6.1 below illustrates an example where the risk variable x is *tumor grade*, taking values for "low," "intermediate," and "high" tumor grade. Here x = "low" is used as the baseline reference profile (a low-grade patient tumor). The HR measures the relative difference in risk between this reference and an intermediate-grade or high-grade patient tumor (with x = "intermediate" and "high," respectively). The case x = "high" yields a HR of 6.22, indicating a (very) large increase in risk for poor outcome compared to the reference case. The variable may also be continuous; for example, if x is (normalized) SUV_{max}, then 0 could be used as the reference value, and the hazard ratio measures the relative change in risk associated with a unit increase in SUV_{max} from a value of 0. In multivariate hazard models, a number of variables are considered together to describe the endpoint of interest. In this context the hazard ratio of a variable quantifies the change in risk for a unit increase of this variable when all other variables are held constant in the model.

The statistical significance of the hazard ratio associated with a risk variable (i.e., of the effect of the risk variable) is often the primary imaging biomarker performance indicator. A statistical test (usually either the Wald or Likelihood Ratio test) is carried out to determine whether the effect of the variable (in other words, the proportional change in risk incurred by a change in this variable) is significantly different from zero. A statistically significant effect indicates that the variable aptly describes some of the risks defined by the endpoint. Statistical significance of a variable is usually determined by its p-value. When the p-value falls below a set significant threshold (usually set at either 1% or 5%), then the variable is deemed a statistically significant risk factor. Although this result is derived from the clinical cohort under study, interpretation applies to the whole population of patients that this cohort represents. In the example of Table 6.1, the p-value for variable x = 'high' is $p = 0.0004$, i.e., $p < 0.01$,

Table 6.1 Left: Cox proportional hazards analysis of tumor grade (low, intermediate, high) effect on overall patient survival duration. The hazard ratios (HR) indicate that the risk of death increases, respectively, by a factor of 2.76 (i.e. a 176% increase) and 6.22 (i.e. a 522% increase) respectively for intermediate- and high-grade tumors, compared to a reference low-grade profile. The p-value smaller than 1% (0.01) for the "high-grade" level confirms that the change in risk in a sarcoma population is statistically significant for high-grade patients, compared to low-grade patients. Right: logistic regression analysis of the effect on the same variable on 2-year survival status (i.e., whether death occurs within 2 years of diagnosis) provides similar assessment. The intercept parameter corresponds to the reference low-grade group, with overall lower risk of death than the other two groups, as indicated by the increase in variable effect across groups. Corresponding p-values indicate that high-grade tumors are associated with a significantly higher risk of death at the 2-year horizon for patients with sarcoma. The corresponding effect (or odds ratio) indicates this increase in risk of death is estimated at 9.39 times the risk for a low-grade patient. Dataset acquired at the University of Washington School of Medicine (August 1993 to January 2003, Dr. Janet F. Eary), after biopsy (202 patients, 91 events; 88 females, 114 males; 52 bone, 17 cartilage, 132 soft-tissue; 32 low-, 69 intermediate-, 101 high-grade)

Cox proportional hazard model (overall survival, continuous endpoint)			Logistic regression model (2-year survival, discrete endpoint)		
Grade level	HR	p-value	Grade level	Effect	p-value
–	–	–	Intercept	0.07	**0.0003**
Intermediate	2.76	0.0593	Intermediate	3.49	0.1154
High	6.22	**0.0004**	High	9.39	**0.0031**

and thus x is deemed a significant risk factor for overall survival of sarcoma patients at the 1% significance level (or "with 99% confidence"), that may be used to classify sarcoma patients into different risk subgroups. From this result we can also infer that any high-grade sarcoma patient has a significantly higher risk of death than a low-grade tumor, whether these patients belong to this cohort or any other.

Statistical reports aiming to validate pseudo-markers or other predictive variables should provide both the p-value and associated variable effect or HR provided by the model, in order to provide both evidence of the statistical significance and an evaluation of the magnitude of the effect of the variable. Confidence intervals for the variable effect or HR are also strongly desired to indicate variability of the statistical assessment.

Multivariate predictive models can also be used for risk stratification for outcome type, based on a single-score summary obtained from them. Risk groups are determined by comparing this score to threshold values, which are set by the analyst according to the context of the cohort, either arbitrarily or based on clinical experience. Survival curve estimates are used to evaluate this stratification, most often by means of a Kaplan-Meier analysis (here, "survival" is used loosely and describes duration-to-event, whatever this endpoint event may be) [6], such as that depicted in Fig. 6.1.

For each risk group, a curve is obtained that starts at 1 and monotonically decreases toward 0 as events occur within that group. One essential advantage of these analyses is that they allow subject censoring, i.e., loss-to-follow-up, to be taken into account. A statistical test (usually the log-rank test) is then used to evaluate the statistical significance of the separation observed between different survival curves. A very small test p-value (at the 1% significance level, any $p < 0.01$) indicates that the survival curves are statistically significantly well separated, i.e., that there are significantly different survival outcomes on average for at least some of the corresponding sub-cohorts.

Risk Characterization for Discrete Endpoints

For discrete endpoints, the problem of interest becomes a classification problem. Duration data for a patient cohort may be available but the goal is to assign patients to different groups, according to risk level, disease stage, disease subtype, etc., on the basis of their information. In this context, statistical models such as logistic regression, decision trees, or more elaborate forms (random forests, support vector machines, neural networks) are used to determine a classification rule based on the available data. The model allows summarizing a patient's multivariate profile into one single-valued score, which is compared

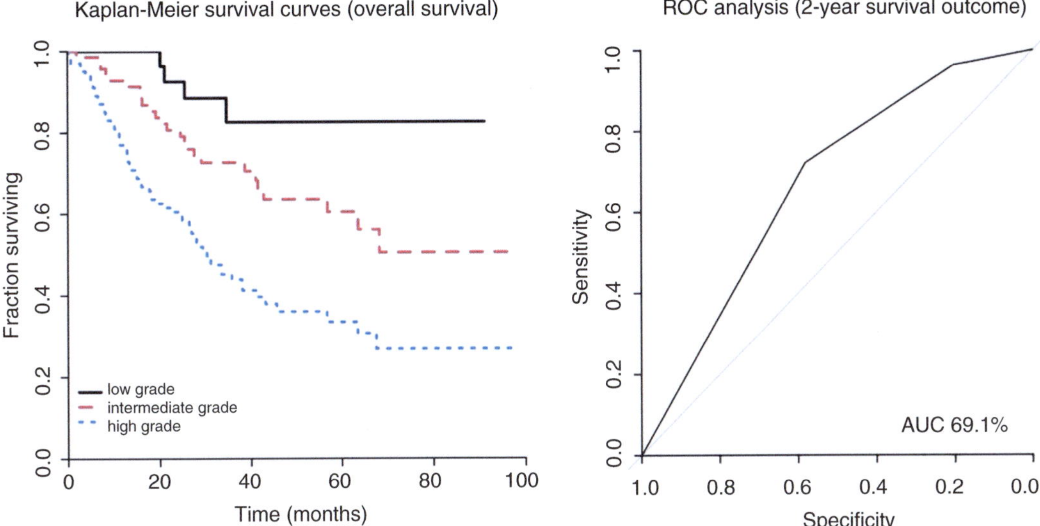

Fig. 6.1 Overall survival risk analysis based on variable grade used in Table 6.1 for the same sarcoma cohort. Left: Kaplan-Meier survival curve estimates as a function of survival duration (a continuous endpoint) obtained for each grade group clearly indicate higher risk (lower chance of survival) as grade increases. The log-rank test p-value $p = 0.000004$ indicates significant difference between the survival curves for each tumor-grade group. Right: ROC analysis of patient survival status (0: dead, 1: alive; a discrete endpoint) predicted by a univariate logistic regression model using the same grade variable. The faint diagonal line indicates the prediction performance obtained by flipping a fair coin. The thick curve indicates the relative gain in prediction accuracy (both in sensitivity and specificity) obtained using the univariate model to predict patient outcome. The associated AUC of 69.1% indicates mediocre overall performance from this model

against a set threshold value in order to classify the case [6, 7]. Just like in a Cox model (which itself relies on a form of linear regression), a classification model yields an assessment of statistical significance for each of its variables. This significance is again evaluated in terms of a p-value compared to a predefined significant threshold, as demonstrated in Table 6.1.

Predictive performance of the classification rule is then evaluated in terms of standard detection theory tools. For binary classification (by far the most common scenario), sensitivity and specificity of the classifier are measured, with values within the [0,1] interval, i.e., between 0% and 100%. Any classification model achieves a trade-off between these two performance metrics and tends to be stronger in one of these two aspects. One controls this trade-off by tuning the above-mentioned classification threshold. Performance of the classifier is commonly assessed by means of an ROC analysis (receiver operating characteristics), which provides a plot of sensitivity (or true positive rate) against 1-specificity (or false-positive rate) for varying classification thresholds, as illustrated in Fig. 6.1. The area under the ROC curve (AUC) yields a single-number summary of the classifier's predictive capacity, but many other related metrics are available for refined performance evaluation. A common rule of thumb is that AUCs between 60–69%, 70–79%, 80–89%, and 90–100%, respectively, indicate poor, fair, good, and excellent model fits, but this is not prescriptive. An AUC of 0.5 (i.e., 50%) corresponds to a decision based on flipping a fair coin [6–8].

Influential Factors in PET-Based Quantitation

Nature of PET Data and Impact of Imaging Protocol

A number of operational parameters such as scanning time, injected dose, patient position, scanner calibration, and other elements of imaging protocols can vary considerably between clinical sites. Some of these aspects directly impact the data quality of the output image. Injected dose is a major contributor to image contrast with some imaging agents resulting in differences in the signal-to-noise ratio in the image. Often with a lower imaging agent dose, there is greater image signal noise. Use and choice of attenuation correction techniques also affect the statistical nature of the final PET imaging data, with significant differences between PET-MR and PET-CT [2, 6, 9]. PET scanners yield different spatial and timing resolutions, depending on manufacturers and especially across generations of tomographs. This can particularly affect the visibility, detection, and characterization of small uptake foci. Slice thickness also has an impact on apparent image noise [10].

PET imaging data consists of reconstructions of photon pairs registered in the scanner detectors. As a result, scanner architectures also have an impact on the image output. PET imaging systems yield lower transverse spatial resolution than MRI and CT systems, due to the nature of the detection mode and information density of each modality. Software treatment of the raw data, either in-built or applied post-acquisition for all these systems, also has an impact. The raw acquired system input are positive integer values, but due to the tomography process, their spatial distribution must be reconstructed in a 3D spatial coordinate domain to produce a final image. During that step, the imaging input events become continuous values as opposed to integers, due to the application of image reconstruction algorithms. Choice and calibration of these algorithms has an impact on the statistical characteristics of the reconstructed image output data. As an example, previous reconstruction methods based on filtered back projection (FBP) produce images where (mostly background) voxels may have negative intensity values, but lower overall bias, whereas more current methods relying on ordered-subset expectation maximization (OSEM) ensure positive uptake values in all areas of the image, but result in larger reconstruc-

tion bias [11]. Image reconstruction may be carried out iteratively over acquired 2D slices or overall across the imaged 3D volume.

Segmentation and Post-Processing

We mentioned earlier that the choice of segmentation algorithm can drastically impact image quantitation. For example, in a case where peak tissue VOI uptake is found at the tumor boundary, improper volume delineation may remove some of the voxels contributing to the 1 cc sphere placed around the VOI designated for determination of tumor SUV_{max}. This would result in an error in SUV_{peak} determination. Tumor of other tissue uptake focus volume assessment and other parameters are also very sensitive to image segmentation approaches.

Image interpolation procedures are also known to have a potentially great influence on analysis output variables [3]. Image interpolation is carried out when the resolution of the image needs to be adapted in order to apply image-based data analysis types such as radiomics, described further in Sect. 3. In some of these schemes, approximate voxel intensities are calculated in tissue locations with a finer or coarser image array size. In a simple example consisting of a function for halving slice thickness, voxel intensities in each slice k in the interpolated image would be predicted on the basis of its neighboring slices $k - 1$ and $k + 1$, e.g., by averaging adjacent voxels.

PET spatial resolution induces another limitation on quantitative image analysis, due to the partial volume effect (PVE) for some tissue uptake foci in various body locations. Large voxel sizes imply that the information contained within a voxel partially captures the activity of its surrounding voxels [12–15]. PVE correction techniques are oftentimes used in order to correct this spillover effect and ensure that the voxel intensity reflects the activity in the tissue at that location only. This correction takes scanner specifications (its point-spread function, PSF) and voxel resolution into account. VOI interpolation should generally also be followed by PVE correction.

Quantitation with Short-Half-Life Tracers Radiotracers

Important considerations in PET imaging are radiotracer physical and biological half-lives. Using radiotracers with short uptake and clearance times often reduces the overall duration of the imaging procedure, resulting in less radio-isotope decay which increases the number of photon-induced count input from each imaging plane. This factor, in turn, can give a positive impact on image quality. Some imaging agents can also result in enhanced image contrast by yielding low tracer uptake in background tissue [16]. Several studies with short half-life tracers have been reported. In melanoma, amino acid imaging agents for tissue protein synthesis radiolabeled with carbon ^{11}C (20.4-minute half-life) have been evaluated for imaging prediction of therapeutic response. ^{11}C-alpha-methyltryptophan (^{11}C-AMT) was evaluated in NIH clinical trials in metastatic melanoma, and ^{11}C-methionine (^{11}C-MET) was studied in patients with mucosal malignant melanoma [17]. Gallium (^{68}Ga) has a 67.7-minute half-life, and imaging agents that use this radiolabel have been considered for study in several cancers including sarcoma [16]. Guidance on image quantitative analysis for these imaging agents is not yet clear, since the statistical characteristics of the PET imaging data output will strongly depend upon imaging agent characteristics, including administered dose.

Quantifying Tumor Heterogeneity

Motivation for PET-Based Heterogeneity Assessment

The level of biologic heterogeneity in subpopulations of cancer cells within a tumor has been identified as a key driver of cancer patient outcome, in many forms of cancer including sarcoma and melanoma [6, 14, 18–20]. Intratumoral biologic heterogeneity is most commonly assessed by tissue biopsy, in a process that requires that the optimal sampling area be identi-fied, and sampled for histopathologic assessment. This is a challenging task, and there is a significant risk that the histopathologic assessment may not represent the underlying phenotypic or genetic landscape of the disease fully or adequately [21].

The promising potential of imaging biological assessment for personalized cancer care motivates the use of noninvasive imaging, and in particular PET, to replace biopsy-based histopathology assessments with a more convenient, faster, reliable, and accurate evaluation process. This approach relies on the assumption that tumor biological heterogeneity drives imaging agent uptake heterogeneity. Results from current work can be interpreted to suggest that macroscopic uptake heterogeneity observable on PET images is likely to reflect the microscopic heterogeneity of cancerous tissue. The prognostic potential of PET tumor uptake heterogeneity has been established for several cancer types, predominantly using FDG-PET imaging [13, 19, 22, 23]. Interpretation of PET-derived heterogeneity quantitation must be made in the context of the PET tracer used [6, 14]. Interpretation of the uptake variations at macroscopic level in the PET tracer uptake pattern must be made in terms of the specific agent used for imaging different tumor biologic parameters such as glycolysis, hypoxia, or cell proliferation. Specific PET agents for imaging these parameters are fluorode-oxyglucose (FDG), fluoromisonidazole (FMISO), and fluorothymidine (FLT).

Heterogeneity Characterization in Sarcoma

The main methodological approaches to image-based evaluation of intratumoral heterogeneity in radiotracer uptake distribution in the literature can be organized into two generic groups [6]. One strategy that has received consideration relies on the analysis of image texture, using well-established tools from the (non-radiological) image processing community. Texture analysis produces a large number of image-derived variables, or features, that capture different aspects of the image content, summarizing variations in image intensity and relief, among other things. Following a trend that started about 15 years ago, a growing number of studies characterize intratumoral radiotracer uptake distribution heterogeneity in terms of combinations of a number of these texture features. Novel multivariate predictive models, or nomograms, for staging and prognosis can be built by incorporating such combinations with existing clinical variables used routinely, such as patient age and tumor SUV_{max} (in FDG-PET imaging) [14]. However, selecting an adequate number and subset of texture variables is a considerable task. This prompts advanced model selection procedures relying on modern statistical learning techniques, and for this reason the underlying concept and use of texture analysis for image heterogeneity assessment is further described in Sect. 3.

The second methodology consists in comparing the observed tracer uptake distribution to reference shapes or patterns. Motivated by clinical experience with sarcoma, intratumoral radiotracer uptake spatial heterogeneity has been measured conceptually as a degree of conformity of the spatial PET tracer uptake distribution with an idealized ellipsoidal pattern. Less conformity of the tumor spatial uptake pattern with the idealized ellipsoidal object implies more heterogeneity in tumor radiotracer spatial uptake [6, 19]. The 3D spatial map of tracer uptake in the tumor VOI can be described using a mathematical model that represents each voxel in terms of its radial position within the idealized ellipsoidal pattern:

$$SUV_{ideal} \approx g\left(\text{voxel radial position}\right)$$

where g is a function of voxel location that represents the uptake profile signature going from the VOI core out toward its boundary. Figure 6.2 illustrates two examples of sarcoma studies acquired at the University of Washington with a GE Advance PET, presenting different levels of tumor FDG spatial uptake heterogeneity, and shows the corresponding uptake profile g obtained following this approach, where the uptake is shown on the y-axis as a function of the radial voxel position on the x-axis. Clinical experience indicates that a tumor mass with an FDG-avid (viable tissue) central region is usually

observed in a histologically low-grade tumor, whereas a tumor that has a photopenic central region that likely represents a necrotic zone is a histologically high-grade tumor. This image analysis spatial model was designed with the purpose of capturing these tumor features and used to derive a measure of conformity to the "idealized" pattern of a homogeneous uptake mass, thus defining FDG uptake spatial heterogeneity in terms of the scaled distance between idealized and observed SUV data:

$$Het \approx \left(SUV_{obs} - SUV_{ideal}\right)^2 / Variance\left(SUV_{obs}\right)$$

Based on the above definition, a low value of Het is assigned to studies for which the difference $SUV_{obs} - SUV_{ideal}$ is small. In the examples of Fig. 6.2, this difference corresponds to the average distance of the dots (the observed uptake data, SUV_{obs}) to the model line (the idealized SUV, SUV_{ideal}).

Baseline prognostic potential of this FDG spatial uptake heterogeneity assessment was validated for sarcoma patient overall survival [6, 19]. This method can be applied to PET/CT and PET/MR data. Variations using a tubular reference structure were also considered, to provide a more flexible structure for characterization [24].

Further Characterization of Spatial Tumor Uptake Patterns

Statistical modeling of intratumoral uptake creates opportunities for a detailed quantitative characterization of tumor imaging agent uptake parameters beyond standard heterogeneity evaluation. In particular, local spatial variations in uptake may also be assessed from modeling of the spatial uptake distribution, to evaluate differences in uptake at any location within the VOI. Mathematically, this difference can be defined as the derivative (or gradient) of the uptake profile function g defined above, and a gradient value can be derived for any voxel:

$$Gradient \approx -g'\left(\text{voxel radial position}\right)$$

This measure quantifies the steepness of the profile uptake curve of Fig. 6.2, along that radial

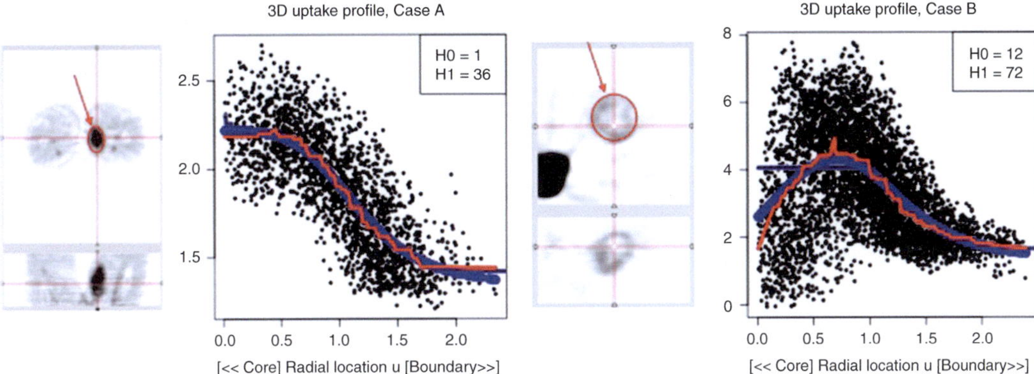

Fig. 6.2 Example of sarcoma studies from the cohort of Table 6.1, with uptake profile curve g and corresponding heterogeneity quantitation indicated in inset (figure adapted from [6]). Input VOIs are segmented as an ellipsoidal volume such as those outlined in red on the transverse views (top). Case A (left): 49-year-old male with upper thigh soft tissue sarcoma with an active, homogeneous core represented by a gradually decreasing uptake profile pattern. Case B (right): 48-year-old male with pelvis soft tissue sarcoma, with a heterogeneous core with low activity captured by a modal uptake profile pattern

position within the VOI. Following the mathematical definition of Wolsztynski et al. [6], a negative gradient value indicates a locally decreasing uptake profile when applied to an FDG-PET image data set (relative to peak activity and when exploring the VOI from the tumor center toward the tumor boundary). A positive gradient value corresponds to an area of increasing uptake signature. Following this representation, higher-grade sarcoma will typically exhibit increased avidity further away from its center, and tumor central uptake would be seen to decrease, resulting in local negative gradients in that area. Whether the gradient is positive or negative, its absolute value indicates the magnitude of the trend of uptake change occurring along a given tumor radius and for all radii between the tumor center and its boundary.

Since this spatial uptake gradient quantitation evaluates average radial differences in uptake throughout the VOI, one can map areas of uptake differences within the tumor, including information on the direction of change. This may be useful, for example, to locate and visualize areas with more significant local variations in uptake. The sample of gradients derived from the image can also be summarized into a single value (e.g., its median value, 95th percentile, or maximum value), to be used in multivariate prognostic models alongside other variables. The prognostic utility of spatial uptake pattern gradient summaries in sarcoma has been demonstrated by Wolsztynski et al. [6].

Tumor Uptake Spatial Heterogeneity Characterization in Melanoma

Early-stage melanoma is associated with favorable outcome following complete resection, but challenges are much greater for effective treatment of advanced disease, including elevated risk of tumor in stage IV. Stage IV melanoma tends to present with a high level of both intratumoral and intertumoral heterogeneity in imaging agent uptake [25, 26], which can increase the mathematical uncertainty associated with baseline tumor and risk characterization. Assessment of these two forms of biologic heterogeneity would be helpful in effective treatment personalization.

Currently, biological and mutation-driven cancer therapies are treatments of choice for a number of malignancies, which explains a predominance of studies focused on tumor genomic and immune heterogeneity assessment, and assessment of metastases. To date, it is however unclear how markers of genetic heterogeneity are captured by PET imaging, and radiological intratumoral heterogeneity assessment in melanoma is not as developed as in sarcoma. Most image quantitation is currently based on FDG PET SUV-type summaries, most often in terms of change in SUV_{max} or SUV_{peak}, SUV_{peak} interquartile range, or sum of SUV summary values measured at the predominant lesion sites [27, 28]. PET image spatial uptake heterogeneity is usually defined as a measure of variability in imaging agent uptake profiles, but with limited spatial relevance.

Artificial Intelligence and Radiomics in PET

The Role of Artificial Intelligence in Radiology

Motivation and Current Uses of Artificial Intelligence in Radiology

In order to improve patient care processes and develop patient-adaptive therapeutic pathways, modern healthcare has turned to artificial intelligence (AI). The term designates a "universal field" aiming to "build intelligent entities" [7]. It consists of integrated processes that have the ability to learn from data and take actions or formulate decisions adequately with respect to the input provided. AI solutions tend to be computationally more effective than conventional human- or computer-based techniques, allowing for efficient processing of large volumes of data at high speeds. They are built to learn continuously and aim to outperform human experts for specific tasks. Well-known universal examples include voice-powered personal assistants available in today's smartphones, driverless robotic vehicles, and the IBM DeepBlue chess-playing computer [7]. In medical environments, AI is considered for a wide range of purposes, such as the analysis of ECG data [29], computer-aided diagnosis (CAD) [30], or management of electronic health records and medical notes available in unstructured formats [31]. One of the most powerful examples of AI in healthcare is the IBM Watson system for diagnosis and adaptive treatment decision-making. However most developments in this field are currently still at the experimentation stage and face limitations in terms of regulations, logistics, and validation [31].

In radiology, current research underway is predominantly focused on AI for tumor screening, characterization, and diagnosis purposes. Applications of AI to radiological data remain experimental or exploratory, although support decision systems were reported in the 1970s [32]. Recent developments include CAD for breast cancer screening [8, 33], aiming to reduce the high false-positive rates of existing exam approaches. Screening processes perform classification of the VOI (for instance, into binary decisions such as disease presence/absence) on the basis of a number of input variables, some from routine clinical investigation, and others extracted from the radiological image. Results to date suggest that current AI practice provides improvement when used as a support tool (i.e., as a second opinion) rather than a standalone solution in this domain and needs further validation.

Image-based tumor segmentation can also benefit from AI technologies, for both tumor delineation and intratumoral parameters profiling. Current advances for these tasks rely on automatic learning techniques (which AI systems heavily rely upon) rather than implement full AI processes. Namely, "machine learning" and "deep learning" frameworks allow building of predictive models based on training data. Advanced automated processes are considered in addressing interuser variability in image segmentation and to speed up this time-consuming task. A broad range of strategies for automatic tumor delineation in images have been explored, some relying heavily on classical image processing tools such as wavelet decomposition. Others involve an elaborate panel of tumor features calculated from the VOI. Researchers report using deep learning techniques for VOI segmentation especially for MRI and CT data [34–36]. Volume delineation based on neural networks could also be applied effectively to PET data [37]. VOI segmentation remains conservative due to its critical impact on subsequent analysis. Implementation of complete AI solutions within commercialized or serialized products (either imaging devices or software) will require considerably more development. Recent efforts have evaluated tumor image segmentation for tumor prognosis potential. This is reflected in recent major community challenges such as the Brain Tumor Segmentation Challenge (BRaTS) for glioma segmentation and prognostic assessment using AI-based techniques on multicentric preoperative MRI data [38].

Tumor characterization and prognosis is the area in which the field of radiology has enjoyed the most progress with the emergence and generalization of AI. In routine practice, translating and interpreting the wealth of information captured by 3D imaging data into precise and reliable clinical assessment and prognosis is challenging. Based on visual or semiquantitative assessment, a radiologist evaluates disease presence/absence, size, and stage and forms an expert opinion on the level of tissue heterogeneity within a tumor, areas of specific interest such as target regions for biopsy, or therapeutic response [1, 39, 40]. For PET imaging data in particular, quantitative assessment as described in Sect. 2 above is often restricted to simple SUV summaries (SUV_{max}, TLG, etc.) that do not usually include heterogeneity valuation. The imaging data, which comprises of thousands of voxels in many cases, provides an opportunity for a much finer characterization of the disease but remains underexploited in clinical settings [1]. This calls for more elaborate image analysis approaches, which can in turn enhance prognostic modeling thanks to a more informed description of the disease process [6]. The accumulation of significant experimental results in this area of investigation has led to the rapidly emerging field of "radiomics," whose principle, described in the next section, is not unlike that of genomics [2, 14, 22, 41].

Radiomics: Machine Learning for Tumor Characterization and Prognosis

A growing number of image-derived variables have been considered in recent research to either replace or complement routine quantitative tumor assessment. Particular emphasis has been placed on capturing various aspects of intratumoral spatial uptake heterogeneity noninvasively, using a subset of dozens, sometimes hundreds, of descriptors of voxel intensity distribution, image texture, and related image processing aspects. Such a collection of metrics are often referred to as "textural parameters" or "radiomic features" and may be divided into groups of image descriptors; Table 6.2 below illustrates some of these groups with examples of well-known features for each [3]. This description is non-exhaustive. A wide range of other metrics is available, e.g., textural descriptors derived from wavelet transforms

Table 6.2 Some of the more common families of radiomic features and examples of features in each family. Figure 6.3 further below illustrates the nature of the representations of VOI uptake distributions used to define feature families (A)–(D)

(A) Morphological features	(B) Intensity features	(C) Spatial textural features	(D) Regional features
Shape and structure descriptors of the volume of interest	*First-order aspects of the distribution of voxel intensity levels (histogram-based, not spatially relevant)*	*Second-order aspects of the spatial distribution of voxel intensity levels (associations of neighboring voxels)*	*Higher-order aspects of spatial distribution of connex groups of voxels (number and size of groups, etc.)*
Examples of features (variables)			
Volume	Mean intensity	Joint average	Long-run emphasis
Surface area	Intensity variance	Joint variance	Run length variance
Sphericity	Maximum intensity	Joint entropy	Small/large zone emphasis
Major axis length	Intensity range	Correlation	Gray-level non-uniformity
Elongation	Intensity uniformity	Homogeneity	...
Flatness	Histogram entropy	Contrast	
...	...	...	

of the image. The variables of Sect. 2 measuring heterogeneity and radial variation in uptake are other candidates.

Figure 6.3 illustrates different summaries of the distribution of gray levels in the VOI in an FDG-PET sarcoma image, aligned with the columns of Table 6.2. The group of first-order metrics (second column in Table 6.2) is not spatially relevant, i.e., these metrics would remain unchanged if the image were scrambled. They are very close in nature to quantitative summaries used routinely such as SUV_{max} or SUV_{mean}. Second-order features summarize how any two voxel intensity levels i and j may be distributed within the image—for example, if it is likely to find a very bright voxel next to a very dark one (image contrast). Higher-order features describe other aspects of the structure of intensity levels within the image after its requantization into a lower number of gray levels (usually 32 or 64), such as the size and number of groups of voxels of comparable intensities, or their homogeneity within the volume.

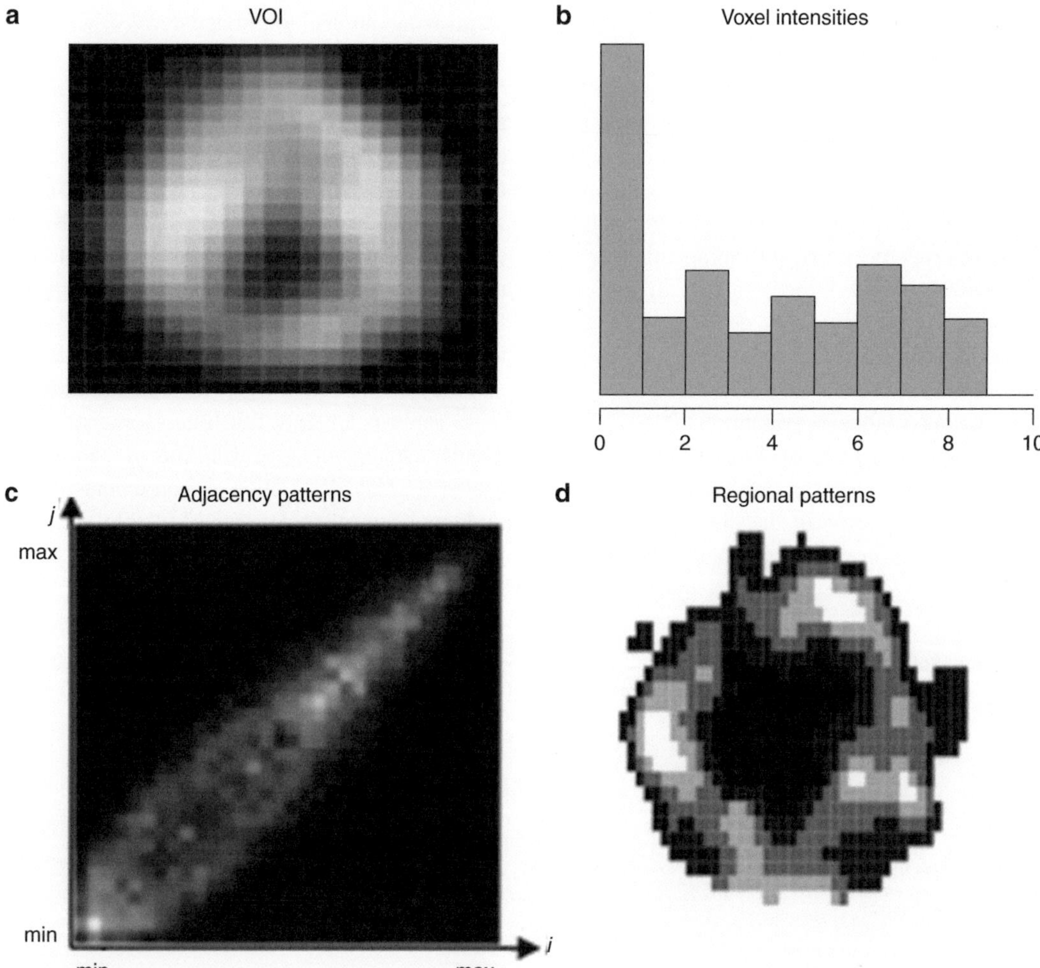

Fig. 6.3 Various distribution summaries of the voxel intensity levels found in a soft-tissue sarcoma volume of interest, of which a transverse slice is shown in (**a**) first-order probabilities of intensity levels (**b**); second-order probabilities of co-occurrences of gray level intensity pairs (i,j) (dark and bright points on this matrix, respectively, indicate low and high probabilities of finding voxels of intensities i and j next to each other within the volume of interest) (**c**); regional patterns in gray level intensities (**d**), obtained following image requantization into a set number of gray level bins (typically into 32 or 64 gray levels). Note this requantization is also used before computing second-order texture features (**c**), and for some of the first-order intensity features (**b**)

A very informative tumor profile can be derived from clinical assessment and patient imaging that includes clinical biomarkers, radiological markers, and other potential risk factors. Radiomics analyses rely on algorithms that have the ability to discover patterns and relationships among this wealth of clinical variables. These pattern-finding techniques belong to a sub-branch of AI called "machine learning" (ML), which greatly overlaps with the statistical learning theory framework—in fact, many data scientists and other analysts who are not involved or interested in AI use ML techniques on a routine basis. These are used to automatically build mathematical (e.g., prognostic or diagnostic) models from sample data, can be used to process very large amounts of information, and require only very mild assumptions and prior knowledge of the data. Various ML techniques can be considered, the most popular of which are named random forests, support vector machines, and artificial neural networks (ANN). The latter attempt to mimic a human brain, and allow for nonlinear interactions between variables, provides an opportunity for deeper exploration of existing patterns in the data. As a result ANN have yielded their own paradigm, termed "deep learning," within the ML framework.

The overall objective of a typical radiomics analytical pipeline is to create, from a dataset of measurable clinical information, a model that will allow predicting a target variable for future patients (patient outcome, disease type, etc., depending on the objective). For tumor characterization this target variable or label could be, e.g., tumor subtype, stage, grade, or biopsy-assessed biologic heterogeneity. For a prognostic model, the goal is usually a clinical endpoint, patient outcome at last follow-up, or duration of patient survival until last follow-up [2, 14, 22, 41].

The following key methodological aspects involved in radiomics analyses are driven by statistical considerations:

(i) Preliminary feature elimination is usually performed in order to "sieve through" the hundreds of input variables, or features, to eliminate redundant information and reduce the size of the dataset to be analyzed. This step is taken to increase pertinence and performance potential of the predictive model being built. It may be performed using a number of statistical techniques such as correlation analysis, multivariate factor analysis, or using an iterative elimination process [42–44].

(ii) Then the predictive model is "trained" on, or fit to the data, so that it learns to use the features together to characterize the target variable. This phase is usually a form of supervised learning, which means that the set of clinical and radiological features is explored retrospectively against the observed value of the target variable for previous clinical patients. It is critical that some form of statistical methodology such as cross-validation is used at this stage in order to avoid model overfitting, a case where the model would describe the known data too well but perform more poorly on independent data [42, 43].

(iii) Ideally, predictive performance of the trained model should be evaluated on independent data, to avoid any statistical bias in this assessment [44]. If this were not the case, predictive assessment of the trained model would likely be overinflated, since the latter would be used to predict values that it has already somehow "seen" during the training process. Because of the requirement to use a sound statistical validation framework, it may be unfeasible to use an independent validation sample when the clinical dataset available for analysis is relatively small (e.g., less than, say, 100 patients). In that case, significant predictive performance may still be indicative of clinical potential but should be validated with follow-on studies on larger sample sizes.

(iv) Final choice of an appropriate predictive model (e.g., a random forest, neural network, etc.) may be made via benchmarking but could also take practical aspects such as clinical interpretation into account. Conventional statistical models used extensively in medical and clinical studies, such

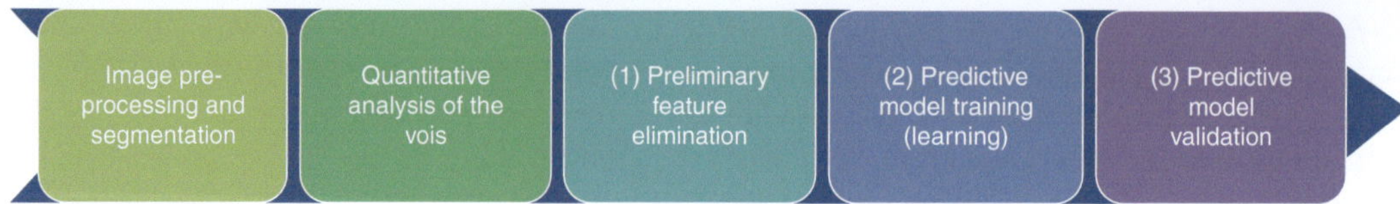

Fig. 6.4 Overall analysis pipeline for the construction of a predictive model from retrospective clinical data

as logistic or Cox proportional hazards models, could also be considered for such applications against more elaborate machine learning techniques, if they were obtained via sound statistical training as described above. Alternatives such as random forests or neural networks are however more appropriate when the data comprises of more variables than patients.

Figure 6.4 illustrates the arrangement of the first three aspects in a typical analytical pipeline. Phases (i)–(iii) of this process can be replicated for different models, and the best model may be selected on the basis of performance indicators that are adequate to the desired application.

Radiomics in Melanoma Imaging

The literature describes uses of radiomics for melanoma mainly for screening and to a smaller extent for classification or prognostic models. The majority of reports explore the use of AI in melanoma characterization from either dermoscopic images or digital photographs [45–49]. Study results were reported over 20 years ago [50]. A consensus is forming that AI methodologies applied to dermoscopic imaging can improve skin screening performance for melanoma.

Although PET/CT has become routine practice for staging and management of malignant melanoma, radiomics analyses of PET imaging data in melanoma have yet to be reported. Some studies have only recently considered radiomics for immunotherapy response assessment in melanoma, using CT data [51]. Currently, radiomic characterization in melanoma primarily targets the prognostic drivers in advanced forms of melanoma. As a result, recent works focused on the

analyses of metastases as opposed to the primary tumor, often using CT or MR imaging data, focusing in particular on regional lymph nodes and brain metastases [52, 53].

Radiomics in Sarcoma Imaging

Only a few studies on radiomics in human sarcoma have been reported to date. Vallières et al. [54] used radiomics to improve prediction of lung metastasis in soft-tissue sarcoma (STS) of the extremities based on joint FDG-PET and MR imaging data. MRI data were also used by Corino et al. [55] for grading of STS tumors. Survival prediction based on a radiomics analysis of baseline CT imaging of high-grade osteosarcoma was also considered by Wu et al. [56]. The only report to date of a radiomics analysis for sarcoma using exclusively FDG-PET data was contributed by Wolsztynski et al. [6], where various ML models were considered for overall survival prediction. The authors demonstrated that prognostic models could be found that yielded effective risk prediction by combining routine clinical information, tumor spatial uptake heterogeneity characterization, and radiomic features.

These scarce explorative works on relatively small clinical cohorts need to be replicated and validated at larger scales. They however have the merit to illustrate the potential of radiomics and machine learning-based methodologies for various aspects of human sarcoma risk characterization, improving upon traditional clinical risk assessment practices. They also highlight how clinical interpretation of radiomic models is more challenging than that of tumor characterization methodologies based on clinical experience. Some recent works [6] indicate that structural modeling of the PET tracer uptake distribution within sarcoma tumors allows capturing some aspects of the PET imaging data that are not exploited by traditional radiomic analyses. Extending the spectrum of features to include these clinically relevant metrics should improve both our clinical understanding of radiomic variables and our interpretation of multivariate predictive models formed on their basis.

Limitations and Future Opportunities

Fully operative AI solutions in radiology are currently not ready for routine implementation. Current research and development efforts mainly make use of elaborate analytical methods such as ML to explore novel risk variables and pseudo-biomarkers and advance academic and clinical understanding of the vastly unexploited potential information contained in radiological imaging data. These efforts however aim at the long-term objective of integrating AI within routine practice.

Limitations of Machine Learning Methodologies in Radiology

Among the main limitations and current challenges faced by AI developers, we can list the following aspects:

- Need for upskilling: AI has matured over decades to yield a broad range of concepts and methodologies. This may put the onus on radiologists to grasp a new paradigm. Data scientists should provide support and expertise, but ideally modern radiologists should acquire a working knowledge of this particular field and what the application to radiology requires.
- Reliance: The assistance provided by AI may result in reduced vigilance and undue trust or reliance on this convenience [29].
- Interpretability: Radiomic tumor analyses usually offer limited clinical interpretability, mainly because of the involvement of textural features that do not have a direct biological or structural meaning. In the same spirit, AI-derived decision-making processes are usually not easily translatable into clinically relevant reasoning. This is without doubt one of the major challenges facing clinical implementation of comprehensive AI decision-making solutions.

- Unbalanced performance: By construction, classification methods operate a trade-off between sensitivity (yielding very few false negatives) and specificity (yielding very few false-positive results). Current AI-based technologies for computer-aided detection (CAD) or automatic tumor segmentation tend to perform well in one of these aspects, to the detriment of the other [46]. Clinical performance is also biased toward particular medical conditions, since by construction a machine learning algorithm is usually only trained effectively to detect or classify one specific characteristic.
- Additional burden: Despite the aim to use AI screening and diagnostic solutions as a second expert opinion to the radiologist's reading of the imaging data, output from current technologies must be cross-examined by the expert, which generates additional workload. Similarly, radiomics analyses for tumor characterization require expert interpretation and clinical confirmation.
- Liability and regulation: Future clinical environments will need to clarify the distribution of legal responsibilities among radiologists, manufacturers, and other AI-related skills providers when AI technologies are involved in medical errors [7]. These technologies will also require approval and regulation by relevant bodies, such as the Food and Drug Administration for the USA, for example.

Opportunities Offered by AI

Despite its inherent challenges, AI provides notable opportunities in all areas of cancer care, including through the following pivotal radiology-based aspects:

- More effective early detection: research has already demonstrated that AI can benefit early detection of cancer from radiological data, which would in turn improve survival rates [57].

- More effective baseline prognostic models, incorporating more insightful tumor descriptors, can enhance characterization and prognostic accuracy [2, 6].
- Patient-adaptive therapy can be facilitated by enabling individualized assessment of therapeutic effectiveness [2].
- Cumbersome workloads and fatigue pertaining to repetitive routine tasks for radiologists can be alleviated by reducing reading times with computer-guided imaging data evaluation [7].

Efforts in the foreseeable future will improve our understanding of the precise nature and magnitude of these opportunities. We already know that different imaging modalities offer different capabilities, and these vary with the disease. For instance, MRI is more sensitive than CT imaging in the diagnosis of non-small cell lung cancer [58]. This is not different for AI methodologies, since they depend on and build upon the nature of the imaging data, and their potential mainly consists in enhancing this information.

The need for a multidisciplinary approach to treating most types of cancers is now universally recognized. Methodological changes in this direction naturally entail the need to exploit and recombine larger volumes of data. This will soon bring traditional statistical models to face their intrinsic limitations, and machine learning will become the only feasible methodological approach for clinical model building in many contexts. Embedding ML techniques is a computationally demanding and conceptually involved task, requiring adequate technological support and extended data manipulation. Meeting these performance requirements with reliable and scalable processes will allow more effective clinical trials support and design of more real-time utilization of radiological information in routine clinical settings. Such technical improvements may be achieved by combining many AI processes into a single treatment unit ("artificial swarm intelligence").

In any case, neither short- nor long-term AI-based innovations in radiology are likely to exclude the expert radiologist. Despite the hype surrounding the recent emergence of high throughput analytical methodologies for various aspects of cancer care (diagnosis, characterization, prognosis, and therapeutic follow-up), intelligent software that can automatically choose or adapt a sarcoma patient's treatment pathway based on their available medical record without any expert (radiologist, oncologist) input is not to be expected in the near future. The most imminent impact of AI in radiology will likely happen with its integration within modern radiological data management systems (such as PACS—picture archiving and communications systems) [29].

In melanoma and sarcoma more specifically, we may expect different directions of development of technological solutions. Based on the current state of the art, AI may more naturally emerge for melanoma with the opportunity to exploit non-radiological imaging data. As for sarcoma, therapeutic processes relying on AI solutions should not be different in nature to those developed for the characterization of more prevalent solid tumors, such as breast or non-small cell lung cancers. As such, methodological progress achieved for these diseases should be directly transferable to sarcoma care. Sarcomas however have image characteristics that may be relevant to the context of modern high throughput analytics. They often present as advanced tumors at time of diagnosis, and there is a larger proportion of tumors with relatively large sizes as a result of this fact, relative to other cancers. Other sarcoma specifics include the fact that the nature of surgical intervention (resection vs amputation) differs drastically with respect to location of the disease and the broad range of subtypes of this disease in contrast to its low prevalence in adults. These tumor specifics will affect and guide future design of intelligent processes for therapeutic decision-making in sarcoma.

Conclusion and Current Perspectives

Current Clinical Practice

Routine clinical protocols—for sarcoma, melanoma, and many other cancers—use simple statistical summaries of the PET imaging data, such as tumor uptake volume and the average or maximum PET uptake value within the tumor VOI. These measures allow for direct image interpretation, and their prognostic potential has been well established. Such summaries however underexploit the wealth of information contained within a PET image dataset, and recent methodological developments indicate that complex tumor biological aspects can be captured noninvasively using more elaborate quantitation techniques. One key target indicator is intratumoral imaging agent spatial uptake heterogeneity (intertumoral heterogeneity is another key marker in stage IV melanoma). Many techniques are currently evaluated by the research community to capture this information, with growing evidence of their effectiveness. Quantitation methodologies relying on modern statistical frameworks can complement routine clinical assessment and provide opportunities for personalized therapy. These advances have prompted the use of machine learning algorithms toward more effective diagnostic and risk predictive models, resulting in the emergence of a whole new area of image analysis in radiology that includes radiomics. On the methodological horizon, these developments pave the way for the integration of complete artificial intelligence solutions within clinical practice.

Limitations and Need for Standardization

These advances globally remain to be validated for larger clinical cohorts and in multicenter studies. Efforts are also required for improved clinical understanding of complex prognostic models derived from radiomics, before these methodologies can be implemented in routine settings. A single reference subset of baseline radiomic variables for cancer prognosis does not yet exist for any cancer; different multivariate prognostic models are proposed with each new study. In fact, technical variations of various image processing parameters can greatly impact some of these complementary predictive variables. Recent efforts in the community, such as the Image Biomarker Standardisation Initiative [3], clearly indicate the need for homogenization and standardization of quantitative practice, a significant challenge yet to be overcome, as the results of many studies indicate (see, for instance, multicenter studies of the American College of Radiology Imaging Network [4, 5]). Reaching colloquial agreement on future predictive models will also be guided by progress in our understanding of how PET-based tumor quantitation maps to phenotypic or genomic signatures.

Multimodality Data

The prevalence of multimodality (PET/MR and PET/CT) scanners has led to a surge in studies combining co-registered (i.e., re-aligned) image signals. For tumor delineation, a VOI mask defined from MR or CT information is often used to guide segmentation of the PET VOI. But tumor characterization can further benefit from combined imaging modality output, in order to align functional information on tumor biological features with the anatomical and physiological nature (bone, soft tissue, etc.) of corresponding areas within the VOI [59–61]. MT or CT information can complement assessment of PET spatial uptake heterogeneity and perhaps guide further understanding or interpretation of biologic descriptors derived from the PET image. A few analyses have been reported that explore various aspects of tumor assessment for sarcoma by analysis of recombined features [54, 62] and none for melanoma.

For multimodal imaging, two options are available. One is to associate scans acquired via several modalities, either by image co-registration or multimodality (e.g., PET/CT–MRI) scanners; these allow for true CT-based attenuation correction and reliably calibrated imaging data but may require higher radiation doses and longer acquisition times [59, 60]. The other option is to carry out separate scans and recombine extracted features postacquisition, during the analytical phase, albeit using image features that may not originate from identical VOIs [54]. How to best combine these technologies and translate them to clinical practice remains an open and challenging question, at both the operational and analytical levels. Multimodality imaging also allows integrating emerging PET technologies, such as activatable targeted nanoparticle probes, to create novel forms of imaging data, and requires the definition of adapted modeling strategies [59–61].

One practical motivation for analyses using two or more tomographs arises from patient assessment involving PET/MR and PET/CT devices (e.g., to optimize resources when both PET/MR and PET/CT scans are available on-site, or if several care centers are involved). In these contexts, direct comparison of the PET images is not guaranteed, as different calibration settings (dose, contrast, resolution, etc.) are likely and would require dedicated pre-processing to correct for statistical discrepancies in image characteristics. Homogeneous scanner characteristics would however allow for both PET images to be used for comparative analyses.

Kinetic Analysis

The methodologies described above only use static image information. They are limited in capturing other aspects of the tumor biology. For example, they do not provide insight on imaging agent vascular delivery and tissue retention, which may be important for disease assessment and treatment. Dynamic (or kinetic) analysis of the information contained in each time frame after injection of the PET radiotracer, and throughout the entire acquisition duration, allows for evaluation of key imaging parameters such as blood flow and tissue retention characteristics. Recent advances in kinetic analysis also suggest that tumor imaging agent spatial uptake heterogeneity may also be evaluated in dynamic PET information [63, 64]. Dynamic imaging data analysis also provides more informed tissue characterization and tumor delineation with reduced bias (compared to static summed PET or anatomical imaging data), which can benefit quantitation [64]. Kinetic analysis for PET dynamic image acquisition protocols remains mainly conducted

in research settings, in part due to its more challenging practical requirements.

References

1. Joo Hyun O, Lodge MA, Wahl RL. Practical PERCIST: a simplified guide to PET response criteria in solid tumors 1.0. Radiology. 2016;280(2):576–84.
2. Gillies RJ, Kinahan PE, Hricak H. Radiomics: images are more than pictures, they are data. Radiology. 2016;278(2):563–77.
3. Zwanenburg A, Abdalah MA, Apte A, Ashrafinia S, Beukinga J, Bogowicz M, et al. Results from the image biomarker standardisation initiative. Radiother Oncol. 2018;127:S543–S4.
4. Gerstner ER, Zhang Z, Fink JR, Muzi M, Hanna L, Greco E, et al. ACRIN 6684: assessment of tumor hypoxia in newly diagnosed Glioblastoma Using 18F-FMISO PET and MRI. Clin Cancer Res. 2016;22(20):5079–86.
5. Ratai EM, Zhang Z, Fink J, Muzi M, Hanna L, Greco E, et al. ACRIN 6684: multicenter, phase II assessment of tumor hypoxia in newly diagnosed glioblastoma using magnetic resonance spectroscopy. PLoS One. 2018;13(6):e0198548.
6. Wolsztynski E, O'Sullivan F, Keyes E, O'Sullivan J, Eary JF. Positron emission tomography-based assessment of metabolic gradient and other prognostic features in sarcoma. J Med Imaging (Bellingham). 2018;5(2):024502.
7. Russell SJ, Norvig P. Artificial intelligence: a modern approach. 3rd ed. Prentice Hall: Upper Saddle River; 2010.
8. Rodriguez-Ruiz A, Krupinski E, Mordang JJ, Schilling K, Heywang-Kobrunner SH, Sechopoulos I, et al. Detection of breast Cancer with mammography: effect of an artificial intelligence support system. Radiology. 2019;290(2):305–14.
9. Al-Nabhani KZ, Syed R, Michopoulou S, Alkalbani J, Afaq A, Panagiotidis E, et al. Qualitative and quantitative comparison of PET/CT and PET/MR imaging in clinical practice. J Nucl Med. 2014;55(1):88–94.
10. Moses WW. Fundamental Limits of Spatial Resolution in PET. Nucl Instrum Methods Phys Res A. 2011;648(Supplement 1):S236–S40.
11. Mou T, Huang J, O'Sullivan F. The gamma characteristic of reconstructed PET images: implications for ROI analysis. IEEE Trans Med Imaging. 2018;37(5):1092–102.
12. Soret M, Bacharach SL, Buvat I. Partial-volume effect in PET tumor imaging. J Nucl Med. 2007;48(6):932–45.
13. Hatt M, Majdoub M, Vallieres M, Tixier F, Le Rest CC, Groheux D, et al. 18F-FDG PET uptake characterization through texture analysis: investigating the complementary nature of heterogeneity and func-

tional tumor volume in a multi-cancer site patient cohort. J Nucl Med. 2015;56(1):38–44.

14. Hatt M, Tixier F, Pierce L, Kinahan PE, Le Rest CC, Visvikis D. Characterization of PET/CT images using texture analysis: the past, the present... any future? Eur J Nucl Med Mol Imaging. 2017;44(1):151–65.

15. Yan J, Lim JC, Townsend DW. MRI-guided brain PET image filtering and partial volume correction. Phys Med Biol. 2015;60(3):961–76.

16. Kratochwil C, Flechsig P, Lindner T, Abderrahim L, Altmann A, Mier W, et al. (68)Ga-FAPI PET/CT: tracer uptake in 28 different kinds of cancer. J Nucl Med. 2019;60(6):801–5.

17. Hasebe M, Yoshikawa K, Nishii R, Kawaguchi K, Kamada T, Hamada Y. Usefulness of (11) C-methionine-PET for predicting the efficacy of carbon ion radiation therapy for head and neck mucosal malignant melanoma. Int J Oral Maxillofac Surg. 2017;46(10):1220–8.

18. Bedard PL, Hansen AR, Ratain MJ, Siu LL. Tumour heterogeneity in the clinic. Nature. 2013;501(7467):355–64.

19. Eary JF, Conrad EU, O'Sullivan J, Hawkins DS, Schuetze SM, O'Sullivan F. Sarcoma mid-therapy [F-18]fluorodeoxyglucose positron emission tomography (FDG PET) and patient outcome. J Bone Joint Surg Am. 2014;96(2):152–8.

20. Grzywa TM, Paskal W, Wlodarski PK. Intratumor and intertumor heterogeneity in melanoma. Transl Oncol. 2017;10(6):956–75.

21. Davnall F, Yip CS, Ljungqvist G, Selmi M, Ng F, Sanghera B, et al. Assessment of tumor heterogeneity: an emerging imaging tool for clinical practice? Insights Imaging. 2012;3(6):573–89.

22. Buvat I, Orlhac F, Soussan M. Tumor texture analysis in PET: where do we stand? J Nucl Med. 2015;56(11):1642–4.

23. Soussan M, Orlhac F, Boubaya M, Zelek L, Ziol M, Eder V, et al. Relationship between tumor heterogeneity measured on FDG-PET/CT and pathological prognostic factors in invasive breast cancer. PLoS One. 2014;9(4):e94017.

24. O'Sullivan F, Wolsztynski E, O'Sullivan J, Richards T, Conrad EU, Eary JF. A statistical modeling approach to the analysis of spatial patterns of FDG-PET uptake in human sarcoma. IEEE Trans Med Imaging. 2011;30(12):2059–71.

25. Yancovitz M, Finelt N, Warycha MA, Christos PJ, Mazumdar M, Shapiro RL, et al. Role of radiologic imaging at the time of initial diagnosis of stage T1b-T3b melanoma. Cancer. 2007;110(5):1107–14.

26. Rajkumar S, Watson IR. Molecular characterisation of cutaneous melanoma: creating a framework for targeted and immune therapies. Br J Cancer. 2016;115(2):145–55.

27. Carlino MS, Saunders CA, Haydu LE, Menzies AM, Martin Curtis C Jr, Lebowitz PF, et al. (18)F-labelled fluorodeoxyglucose-positron emission tomography (FDG-PET) heterogeneity of response is prognostic in dabrafenib treated BRAF mutant metastatic melanoma. Eur J Cancer. 2013;49(2):395–402.

28. Mena E, Sanli Y, Marcus C, Subramaniam RM. Precision medicine and PET/computed tomography in melanoma. PET Clin. 2017;12(4):449–58.

29. Fazal MI, Patel ME, Tye J, Gupta Y. The past, present and future role of artificial intelligence in imaging. Eur J Radiol. 2018;105:246–50.

30. Zhang Z, Chen P, McGough M, Xing F, Wang C, Bui M, et al. Pathologist-level interpretable whole-slide cancer diagnosis with deep learning. Nat Mach Intell. 2019;1(5):236–45.

31. Jiang F, Jiang Y, Zhi H, Dong Y, Li H, Ma S, et al. Artificial intelligence in healthcare: past, present and future. Stroke Vasc Neurol. 2017;2(4):230–43.

32. Kahn CE Jr. Artificial intelligence in radiology: decision support systems. Radiographics. 1994;14(4):849–61.

33. Rodriguez-Ruiz A, Lang K, Gubern-Merida A, Broeders M, Gennaro G, Clauser P, et al. Stand-alone artificial intelligence for breast cancer detection in mammography: comparison with 101 radiologists. J Natl Cancer Inst. 2019;111(9):916–22.

34. Christ PF, Elshaer MEA, Ettlinger F, Tatavarty S, Bickel M, Bilic P, et al. Automatic liver and lesion segmentation in CT using cascaded fully convolutional neural networks and 3D conditional random fields. arXiv e-prints [Internet]. October 1, 2016. Available from: https://ui.adsabs.harvard.edu/abs/2016arXiv161002177C.

35. Havaei M, Davy A, Warde-Farley D, Biard A, Courville A, Bengio Y, et al. Brain tumor segmentation with deep neural networks. Med Image Anal. 2017;35:18–31.

36. Savadjiev P, Chong J, Dohan A, Agnus V, Forghani R, Reinhold C, et al. Image-based biomarkers for solid tumor quantification. Eur Radiol. 2019;29(10):5431–40.

37. Berthon B, Evans M, Marshall C, Palaniappan N, Cole N, Jayaprakasam V, et al. Head and neck target delineation using a novel PET automatic segmentation algorithm. Radiother Oncol. 2017;122(2):242–7.

38. Bakas S, Reyes M, Jakab A, Bauer S, Rempfler M, Crimi A, et al. Identifying the best machine learning algorithms for brain tumor segmentation, progression assessment, and overall survival prediction in the BRATS challenge. arXiv e-prints [Internet]. November 1, 2018. Available from: https://ui.adsabs.harvard.edu/abs/2018arXiv181102629B.

39. Pirotte B, Goldman S, Massager N, David P, Wikler D, Vandesteene A, et al. Comparison of 18F-FDG and 11C-methionine for PET-guided stereotactic brain biopsy of gliomas. J Nucl Med. 2004;45(8):1293–8.

40. Schwartz LH, Litiere S, de Vries E, Ford R, Gwyther S, Mandrekar S, et al. RECIST 1.1-update and clarification: from the RECIST committee. Eur J Cancer. 2016;62:132–7.

41. Lambin P, Rios-Velazquez E, Leijenaar R, Carvalho S, van Stiphout RG, Granton P, et al. Radiomics:

extracting more information from medical images using advanced feature analysis. Eur J Cancer. 2012;48(4):441–6.

42. Guyon I, Elisseeff A. An introduction to variable and feature selection. J Mach Learn Res. 2003;3(7–8):1157–82.

43. Ambroise C, McLachlan GJ. Selection bias in gene extraction on the basis of microarray gene-expression data. Proc Natl Acad Sci U S A. 2002;99(10):6562–6.

44. Hastie T, Tibshirani R, Friedman JH. The elements of statistical learning: data mining, inference, and prediction. 2nd ed. New York: Springer; 2009. xxii, 745 p.

45. Magalhaes C, Mendes J, Vardasca R. The role of AI classifiers in skin cancer images. Skin Res Technol. 2019;25(5):750–7.

46. Hosny A, Parmar C, Quackenbush J, Schwartz LH, Aerts H. Artificial intelligence in radiology. Nat Rev Cancer. 2018;18(8):500–10.

47. Bhattacharya A, Young A, Wong A, Stalling S, Wei M, Hadley D. Precision diagnosis of melanoma and other skin lesions from digital images. AMIA Jt Summits Transl Sci Proc. 2017;2017:220–6.

48. Esteva A, Kuprel B, Novoa RA, Ko J, Swetter SM, Blau HM, et al. Corrigendum: dermatologist-level classification of skin cancer with deep neural networks. Nature. 2017;546(7660):686.

49. Gareau DS, Correa da Rosa J, Yagerman S, Carucci JA, Gulati N, Hueto F, et al. Digital imaging biomarkers feed machine learning for melanoma screening. Exp Dermatol. 2017;26(7):615–8.

50. Dreiseitl S, Ohno-Machado L, Kittler H, Vinterbo S, Billhardt H, Binder M. A comparison of machine learning methods for the diagnosis of pigmented skin lesions. J Biomed Inform. 2001;34(1):28–36.

51. Sun R, Limkin EJ, Vakalopoulou M, Dercle L, Champiat S, Han SR, et al. A radiomics approach to assess tumour-infiltrating CD8 cells and response to anti-PD-1 or anti-PD-L1 immunotherapy: an imaging biomarker, retrospective multicohort study. Lancet Oncol. 2018;19(9):1180–91.

52. Giesel FL, Schneider F, Kratochwil C, Rath D, Moltz J, Holland-Letz T, et al. Correlation between SUVmax and CT radiomic analysis using lymph node density in PET/CT-based lymph node staging. J Nucl Med. 2017;58(2):282–7.

53. Kniep HC, Madesta F, Schneider T, Hanning U, Schonfeld MH, Schon G, et al. Radiomics of brain MRI: utility in prediction of metastatic tumor type. Radiology. 2019;290(2):479–87.

54. Vallieres M, Freeman CR, Skamene SR, El Naqa I. A radiomics model from joint FDG-PET and MRI texture features for the prediction of lung metastases in soft-tissue sarcomas of the extremities. Phys Med Biol. 2015;60(14):5471–96.

55. Corino VDA, Montin E, Messina A, Casali PG, Gronchi A, Marchiano A, et al. Radiomic analysis of soft tissues sarcomas can distinguish intermediate from high-grade lesions. J Magn Reson Imaging. 2018;47(3):829–40.

56. Wu Y, Xu L, Yang P, Lin N, Huang X, Pan W, et al. Survival prediction in high-grade osteosarcoma using radiomics of diagnostic computed tomography. EBioMedicine. 2018;34:27–34.

57. Ardila D, Kiraly AP, Bharadwaj S, Choi B, Reicher JJ, Peng L, et al. Author correction: end-to-end lung cancer screening with three-dimensional deep learning on low-dose chest computed tomography. Nat Med. 2019;25(8):1319.

58. Planchard D, Popat S, Kerr K, Novello S, Smit EF, Faivre-Finn C, et al. Metastatic non-small cell lung cancer: ESMO Clinical Practice Guidelines for diagnosis, treatment and follow-up. Ann Oncol. 2018;29(Supplement_4):iv192–237.

59. Chetty IJ, Martel MK, Jaffray DA, Benedict SH, Hahn SM, Berbeco R, et al. Technology for innovation in radiation oncology. Int J Radiat Oncol Biol Phys. 2015;93(3):485–92.

60. Veit-Haibach P, Kuhn FP, Wiesinger F, Delso G, von Schulthess G. PET–MR imaging using a tri-modality PET/CT–MR system with a dedicated shuttle in clinical routine. MAGMA. 2013;26(1):25–35.

61. Kircher MF, Hricak H, Larson SM. Molecular imaging for personalized cancer care. Mol Oncol. 2012;6(2):182–95.

62. Vallieres M, Zwanenburg A, Badic B, Cheze Le Rest C, Visvikis D, Hatt M. Responsible radiomics research for faster clinical translation. J Nucl Med. 2018;59(2):189–93.

63. Asselin M-C, O'Connor JPB, Boellaard R, Thacker NA, Jackson A. Quantifying heterogeneity in human tumours using MRI and PET. Eur J Cancer. 2012;48(4):447–55.

64. Muzi M, O'Sullivan F, Mankoff DA, Doot RK, Pierce LA, Kurland BF, et al. Quantitative assessment of dynamic PET imaging data in cancer imaging. Magn Reson Imaging. 2012;30(9):1203–15.

Ea-sle Chang, Eddy C. Hsueh, and David W. Ollila

Introduction

Surgeons have long been dependent upon radiologic imaging for staging cancer patients, for surgical planning to determine resectability of a malignancy and for surveillance of cancer survivors after their cancer treatment has been completed. Various radiologic imaging modalities have been used, but none took advantage of the functional aspect of malignant cells which have high metabolic needs for lipids, amino acids, and especially glucose. Thus, a glucose analog, 18F-fluorodeoxyglucose [FDG] used in positron emission tomography (PET), can detect glucose-avid neoplasms [1] (Fig. 7.1). Combined with anatomic imaging, computed tomography (CT), utilizing FDG PET/CT for staging, treatment decision-making, and surveillance, is well-established for neoplasms with "high" metabolic rate such as lymphoma, breast, head/neck, colorectal, and lung cancers [2]. This chapter will provide a surgical perspective of the combined functional imaging and cross-sectional imaging, FDG PET/CT, in melanoma patients.

Basic Understanding of FDG PET/CT

The use of PET scan in metastatic melanoma patients has increased dramatically from 4.2% in 2000 to 12.1% in 2007 [3]. As with any diagnostic test, the information gained from FDG PET/CT needs to be considered in conjunction with clinical information to make informed decisions in the management of patients with melanoma. As detailed in previous chapters, nonspecific uptake of FDG can occur in areas with inflamed tissues during infection or inflammation. Bacterial and fungal infections increase the likelihood of false-positive findings, more so than in parasitic or viral infections. Nonspecific uptake of FDG can also occur in certain types of normal tissue such as reactive lymphoid tissue or brown adipose tissue [4] (Fig. 7.2). Clinical interventions such as radiation or surgery can cause inflammatory changes that may increase background FDG uptake and diminish the sensitivity of tumors detection. Conversely, chemotherapy has been shown to increase the false-negative findings on PET, due to its cytotoxic and cytostatic effect on tumor cells [5]. Furthermore, PET has a limited ability to detect for lesions ≤ 5 mm [6].

E.-s. Chang · E. C. Hsueh
Department of Surgery, St. Louis University,
St. Louis, MO, USA
e-mail: iris.chang@health.slu.edu;
eddy.hsueh@health.slu.edu

D. W. Ollila (✉)
Department of Surgery, Division of Surgical
Oncology, University of North Carolina at Chapel
Hill, Chapel Hill, NC, USA
e-mail: david_ollila@med.unc.edu

© Springer Nature Switzerland AG 2021
A. H. Khandani (ed.), *PET/CT and PET/MR in Melanoma and Sarcoma*,
https://doi.org/10.1007/978-3-030-60429-5_7

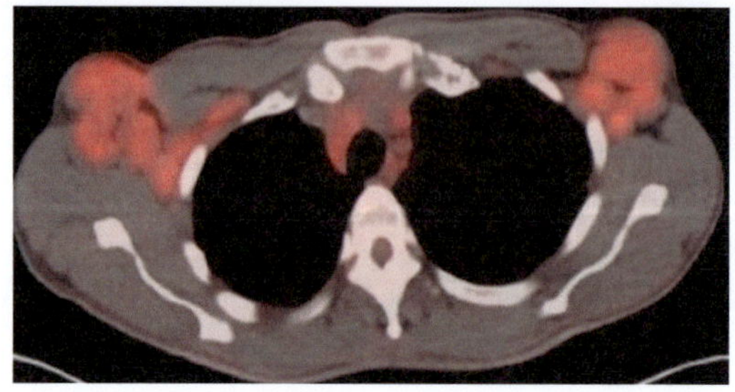
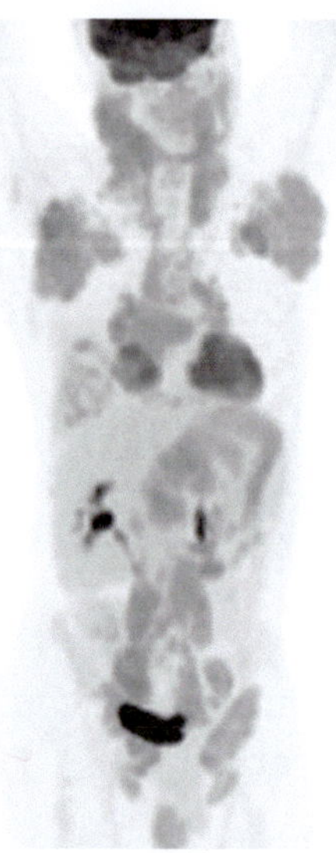

Fig. 7.1 FDG PET/CT demonstrating widely disseminate FDG-avid malignancy

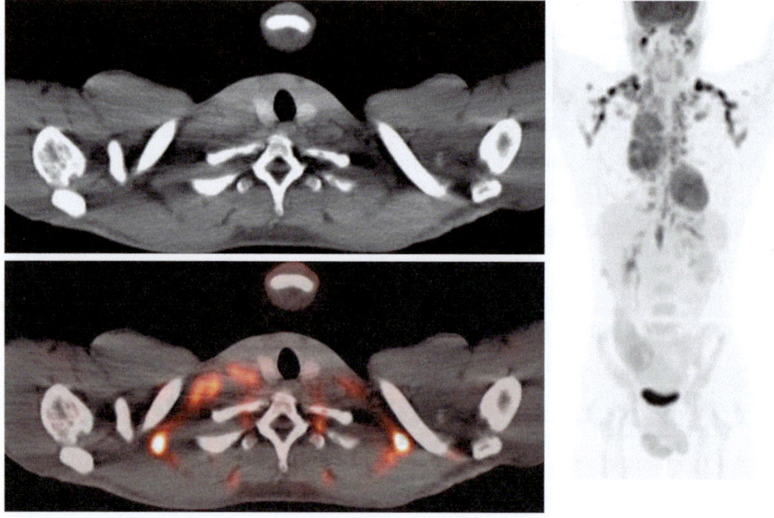

Fig. 7.2 An experienced nuclear medicine physician can easily determine brown adipose tissue, and this does not require a confirmatory biopsy. Right lower neck lymph node. Otherwise, brown fat

Combining anatomic cross-sectional imaging, i.e., CT, with PET was first introduced in 1998 [7]. This has led to more accurate cancer staging preoperatively, improved evaluation of tumors for resectability, and a surveillance strategy with combined metabolic and anatomical characteristics of tumors. Since metabolic changes in a malignancy often occur much earlier than anatomical changes, PET/CT has the advantage of detecting lesions earlier than conventional imaging [8] (Fig. 7.3). When compared with conventional CT imaging, PET/CT offers larger imaging field, superior detection of intramuscular and bone metastases, and ability to identify lesions in previous operated areas [9]. A prospective study by Bastiaannet and colleagues showed sensitivity, specificity, positive predictive value, and negative predictive value, at 86.1%, 93.1%, 85.0%, and 93.6%, respectively, for detecting melanoma metastases with FDG PET/CT [10]. This chapter will focus on the advantages FDG PET/CT has in melanoma staging, metastasectomy, and melanoma survivor surveillance.

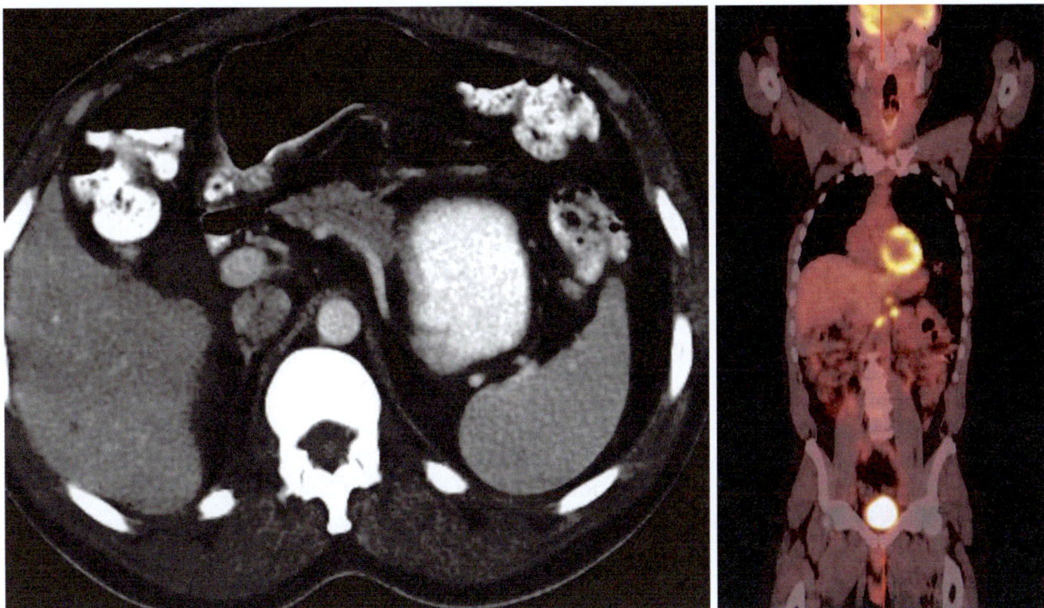

Fig. 7.3 A metastasis which is FDG-avid, but very difficult to identify with just cross-sectional imaging

Table 7.1 Utility of PET and PET/CT in detecting melanoma metastasis

	Stage	N	Modality	Sensitivity	Specificity	Positive PV	Negative PV
Holder et al., 1998 [81]	2–4	76	PET	94.2	83.3	86	93
Rinne et al., 1998 [82]	1–4	100	PET	91.8	94.4		
Eigtved et al., 2000 [83]	2–3	38	PET	97	56	86	83
Tyler et al., 2000 [84]	3	95	PET	87.3	43.5	78.6	58.8
Fuster et al., 2004 [85]	1–4	156	PET	74	86		
Bastiaannet et al., 2006 [60]	1–4	257	PET	84.2	71.3		
Reinhardt et al., 2006	1–4	250	PET/CT	98.8	97.6	95.3	99.4
Iagaru et al., 2007 [86]	1–4	106	PET/CT	89.3	88		
Pfannenberg et al., 2007 [87]	3–4	64	PET/CT	90.6	77.2	90.6	77.2
Peric et al., 2011 [88]	1–4	115	PET/CT	98.5	90.9	98.5	90.9
Aukema et al., 2010 [89]	3	70	PET/CT	87	98	96	91
Gellen et al., 2015 [90]	1–4	97	PET/CT	98	89.7	83.3	98.9
Chandra et al., 2017 [91]	3–4	70	PET/CT	87	100	100	93

FDG PET/CT and Staging Metastatic Melanoma Patients

As with ordering any diagnostic study, the ordering healthcare provider, not just the nuclear medicine physician, needs to know the sensitivities and specificity of the test being ordered. This is very important for the surgeon ordering a FDG PET/CT. The sensitivities and specificities of PET in detecting melanoma range between 74–99% and 43–100%, respectively (Table 7.1).

A meta-analysis by Xing et al. demonstrated that FDG PET/CT has sensitivity of 80% and specificity of 87% for detecting distant metastases, in comparison to 51% and 69%, respectively, for conventional CT [11]. Other studies have also shown that FDG PET/CT has higher sensitivity and accuracy as compared to CT, 85.1% vs. 78.2% and 91% vs. 89%, respectively [10, 12]. In contrast, Bastiaannet et al. noted that a dedicated chest CT was superior in detecting lung metastases with higher sensitivity [13]. For lesions larger than 1 cm, positive predictive value of detecting metastases was 100% [14]. Similarly, Crippa and colleagues analyzed the sensitivity of PET based on the size of the metastatic lesions. Lesions ≥ 10 mm were detected 100%, while 6–10 mm and ≤ 5 mm were detected 83% and 23% of the time, respectively [15]. Furthermore, Damian et al. observed that 15 of the 16 lesions that failed to be detected on PET were smaller than 1 cm [16]. Detection rate further deteriorated in areas with known high background FDG uptake, e.g., brain, heart, kidneys, and bladder. The sensitivity of detecting brain metastasis on PET/CT is low, ranging from 60% to 68% [17]. Therefore, melanoma patients undergoing imaging evaluation with PET/CT should also undergo brain MRI.

There are conflicting studies on the efficacy of PET/CT in staging melanoma patients. The majority of studies have shown that PET/CT can change the stage of disease with 18–22% patients upstaged from M0 to M1 (Table 7.2). This is a critically important staging distinction, espe-cially in the era of efficacious checkpoint inhibi-tors for stage IV metastatic melanoma patients [18–20]. For high-risk melanoma patients, Danielsen and colleagues proposed four qualities that predicted a true-positive PET/CT scan: increased mitotic rate, tumor thickness >4 mm, bleeding, and lymphadenopathy. They demon-strated that patients with 0 to 2 factors had true-positive PET/CT in 5.8% of the time, while having 3 or all 4 factors led to true positive scans in 47.4% and 100%, respectively [21].

Following diagnosis of a melanoma, PET/CT can provide useful information regarding the extent of disease for treatment decision-making. Detection of distant metastases will change the treatment plan for metastatic melanoma patients. Thus, accurate staging is very important for these patients. Schule et al. demonstrated that accurate staging with PET/CT led to major therapy change in 52% of patients, with 20% of patients avoiding unnecessary surgery [22]. This finding was sup-ported by other studies (ranging 6–69%) demon-strating a significant alteration in their treatment

Table 7.2 Change of melanoma management as result of PET and PET/CT

	Stage	N	% upstaged	% change in management	Intermodal change in management[a]	Intramodal change in management[b]
Tyler et al., 2000 [84]	3	95		15%	14/15 (93%)	1/15 (7%)
Stas et al., 2002 [92]	3–4	100		26%	23/26 (88%)	3/26 (12%)
Gulec et al., 2003 [14]	2–4	49		49%	18/24 (75%)	6/24 (25%)
Fuster et al., 2004 [85]	1–4	156		36%		
Harris, et al., 2005 [93]	1–4	126		34%	38/43 (88%)	5/43 (12%)
Bastiaannet et al., 2006 [60]	1–4	257	21.8%	17.1%	40/46 (87%)	6/46 (13%)
Reinhardt et al., 2006 [18, 94]	1–4	250		48.4%	100/121 (83%)	21/121 (17%)
Falk et al., 2007 [95]	1–4	60		27.6%		
Pfannenberg et al., 2007 [87]	3–4	64		64%		
Aukema et al., 2010 [89]	3	70		37%	20/26 (77%)	6/26 (23%)
Etchebehere et al., 2010 [96]	3–4	78	22%	24.4%	17/19 (89%)	2/19 (11%)
Bronstein et al., 2012 [9]	3–4	32		12.5%	3/4 (75%)	1/4 (25%)
Koskivuo et al., 2016 [6]	2–3	110		6.3%		
Singnurkar et al., 2016 [97]	2–4	319	17.6%	28%		
Chandra et al., 2017 [91]	3–4	70	23%	38.6%		
Forschner et al., 2017 [98]	1–4	107		73.8%	55/79 (70%) – From surgery to non-surgical management	24/79 (30%) – Change in surgical approach
Pfannenberg et al., 2019 [99]	1–4	750		46%		

[a]Intermodal change denotes change from surgery, radiation, or systemic therapy to other mode of therapy including no therapy or addition of other mode of therapy
[b]Intramodal change denotes change in planning for intended mode of treatment

plan following PET/CT (Table 7.2). Gulec and colleagues compared PET/CT to conventional CT imaging of the chest, abdomen, and pelvis and MRI of the brain in patients with suspected metastatic melanoma [14]. They noted that PET/CT led to change in management in 49% of the patients, with 24% avoiding surgery and 12% qualifying for surgical resection [14]. PET/CT was able to detect additional lesions in 55% of the study patients with 22% of these lesions not in the field of conventional CT imaging (Fig. 7.4). Studies have demonstrated detection of lesions in the extremities (2.7–6%) that would not be evident on conventional imaging [9, 23].

In contrast, a few other studies have not shown PET/CT to be an accurate staging modality. Frary et al. utilized PET/CT on patients with known positive sentinel node and observed that 13% of patients had false-positive findings subsequently leading to additional imaging studies and/or invasive procedures [24]. Similarly, Scheier and colleagues showed that despite 33% of patients having FDG-avid lesions on PET/CT, only 7% were confirmed as metastasis [25]. Wagner et al. observed 13% of patients having abnormal uptake on imaging, of which none were metastatic [26]. Barsky et al. observed an 85% false-positive rate leading to 44% of patients undergoing additional procedures/tests [27]. Despite these contradictory studies, the overwhelming majority of the current literature demonstrates FDG PET/CT is the most accurate staging test available for metastatic melanoma patients, but it does have drawbacks. To be a more accurate and reliable imaging modality, the sensitivity of FDG PET/CT needs to be increased, and the false-positive rate, which leads to additional procedures/tests, needs to be decreased.

FDG PET/CT and Metastasectomy

While staging is important in metastatic melanoma patients, metastasectomy can actually improve survival [28–31]. While this may not be intuitive for a hematogenous metastasis, there is data to suggest there is an overall survival advantage [32]. Metastasectomy is defined as surgical resection of all radiographic and clinical lesions. Metastatic melanoma patients derive an overall survival benefit from a complete metastasectomy. An incomplete metastasectomy does not improve overall survival and should only be used as a palliative procedure [33]. Prior to advent of FDA-approved immunotherapy [34–36], targeted therapy [37, 38], and oncolytic virus therapy [39, 40], the senior authors (ECH, DWO) would recommend a metastasectomy for oligometastatic disease or a clinical trial for disseminated stage

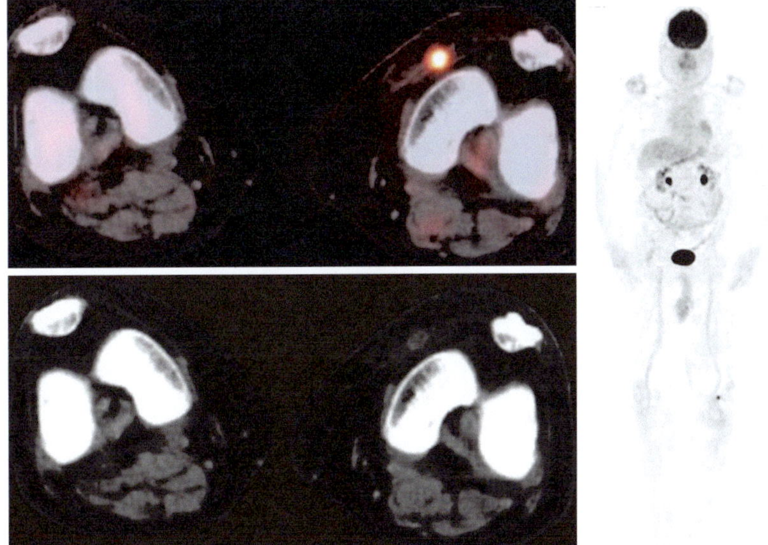

Fig. 7.4 Dedicated imaging of the entire extremity can detect metastatic melanoma not seen on conventional CT scans of the chest, abdomen, and pelvis

IV disease. However, with the introduction of all the new drugs, the 5-year survival for stage IV melanoma patients now ranges from 39% to 52% depending upon the therapy [18–20]. The development of these treatments not only improved overall survival by effectively treating disseminated metastatic melanoma, but it further improved survival by increasing the number of patients who can qualify for a complete metastasectomy once maximal response has been achieved. In other words, for patients who do not achieve a radiologic complete response, the residual disease can still be considered for a complete metastasectomy.

PET/CT can have significant impact in treatment planning for patients undergoing neoadjuvant therapy with immunotherapy, targeted therapy, and oncolytic virus therapy. When utilizing PET/CT for surgical planning, a phenomenon of "pseudoprogression" has to be considered (Fig. 7.5). Immunotherapy augments the host's immune response against cancer cells, which elicit inflammation. The increased inflammatory responses may falsely increase FDG uptake, making it difficult to differentiate between response to therapy or progression of disease with new lesions [41]. Patients with pseudoprogression typically have enlargement of the lesions prior to reduction due to the atypical immune response. When these lesions were biopsied, they were noted to have inflammatory cell infiltration and necrosis, rather than tumor progression [42]. Patients who experience "pseudoprogression" had similar survival rate as those who experienced radiographic regression during treatment. It is crucial that treatment is not discontinued prematurely due to these pseudoprogression radiographic changes.

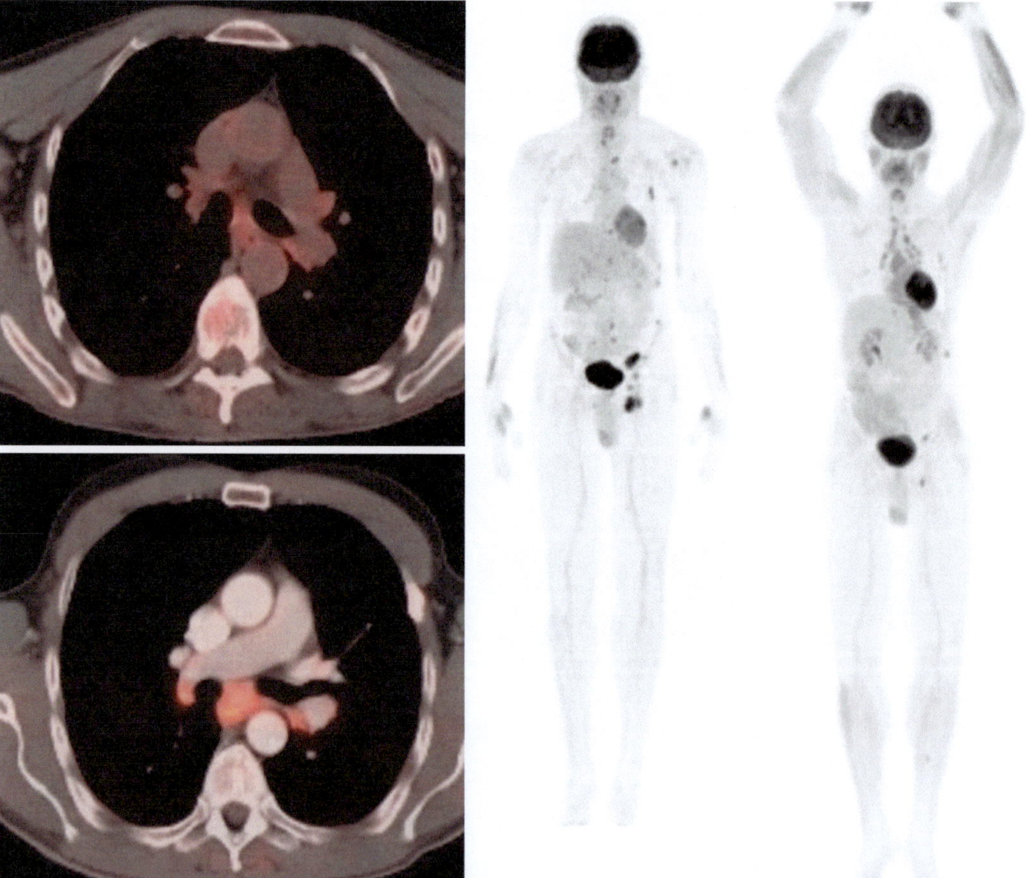

Fig. 7.5 "Pseudoprogression" observed during PD1 inhibitor therapy

Metastatic melanoma patients derive an organic specific survival benefit based upon the anatomic site resected. M1a (metastasis to the skin, soft tissue, and distant nodes) (Fig. 7.6) is the most common anatomic site of stage IV melanoma and comprises approximately 40% of all stage IV melanoma patients. Currently, these patients have a median survival ranging from 10 to 18 months [43], while those who underwent a complete metastasectomy had median survival of 24 months [12, 32, 44–49]. Examining the visceral metastases sites, pulmonary metastases (M1b) (Fig. 7.7) are the most common, comprising approximately 12–36% of patients [43].

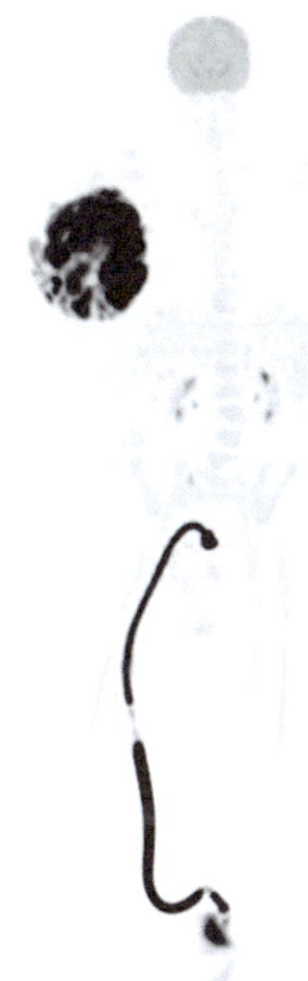

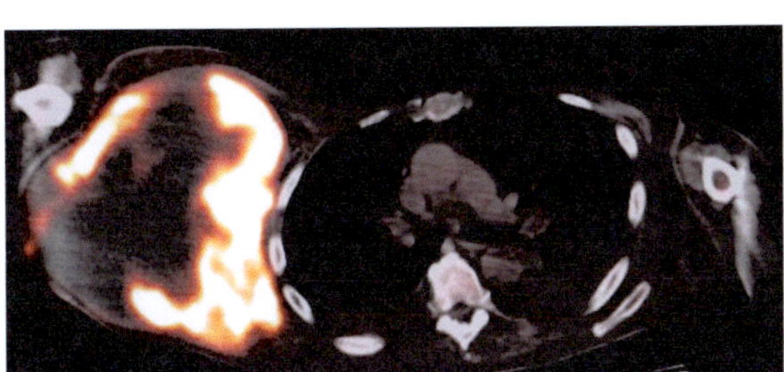

Fig. 7.6 Metastatic melanoma to a distant lymph node

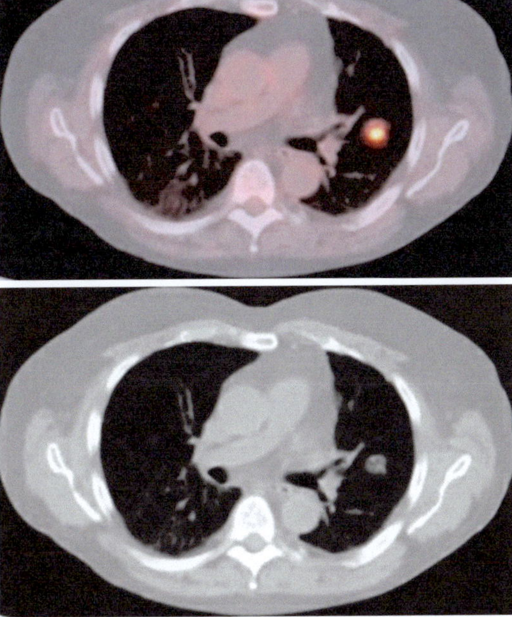

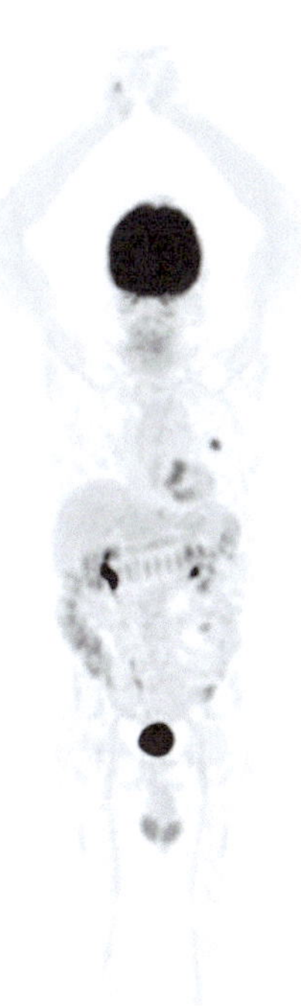

Fig. 7.7 Example of metastatic melanoma to the lung

Bilateral lung involvement and multiple pulmonary nodules are not absolute contraindication for surgical resection. Studies have shown that the 5-year overall survival ranges from 20% to 27% after surgical intervention as opposed to 3% in those deemed surgically unresectable [50, 51]. Despite having only 2–4% of patients having metastasis to the gastrointestinal tract, approximately 50% of patients who die with stage IV disease have gastrointestinal involvement [43, 52]. Median survival following complete metastasectomy of GI metastases (Fig. 7.8) ranged from 15 to 28 months as compared to 5–8 months for those who did not [12, 53–58].

To understand the importance of FDG PET/CT in metastatic melanoma patients, a brief overview of the metastasectomy literature is necessary. Critics of metastasectomy in stage IV patients rightly point out that these are highly selected patients with data derived from single institution series. There is scant prospective randomized trial data supporting metastasectomy. Proponents of metastasectomy cite three trials that support resection [12, 28–30]. The first, a prospective, multicenter trial for metastasectomy in stage IV melanoma patients, was started by the Southwest Oncology Group (SWOG) (A Phase II Trial of Complete Surgical Resection For Stage IV Melanoma – Surgical Resection With Biological Evaluation and Clinical Follow-Up, NCT00002860) [28]. Sixty-four patients met the standard of a complete metastasectomy with tumor-free surgical margins. Although the trial closed prior to reaching accrual goals, the median overall survival was 21 months, and overall survival at 3 and 4 years was 36% and 31%, respectively.

The second trial of metastasectomy in stage IV patients (A Phase III, Randomized, Double-Blind, Placebo-Controlled Trial of Immunotherapy with a Polyvalent Melanoma Vaccine, Canvaxin™ plus BCG vs. Placebo plus BCG as a Post-Surgical Treatment for Stage IV Melanoma, NCT00052156) required all patients ($n = 496$) to have had a complete metastasectomy with tumor-free surgical margins. Although onamelatucel-L (Canvaxin™) as an adjuvant therapy did not demonstrate an overall survival benefit, there was a 5-year overall survival rate of 40% for the entire study cohort [29, 30]. This 5-year survival rate, with surgical metastasectomy, had never been achieved in any random-

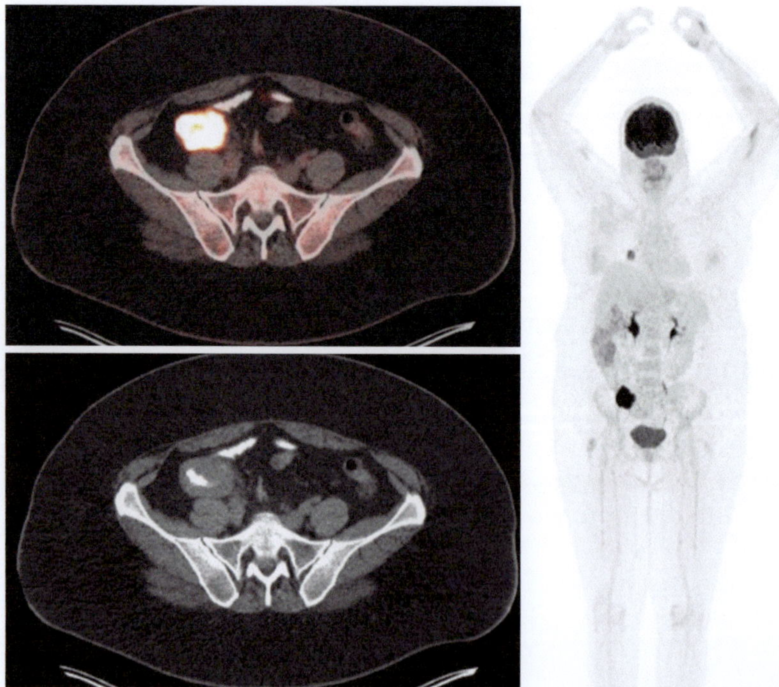

Fig. 7.8 Gastrointestinal metastasis which was completely resected

ized stage IV melanoma trial, prior to the recent immunotherapy trials [18–20].

The third trial, a secondary analysis of the Multicenter Selective Lymphadenectomy Trial (MSLT-I) (A Clinical Study of Wide Excision Alone Versus Wide Excision With Intraoperative Lymphatic Mapping and Selective Lymph Node Dissection in the Treatment of Patients With Cutaneous Invasive Melanoma, NCT00275496), demonstrated that a 4-year survival rate was significantly higher for patients undergoing metastasectomy (20.8%) vs. best available systemic therapy (7%) [12]. Collectively, these three trials demonstrate that in patients with oligometastatic disease, complete metastasectomy can improve overall survival. It is important to note, however, that the overall survival does not change in simply decreasing tumor burden with a partial or incomplete metastasectomy, but rather a complete metastasectomy must be performed [31]. FDG PET/CT can provide an accurate roadmap for identifying which patients can undergo a complete metastasectomy.

Incidental Findings of FDG PET/CT

As FDG PET/CT provides a set of whole body head to toe imaging, incidental findings, unrelated to the patient's melanoma, have been reported. Conrad et al. found that approximately 20% of the melanoma patients have incidental findings on the PET/CT, including 4 colorectal cancers and 1 prostate cancer and 11 tumors, which required an invasive procedure to prove benign [59]. Similarly, Bastiaannet and colleagues found 4.3% of patients had incidental findings, mostly colorectal in origin, and Koskivuo et al. found 4% with incidental malignancies, three thyroid, one breast, and one kidney [6, 60]. Collectively, incidental primary malignancies have been reported at incidences ranging from 1.7% to 11%, most often colorectal cancer, thyroid cancer, and renal cell carcinoma (Table 7.3) (Fig. 7.9).

Surveillance After Surgical Resection

Post-surgical surveillance is crucial and should be comprehensive as the location of melanoma metastases is unpredictable. The 5- and 10-year melanoma-specific survival probability for stage IIIA is 93% and 88%, for stage IIIB is 83% and 77%, for stage IIIC is 69% and 60%, and for stage IID is 32% and 24% [61]. When selecting surveillance regimen, factors such as life expectancy, quality of life, and cost-effectiveness of imaging methods should be considered. Close clinical surveillance, with/without radiographic studies, will allow detection of second primary

Table 7.3 Incidental tumors noted on PET and PET/CT workup of melanoma patients

	N	% unexpected tumors	Tumor type
Holder et al., 1998 [81]	76	7.9%	Thyroid cancer- 1, bronchogenic carcinoma- 1, Warthin's tumor- 1, suture granuloma-1, endometriosis- 1, inflamed epidermal cyst- 1
Stas et al., 2002 [92]	100	11%	Goiter- 5, colon tumor- 2, Schwannoma- 2, neuroma- 1, venous thrombus- 1
Bastiaannet et al., 2006 [60]	257	4.3%	Colorectal polyp- 5, colorectal cancer- 3, pituitary adenoma- 1, unspecified- 2
Gold et al., 2007 [100]	181	1.7%	Renal cell cancer- 2, lymphoma- 1
Constantinidou et al., 2008 [101]	30	6%	Neuroendocrine thyroid tumor- 1, granuloma- 1
Conrad et al., 2016 [59]	181	8.8%	Colorectal cancer- 4, prostate cancer- 1, colorectal adenoma- 6, thyroid adenoma- 1, thyroid nodule- 1, Warthin's tumor- 1, unspecified- 2
Koskivuo et al., 2016 [6]	110	4%	Thyroid cancer- 3, breast cancer- 1, renal cell cancer- 1

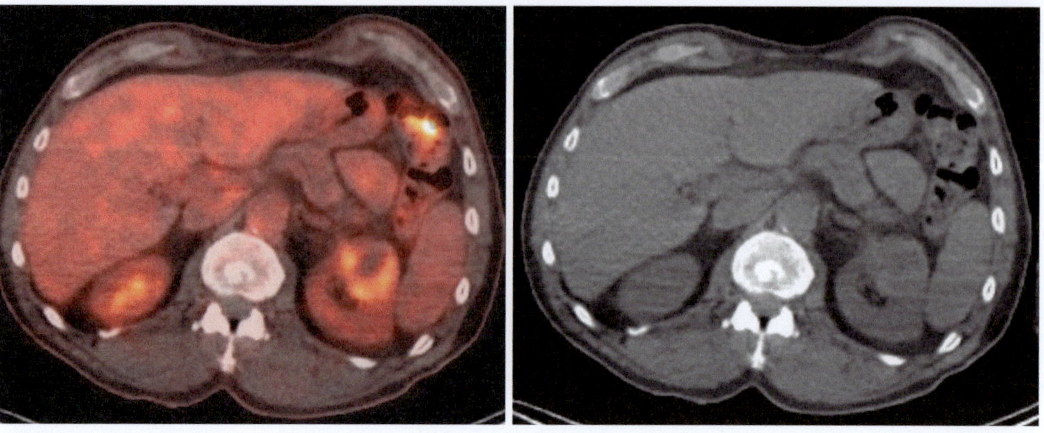

Fig. 7.9 Incidental finding of an asymptomatic left renal lesion which is a biopsy-proven renal cell carcinoma

melanomas, other cutaneous malignancies, locoregional recurrences, and distant recurrences. The highest risk of local recurrences is noted to be within the first 2–3 years of diagnosis [62]. For patients who have undergone resection of high-risk melanoma, routine imaging surveillance can play an essential role in identifying the patients who may be qualified to undergo further salvage resection and be potentially cured with select locoregional or oligometastatic recurrences [63].

Surveillance must be risk-adjusted for risks of subsequent primary melanomas [64], locoregional recurrences, and distant metastases. There is clearly additional benefit from educating patients to do self-exams. Routine surveillance can also identify patients with disseminated stage IV disease who can benefit from immunotherapy [18–20]. Patient detected recurrences occur 17–47% of the time [65, 66]. The higher proportion of patients with recurrences have clinically occult asymptomatic disease (range 50–80%) [63, 67–70]. Lewin et al. also found that PET was able to detect approximately 70% of asymptomatic recurrences [70]. Just as the recurrences detected by the patients and routine physical examinations were noted to be more superficial, the occult recurrent lesions detected by FDG PET/CT involved visceral organs and deeper anatomical structures, thus emphasizing the need for combination of patient and radiologic surveillance schemes.

Routine surveillance FDG PET/CT has an associated psychological and financial burden. Vensby and colleagues demonstrated the high negative predictive value of 97% in PET/CT in detecting relapses, which allows a negative scan to effectively assure patients and clinicians of disease-free status [71]. The lower positive predictive value of 71% showed that almost 30% of patients were incorrectly suspected to have recurrence. These findings were mostly attributed to the uptake of FDG by inflammatory cells, most often located in the lymph nodes. Utilizing cross sectional imaging to rule out relapse during surveillance may help to decrease the anxiety and reassure patients, but this comes at a high cost. For patients with false-positive findings, further diagnostic procedures or imaging tests add to their healthcare costs.

Patients undergoing routine surveillance PET/CT were found to have undergone a median of two imaging studies prior to their first recurrence and a median of nine imaging studies for those without a recurrence [63]. Leon-Ferre et al. predicted that this would be an added cost of $3728/patient with recurrence and $16,776/patient without recurrence [63]. To optimize the cost-effectiveness of surveillance, the total duration of imaging surveillance should be determined for each stage of melanoma patient. Ideally, this would be longer for those at higher risk and shorter for those at lower risk. Ultimately, high-risk and low-risk melanoma patients have the same risk for a recurrence 8 years following a melanoma resection [62]. Thus, since there is no benefit to routine radiologic surveillance in low-risk patients, there is no justification in high-risk patients after year 8. Imaging surveillance would provide the most benefit up to 3 years after resection, as 90% of recurrences were noted to occur within the first 3 years. Koskivuo and colleagues demonstrated that the sensitivity of PET/CT in detecting occult recurrence was 78.5% with follow-up at 6 months, but this drastically decreased to 29.5% with 5 year follow-up [6].

FDG PET/CT vs. Sentinel Node Biopsy

Sentinel node biopsy (SNB) is considered to be the golden standard for nodal staging in patients with primary cutaneous melanoma [72]. Although SNB is a minimally invasive procedure, complications related to the procedure have been reported including common surgical complications such as surgical site infection, seroma, and hematomas and those unique to the radiotracer and/or isosulfan blue dye (Lymphasurin, Hirsch Industries, Inc.): skin necrosis, blue urticaria, angioedema, and anaphylaxis to name a few [73]. Evaluation of PET vs. SNB has been performed. Schaarschmidt et al. showed that sensitivities for detecting sentinel lymph nodes were too low for both PET/CT and PET/MR, 17.7% and 23.5%, respectively [74], so that the low sensitivity makes the imaging modality a poor alternative to SNB. This finding was supported by Chessa et al., with similarly low sensitivity of 25%, but higher specificity of 98% for PET/CT [75]. Collectively, the low sensitivity and specificity of FDG PET/CT does not allow the modality to supplant the gold standard, sentinel node biopsy.

Novel Applications: Intraoperative PET Probe

With the wide acceptance of PET as an accurate imaging study for melanoma and the application of gamma probe in sentinel node detection, the concept of utilizing FDG as radiotracer and a hand-held probe for detected FDG-avid lesions found on PET has been explored. The probe used in sentinel node biopsy is a low energy (approximately 140 keV gamma probe), while FDG has an energy of 511 keV [76]. Therefore, probe used for FDG should have a shield for high energy (511 keV) photons. Since the metabolism and clearance of FDG in normal cells is faster than tumor cells, the tumor-to-background ratio (TBR) is higher when there is a longer waiting period after injection of FDG [77]. After intravenous injection of FDG, TBR must be 1.5:1 or greater in order for a lesion to be deemed FDG positive. After injection, 1–6 hours wait time must occur before surgery can proceed [78, 79].

In a feasibility study, Molina and colleagues demonstrated that the FDG probe had 100% accuracy identifying FDG avid lesions seen on the PET scans for various tumors, including gastric cancer, melanomas, breast cancer, and lymphoma [76]. Patient selection was limited to those who would be able to attain complete disease-free status after the surgery. Similar success was noted in a study by Gulec and colleagues, where all of the lesions noted on FDG PET were detected by the handheld FDG probe, with the smallest lesion measuring 0.5 cm [77]. They were able to identify lesions that were not demonstrated on the PET. A study published by Franc and colleagues specifically looked at patient population with melanomas and were able to demonstrate a sensitivity of 89% and specificity of 100% [79]. Multiple studies published with utilizing handheld PET probes were able to demonstrate the benefit of detecting lesions in scar tissue or occult lesions [76–80].

The gamma probes have also been shown to be an asset in detecting occult lesions that are difficult to distinguish even during surgical exploration. Even with the development of new gamma probes, the effectiveness of detecting FDG lesions in proximity to the organs with high FDG activity would be difficult and less accurate. In order to optimize detecting the lesions, a Foley catheter should be placed to minimize the urine volume in the bladder. This would also decrease the radiation exposure to others. Diabetic patients should have their blood glucose checked prior to

FDG injection to ensure a level ≤140, if possible, as discussed in previous chapters. Intravenous fluid administration during the NPO status should not contain glucose, and no insulin should be injected in order to minimize FDG uptake in muscles and fat [78]. For more accurate results, patients with lesions in the thorax are encouraged to adapt a low-carbohydrate diet 1 week prior to surgery to minimize FDG uptake in the myocardium [79]. Multiple factors, including the FDG uptake of the lesion, its anatomic location, proximity to organs with high FDG avidity, or timing of surgery after injection of FDG, can influence the success of the gamma probes in detection of tumors. With set guidelines and further experience, handheld gamma probes may improve the outcomes of patients with recurrent and metastatic melanoma.

Conclusion

From a surgical perspective, there are several advantages for FDG PET/CT compared to anatomic imaging modalities such as CT in metastatic melanoma patients. On balance, PET/CT is the superior radiologic imaging study, giving the melanoma surgeons as complete staging information as possible concerning the extent of the disease. PET/CT also offers the best radiologic evaluation for a metastatic melanoma patient being considered for a complete metastasectomy. Finally, as we are observing more and more survivors of metastatic melanoma because of surgery, checkpoint inhibitors, and targeted therapy, accurate, risk-adjusted surveillance strategies, which include PET/CTs, are necessary and needed.

References

1. Gritters LS, Francis IR, Zasadny KR, Wahl RL. Initial assessment of positron emission tomography using 2-fluorine-18-fluoro-2-deoxy-D-glucose in the imaging of malignant melanoma. J Nucl Med. 1993;34(9):1420–7.
2. Gambhir SS. Molecular imaging of cancer with positron emission tomography. Nat Rev Cancer. 2002;2(9):683–93.
3. Wasif N, Etzioni D, Haddad D, Gray RJ, Bagaria SP, Pockaj BA. Staging studies for cutaneous melanoma in the United States: a population-based analysis. Ann Surg Oncol. 2015;22(4):1366–70.
4. Tchernev G, Popova LV. PET scan misses cutaneous melanoma metastasis with significant tumour size and tumour thickness. Open Access Maced J Med Sci. 2017;5(7):963–6.
5. Keu KV, Iagaru AH. The clinical use of PET/CT in the evaluation of melanoma. Methods Mol Biol. 2014;1102:553–80.
6. Koskivuo I, Kemppainen J, Giordano S, Seppanen M, Verajankorva E, Vihinen P, et al. Whole body PET/CT in the follow-up of asymptomatic patients with stage IIB-IIIB cutaneous melanoma(). Acta Oncol. 2016;55(11):1355–9.
7. Townsend DW, Beyer T. A combined PET/CT scanner: the path to true image fusion. Br J Radiol. 2002;75:S24–30.
8. James ML, Gambhir SS. A molecular imaging primer: modalities, imaging agents, and applications. Physiol Rev. 2012;92(2):897–965.
9. Bronstein Y, Ng CS, Rohren E, Ross MI, Lee JE, Cormier J, et al. PET/CT in the management of patients with stage IIIC and IV metastatic melanoma considered candidates for surgery: evaluation of the additive value after conventional imaging. AJR Am J Roentgenol. 2012;198(4):902–8.
10. Bastiaannet E, Uyl-de Groot CA, Brouwers AH, van der Jagt EJ, Hoekstra OS, Oyen W, et al. Cost-effectiveness of adding FDG-PET or CT to the diagnostic work-up of patients with stage III melanoma. Ann Surg. 2012;255(4):771–6.
11. Xing Y, Bronstein Y, Ross MI, Askew RL, Lee JE, Gershenwald JE, et al. Contemporary diagnostic imaging modalities for the staging and surveillance of melanoma patients: a meta-analysis. J Natl Cancer Inst. 2011;103(2):129–42.
12. Howard JH, Thompson JF, Mozzillo N, Nieweg OE, Hoekstra HJ, Roses DF, et al. Metastasectomy for distant metastatic melanoma: analysis of data from the first multicenter selective lymphadenectomy trial (MSLT-I). Ann Surg Oncol. 2012;19(8):2547–55.
13. Bastiaannet E, Wobbes T, Hoekstra OS, van der Jagt EJ, Brouwers AH, Koelemij R, et al. Prospective comparison of [18F]fluorodeoxyglucose positron emission tomography and computed tomography in patients with melanoma with palpable lymph node metastases: diagnostic accuracy and impact on treatment. J Clin Oncol. 2009;27(28):4774–80.
14. Gulec SA, Faries MB, Lee CC, Kirgan D, Glass C, Morton DL, et al. The role of fluorine-18 deoxyglucose positron emission tomography in the management of patients with metastatic melanoma: impact on surgical decision making. Clin Nucl Med. 2003;28(12):961–5.
15. Crippa F, Leutner M, Belli F, Gallino F, Greco M, Pilotti S, et al. Which kinds of lymph node metastases can FDG PET detect? A clinical study in melanoma. J Nucl Med. 2000;41(9):1491–4.

16. Damian DL, Fulham MJ, Thompson E, Thompson JF. Positron emission tomography in the detection and management of metastatic melanoma. Melanoma Res. 1996;6(4):325–9.

17. Webb HR, Latifi HR, Griffeth LK. Utility of whole-body (head-to-toe) PET/CT in the evaluation of melanoma and sarcoma patients. Nucl Med Commun. 2018;39(1):68–73.

18. Wolchok JD, Chiarion-Sileni V, Gonzalez R, Rutkowski P, Grob JJ, Cowey CL, et al. Overall survival with combined nivolumab and ipilimumab in advanced melanoma. N Engl J Med. 2017;377(14):1345–56.

19. Hodi FS, Chiarion-Sileni V, Gonzalez R, Grob JJ, Rutkowski P, Cowey CL, et al. Nivolumab plus ipilimumab or nivolumab alone versus ipilimumab alone in advanced melanoma (CheckMate 067): 4-year outcomes of a multicentre, randomised, phase 3 trial. Lancet Oncol. 2018;19(11):1480–92.

20. Larkin J, Chiarion-Sileni V, Gonzalez R, Grob JJ, Rutkowski P, Lao CD, et al. Five-year survival with combined nivolumab and ipilimumab in advanced melanoma. N Engl J Med. 2019;381(16):1535–46.

21. Danielsen M, Kjaer A, Wu M, Martineau L, Nosrati M, Leong SP, et al. Prediction of positron emission tomography/computed tomography (PET/CT) positivity in patients with high-risk primary melanoma. Am J Nucl Med Mol Imaging. 2016;6(5):277–85.

22. Schule SC, Eigentler TK, Garbe C, la Fougere C, Nikolaou K, Pfannenberg C. Influence of (18) F-FDG PET/CT on therapy management in patients with stage III/IV malignant melanoma. Eur J Nucl Med Mol Imaging. 2016;43(3):482–8.

23. Niederkohr RD, Rosenberg J, Shabo G, Quon A. Clinical value of including the head and lower extremities in 18F-FDG PET/CT imaging for patients with malignant melanoma. Nucl Med Commun. 2007;28(9):688–95.

24. Frary EC, Gad D, Bastholt L, Hess S. The role of FDG-PET/CT in preoperative staging of sentinel lymph node biopsy-positive melanoma patients. EJNMMI Res. 2016;6(1):73.

25. Scheier BY, Lao CD, Kidwell KM, Redman BG. Use of preoperative PET/CT staging in sentinel lymph node-positive melanoma. JAMA Oncol. 2016;2(1):136–7.

26. Wagner T, Meyer N, Zerdoud S, Julian A, Chevreau C, Payoux P, et al. Fluorodeoxyglucose positron emission tomography fails to detect distant metastases at initial staging of melanoma patients with metastatic involvement of sentinel lymph node. Br J Dermatol. 2011;164(6):1235–40.

27. Barsky M, Cherkassky L, Vezeridis M, Miner TJ. The role of preoperative positron emission tomography/computed tomography (PET/CT) in patients with high-risk melanoma. J Surg Oncol. 2014;109(7):726–9.

28. Sondak VK, Liu PY, Warneke J. Surgical Resection for Stage IV melanoma: A southwest Oncology Group trial. J Clin Oncol. 2006;24(Sppl):4575.

29. Morton DL, Mozzillo N, Thompson JF, Kelley MC, Faries M, Wagner J, et al. MMAIT Clinical Trials Group. An international, randomized, phase III trial of bacillus Calmette-Guerin (BCG) plus allogeneic melanoma vaccine (MCV) or placebo after complete resection of melanoma metastatic to regional or distant sites. J Clin Oncol. 2007;25(18_Suppl):8508.

30. Morton DL, Mozzillo N, Thompson JF, Kashani-Sabet M, Kelley M, Gammon G, editors. MMAIT-IV Clinical Trial Group. Multicenter double-blind phase 3 trial of Canvaxin vs. placebo as post surgical adjuvant in metastatic melanoma. Society of Surgical Oncology 59th Annual Cancer Symposium; San Diego, CA; 2006.

31. Caudle AS, Ross MI. Metastasectomy for stage IV melanoma: for whom and how much? Surg Oncol Clin N Am. 2011;20(1):133–44.

32. Essner R, Lee JH, Wanek LA, Itakura H, Morton DL. Contemporary surgical treatment of advanced-stage melanoma. Arch Surg. 2004;139(9):961–6; discussion 6–7.

33. Ollila DW, Laks S, Hseuh EC. Surgery for stage IV metastatic melanoma. In: Melanoma: a modern multidisciplinary approach [internet]. Cham: Springer International Publishing; 2018. p. 467–71.

34. Hodi FS, O'Day SJ, McDermott DF, Weber RW, Sosman JA, Haanen JB, et al. Improved survival with ipilimumab in patients with metastatic melanoma. N Engl J Med. 2010;363(8):711–23.

35. Topalian SL, Sznol M, McDermott DF, Kluger HM, Carvajal RD, Sharfman WH, et al. Survival, durable tumor remission, and long-term safety in patients with advanced melanoma receiving nivolumab. J Clin Oncol. 2014;32(10):1020–30.

36. Ribas A, Hamid O, Daud A, Hodi FS, Wolchok JD, Kefford R, et al. Association of pembrolizumab with tumor response and survival among patients with advanced melanoma. JAMA. 2016;315(15):1600–9.

37. Long GV, Flaherty KT, Stroyakovskiy D, Gogas H, Levchenko E, de Braud F, et al. Dabrafenib plus trametinib versus dabrafenib monotherapy in patients with metastatic BRAF V600E/K-mutant melanoma: long-term survival and safety analysis of a phase 3 study. Ann Oncol. 2017;28(7):1631–9.

38. Flaherty KT, Infante JR, Daud A, Gonzalez R, Kefford RF, Sosman J, et al. Combined BRAF and MEK inhibition in melanoma with BRAF V600 mutations. N Engl J Med. 2012;367(18):1694–703.

39. Andtbacka RH, Kaufman HL, Collichio F, Amatruda T, Senzer N, Chesney J, et al. Talimogene laherparepvec improves durable response rate in patients with advanced melanoma. J Clin Oncol. 2015;33(25):2780–8.

40. Louie RJ, Perez MC, Jajja MR, Sun J, Collichio F, Delman KA, et al. Real-world outcomes of talimogene laherparepvec therapy: a multi-institutional experience. J Am Coll Surg. 2019;228(4):644–9.

41. Anwar H, Sachpekidis C, Winkler J, Kopp-Schneider A, Haberkorn U, Hassel JC, et al. Absolute number of new lesions on (18)F-FDG PET/CT is more pre-

dictive of clinical response than SUV changes in metastatic melanoma patients receiving ipilimumab. Eur J Nucl Med Mol Imaging. 2018;45(3):376–83.

42. Wong ANM, McArthur GA, Hofman MS, Hicks RJ. The advantages and challenges of using FDG PET/CT for response assessment in melanoma in the era of targeted agents and immunotherapy. Eur J Nucl Med Mol Imaging. 2017;44(Suppl 1):67–77.

43. Ollila DW. Complete metastasectomy in patients with stage IV metastatic melanoma. Lancet Oncol. 2006;7(11):919–24.

44. Feun L, Gutterman J, Burgess M, et al. The natural history of resectable metastatic melanoma (stage IV a melanoma). Cancer. 1982;50:1656–63.

45. Overett TK, Shiu MH. Surgical treatment of distant metastatic melanoma. Indications and results. Cancer. 1985;56(5):1222–30.

46. Meyer T, Merkel S, Goehl J, Hohenberger W. Surgical therapy for distant metastases of malignant melanoma. Cancer. 2000;89(9):1983–91.

47. Markowitz J, Cosimi L, Carey R, et al. Prognosis after initial recurrence of cutaneous melanoma. Ann Surg. 1991;214:70–707.

48. Karakousis C, Velez A, Driscoll B, et al. Metastasectomy in malignant melanoma. Surgery. 1994;115:295–302.

49. Gadd M, Coit D. Recurrence patterns and outcome in 1019 patients undergoing axillary or inguinal lymphadenopathy for melanoma. Arch Surg. 1992;127:1412–6.

50. Harpole DH Jr, Johnson CM, Wolfe WG, George SL, Seigler HF. Analysis of 945 cases of pulmonary metastatic melanoma. J Thorac Cardiovasc Surg. 1992;103(4):743–8; discussion 8–50.

51. Tafra L, Dale PS, Wanek LA, Ramming KP, Morton DL. Resection and adjuvant immunotherapy for melanoma metastatic to the lung and thorax. J Thorac Cardiovasc Surg. 1995;110(1):119–28; discussion 29.

52. Ollila DW, Gleisner AL, Hsueh EC. Rationale for complete metastasectomy in patients with stage IV metastatic melanoma. J Surg Oncol. 2011;104(4):420–4.

53. Ollila D, Essner R, Wanek L, et al. Surgical resection for melanoma metastatic to the gastrointestinal tract. Arch Surg. 1996;131:975–9.

54. Ricaniadis N, Konstadoulakis M, Walsh D, et al. Gastrointestinal metastases from malignant melanoma. Surg Oncol. 1995;4:105–10.

55. Agrawal S, Yao T, Coit D. Surgery for melanoma metastatic to the gastrointestinal tract. Ann Surg Oncol. 1999;6:336–44.

56. Klaase JM, Kroon BB. Surgery for melanoma metastatic to the gastrointestinal tract. Br J Surg. 1990;77(1):60–1.

57. Gutman H, Hess K, Kokoysakis J, et al. Surgery for abdominal metastases of cutaneous melanoma. World J Surg. 2001;25:750–8.

58. Sosman JA, Moon J, Tuthill RJ, Warneke JA, Vetto JT, Redman BG, et al. A phase 2 trial of complete resection for stage IV melanoma: results of Southwest Oncology Group Clinical Trial S9430. Cancer. 2011;117(20):4740–06.

59. Conrad F, Winkens T, Kaatz M, Goetze S, Freesmeyer M. Retrospective chart analysis of incidental findings detected by (18) F-fluorodeoxyglucose-PET/CT in patients with cutaneous malignant melanoma. J Dtsch Dermatol Ges. 2016;14(8):807–16.

60. Bastiaannet E, Oyen WJ, Meijer S, Hoekstra OS, Wobbes T, Jager PL, et al. Impact of [18F]fluorodeoxyglucose positron emission tomography on surgical management of melanoma patients. Br J Surg. 2006;93(2):243–9.

61. Gershenwald JE, Scolyer RA, Hess KR, Sondak VK, Long GV, Ross MI, et al. Melanoma staging: evidence-based changes in the American Joint Committee on Cancer eighth edition cancer staging manual. CA Cancer J Clin. 2017;67(6):472–92.

62. Goel N, Ward WH, Yu JQ, Farma JM. Short-term and long-term management of melanoma. In: Ward WH, Farma JM, editors. Cutaneous melanoma: etiology and therapy. Brisbane: Codon Publications; 2017.

63. Leon-Ferre RA, Kottschade LA, Block MS, McWilliams RR, Dronca RS, Creagan ET, et al. Association between the use of surveillance PET/CT and the detection of potentially salvageable occult recurrences among patients with resected high-risk melanoma. Melanoma Res. 2017;27(4):335–41.

64. Cust AE, Badcock C, Smith J, Thomas NE, Haydu LE, Armstrong BK, et al. A risk prediction model for development of subsequent primary melanoma in a population-based cohort. Br J Dermatol. 2020;182(5):1148–57.

65. Romano E, Scordo M, Dusza SW, Coit DG, Chapman PB. Site and timing of first relapse in stage III melanoma patients: implications for follow-up guidelines. J Clin Oncol. 2010;28(18):3042–7.

66. Garbe C, Paul A, Kohler-Spath H, Ellwanger U, Stroebel W, Schwarz M, et al. Prospective evaluation of a follow-up schedule in cutaneous melanoma patients: recommendations for an effective follow-up strategy. J Clin Oncol. 2003;21(3):520–9.

67. Lewin JH, Sanelli A, Walpole I, Kee D, Henderson MA, Speakman D, et al. Surveillance imaging with FDG-PET in the follow-up of melanoma patients at high risk of relaps. JCO. 2015;20(33(15_suppl)):151–7.

68. Hofmann U, Szedlak M, Rittgen W, Jung EG, Schadendorf D. Primary staging and follow-up in melanoma patients--monocenter evaluation of methods, costs and patient survival. Br J Cancer. 2002;87(2):151–7.

69. Kurtz J, Beasley GM, Agnese D, Kendra K, Olencki TE, Terando A, et al. Surveillance strategies in the follow-up of melanoma patients: too much or not enough? J Surg Res. 2017;214:32–7.

70. Lewin J, Sayers L, Kee D, Walpole I, Sanelli A, Te Marvelde L, et al. Surveillance imaging with FDG-

PET/CT in the post-operative follow-up of stage 3 melanoma. Ann Oncol. 2018;29(7):1569–74.

71. Vensby PH, Schmidt G, Kjaer A, Fischer BM. The value of FDG PET/CT for follow-up of patients with melanoma: a retrospective analysis. Am J Nucl Med Mol Imaging. 2017;7(6):255–62.

72. Wong SL, Faries MB, Kennedy EB, Agarwala SS, Akhurst TJ, Ariyan C, et al. Sentinel lymph node biopsy and management of regional lymph nodes in melanoma: American Society of Clinical Oncology and Society of Surgical Oncology clinical practice guideline update. Ann Surg Oncol. 2018;25(2):356–77.

73. Khan SA, Bank J, Song DH, Choi EA. The skin and subcutaneous tissue. In: Brunicardi FC, Andersen DK, Billiar TR, Dunn DL, Hunter JG, Matthews JB, editors. Schwartz's principles of surgery [Internet]. 10th ed. New York: McGraw-Hill Education; 2014. Available from: accessmedicine.mhmedical.com/content.aspx?aid=1117743615.

74. Schaarschmidt BM, Grueneisen J, Stebner V, Klode J, Stoffels I, Umutlu L, et al. Can integrated 18F-FDG PET/MR replace sentinel lymph node resection in malignant melanoma? Eur J Nucl Med Mol Imaging. 2018;45(12):2093–102.

75. Chessa MA, Dika E, Patrizi A, Fanti PA, Piraccini BM, Veronesi G, et al. Sentinel lymph node biopsy versus PET-CT in AJCC stages I and II of melanoma. J Eur Acad Dermatol Venereol. 2017;31(1):e54–e5.

76. Molina MA, Goodwin WJ, Moffat FL, Serafini AN, Sfakianakis GN, Avisar E. Intra-operative use of PET probe for localization of FDG avid lesions. Cancer Imaging. 2009;9:59–62.

77. Gulec SA, Daghighian F, Essner R. PET-probe: evaluation of technical performance and clinical utility of a handheld high-energy gamma probe in oncologic surgery. Ann Surg Oncol. 2016;23(Suppl 5):9020–7.

78. Gulec SA, Hoenie E, Hostetter R, Schwartzentruber D. PET probe-guided surgery: applications and clinical protocol. World J Surg Oncol. 2007;5:65.

79. Franc BL, Mari C, Johnson D, Leong SP. The role of a positron- and high-energy gamma photon probe in intraoperative localization of recurrent melanoma. Clin Nucl Med. 2005;30(12):787–91.

80. Essner R, Hsueh EC, Haigh PI, Glass EC, Huynh Y, Daghighian F. Application of an [(18)F] fluorodeoxyglucose-sensitive probe for the intra-operative detection of malignancy. J Surg Res. 2001;96(1):120–6.

81. Holder WD Jr, White RL Jr, Zuger JH, Easton EJ Jr, Greene FL. Effectiveness of positron emission tomography for the detection of melanoma metastases. Ann Surg. 1998;227(5):764–9; discussion 9–71.

82. Rinne D, Baum RP, Hor G, Kaufmann R. Primary staging and follow-up of high risk melanoma patients with whole-body 18F-fluorodeoxyglucose positron emission tomography: results of a prospective study of 100 patients. Cancer. 1998;82(9):1664–71.

83. Eigtved A, Andersson AP, Dahlstrom K, Rabol A, Jensen M, Holm S, et al. Use of fluorine-18 fluorodeoxyglucose positron emission tomography in the detection of silent metastases from malignant melanoma. Eur J Nucl Med. 2000;27(1):70–5.

84. Tyler DS, Onaitis M, Kherani A, Hata A, Nicholson E, Keogan M, et al. Positron emission tomography scanning in malignant melanoma. Cancer. 2000;89(5):1019–25.

85. Fuster D, Chiang S, Johnson G, Schuchter LM, Zhuang H, Alavi A. Is 18F-FDG PET more accurate than standard diagnostic procedures in the detection of suspected recurrent melanoma? J Nucl Med. 2004;45(8):1323–7.

86. Iagaru A, Quon A, Johnson D, Gambhir SS, McDougall IR. 2-Deoxy-2-[F-18]fluoro-D-glucose positron emission tomography/computed tomography in the management of melanoma. Mol Imaging Biol. 2007;9(1):50–7.

87. Pfannenberg C, Aschoff P, Schanz S, Eschmann SM, Plathow C, Eigentler TK, et al. Prospective comparison of 18F-fluorodeoxyglucose positron emission tomography/computed tomography and whole-body magnetic resonance imaging in staging of advanced malignant melanoma. Eur J Cancer. 2007;43(3):557–64.

88. Peric B, Zagar I, Novakovic S, Zgajnar J, Hocevar M. Role of serum S100B and PET-CT in follow-up of patients with cutaneous melanoma. BMC Cancer. 2011;11:328.

89. Aukema TS, Valdes Olmos RA, Wouters MW, Klop WM, Kroon BB, Vogel WV, et al. Utility of preoperative 18F-FDG PET/CT and brain MRI in melanoma patients with palpable lymph node metastases. Ann Surg Oncol. 2010;17(10):2773–8.

90. Gellen E, Santha O, Janka E, Juhasz I, Peter Z, Erdei I, et al. Diagnostic accuracy of (18)F-FDG-PET/CT in early and late stages of high-risk cutaneous malignant melanoma. J Eur Acad Dermatol Venereol. 2015;29(10):1938–44.

91. Chandra P, Purandare N, Shah S, Agrawal A, Puri A, Gulia A, et al. Diagnostic accuracy and impact of fluorodeoxyglucose positron emission tomography/computed tomography in preoperative staging of cutaneous malignant melanoma: results of a prospective study in Indian population. World J Nucl Med. 2017;16(4):286–92.

92. Stas M, Stroobants S, Dupont P, Gysen M, Hoe LV, Garmyn M, et al. 18-FDG PET scan in the staging of recurrent melanoma: additional value and therapeutic impact. Melanoma Res. 2002;12(5):479–90.

93. Harris MT, Berlangieri SU, Cebon JS, Davis ID, Scott AM. Impact of 2-deoxy-2[F-18]fluoro-D-glucose positron emission tomography on the management of patients with advanced melanoma. Mol Imaging Biol. 2005;7(4):304–8.

94. Reinhardt MJ, Joe AY, Jaeger U, Huber A, Matthies A, Bucerius J, et al. Diagnostic performance of whole body dual modality 18F-FDG PET/CT imaging for N- and M-staging of malignant melanoma:

experience with 250 consecutive patients. J Clin Oncol. 2006;24(7):1178–87.

95. Falk MS, Truitt AK, Coakley FV, Kashani-Sabet M, Hawkins RA, Franc B. Interpretation, accuracy and management implications of FDG PET/CT in cutaneous malignant melanoma. Nucl Med Commun. 2007;28(4):273–80.

96. Etchebehere EC, Romanato JS, Santos AO, Buzaid AC, Camargo EE. Impact of [F-18] FDG-PET/CT in the restaging and management of patients with malignant melanoma. Nucl Med Commun. 2010;31(11):925–30.

97. Singnurkar A, Wang J, Joshua AM, Langer DL, Metser U. 18F-FDG-PET/CT in the staging and Management of Melanoma: a prospective Multicenter Ontario PET Registry Study. Clin Nucl Med. 2016;41(3):189–93.

98. Forschner A, Olthof SC, Guckel B, Martus P, Vach W, la Fougere C, et al. Impact of (18)F-FDG-PET/CT on surgical management in patients with advanced melanoma: an outcome based analysis. Eur J Nucl Med Mol Imaging. 2017;44(8):1312–8.

99. Pfannenberg C, Gueckel B, Wang L, Gatidis S, Olthof SC, Vach W, et al. Practice-based evidence for the clinical benefit of PET/CT-results of the first oncologic PET/CT registry in Germany. Eur J Nucl Med Mol Imaging. 2019;46(1):54–64.

100. Gold JS, Jaques DP, Busam KJ, Brady MS, Coit DG. Yield and predictors of radiologic studies for identifying distant metastases in melanoma patients with a positive sentinel lymph node biopsy. Ann Surg Oncol. 2007;14(7):2133–40.

101. Constantinidou A, Hofman M, O'Doherty M, Acland KM, Healy C, Harries M. Routine positron emission tomography and positron emission tomography/computed tomography in melanoma staging with positive sentinel node biopsy is of limited benefit. Melanoma Res. 2008;18(1):56–60.

PET in Sarcoma: Surgeons Point of View

Brett L. Hayden, Adeet Amin,
and Ernest U. Conrad III

Sarcoma Diagnostic and Treatment Challenges

Sarcomas in adults and pediatric patients are a rare malignancy of mesenchymal, non-glandular, connective tissue. They carry an incidence of 15,000–20,000 new cases per year in the United States, if all subtypes and grades are included [1]. Diagnosing soft tissue tumors has historically proven challenging, and many patients present in a delayed fashion after many months of symptoms. Many benign, degenerative, and inflammatory processes serve as alternative diagnoses and distractions in the evaluation of patients with a possible soft tissue sarcoma, making the diagnostic process challenging.

Compared to carcinomas and other solid tumors, primary soft tissue sarcomas are the only soft tissue malignancy of any type that can occur in patients of any age and in any anatomic location (commonly found in the extremities, pelvis, head and neck, as well as spine). The early imaging of sarcomas is accurately defined with both MRI and PET scans, although often misinterpreted and the diagnostic histopathology remains challenging, even for the most experienced pathologists. Diagnostic errors in the assessment of the tumor grade and tumor subtype occur commonly, in spite of the promising development of sarcoma-specific molecular markers [2]. Given the challenges of assessing tumor malignancy and grade that exists for sarcomas, FDG-PET as a metabolic early diagnostic imaging modality for sarcomas appears to have significant accuracy in predicting initial tumor grade, response to neoadjuvant treatment (chemotherapy and/or radiation therapy), and local recurrence or metastasis [3, 4].

The value of PET imaging for most sarcomas is its capability to identify high-grade tumors by their metabolic activity, as reflected by the PET standard uptake value (SUV) before making decisions about systemic or local, primary treatment. Imaging with PET scans may be able to differentiate high-grade sarcomas from their intermediate and low-grade counterparts in the setting of equivocal or indeterminate microscopic pathology [5]. Additionally, PET provides the ability to identify an early response or lack of response to preoperative neoadjuvant chemotherapy with serial scans. Identifying early chemotherapy response, local recurrence, and/or the presence of metastatic disease with PET scanning allows more accurate and quicker decision-making in the treatment of many sarcomas. PET imaging is best initiated before or after the patient's initial biopsy as it can supplement, confirm, or challenge the biopsy determination in high- vs low-grade sarcomas (Fig. 8.1 Staging for musculoskeletal tumors). As new molecular

B. L. Hayden · A. Amin · E. U. Conrad III (✉)
UTHealth Department of Orthopaedics, McGovern
School of Medicine, Houston, TX, USA
e-mail: Adeet.Amin@uth.tmc.edu

© Springer Nature Switzerland AG 2021
A. H. Khandani (ed.), *PET/CT and PET/MR in Melanoma and Sarcoma*,
https://doi.org/10.1007/978-3-030-60429-5_8

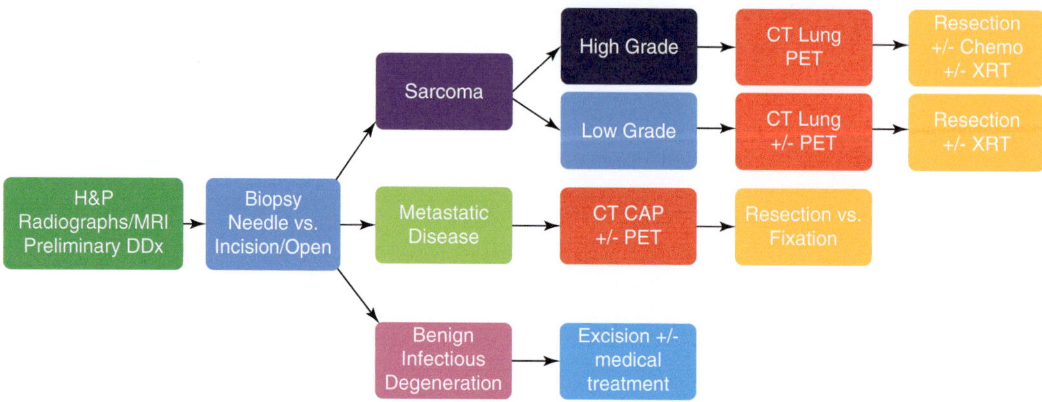

Fig. 8.1 "Staging" model for musculoskeletal tumors. Algorithm for the staging and work-up of bone and soft tissue sarcomas, metastatic disease, and other non-neoplastic lesions. (CAP Chest, abdomen, and pelvis)

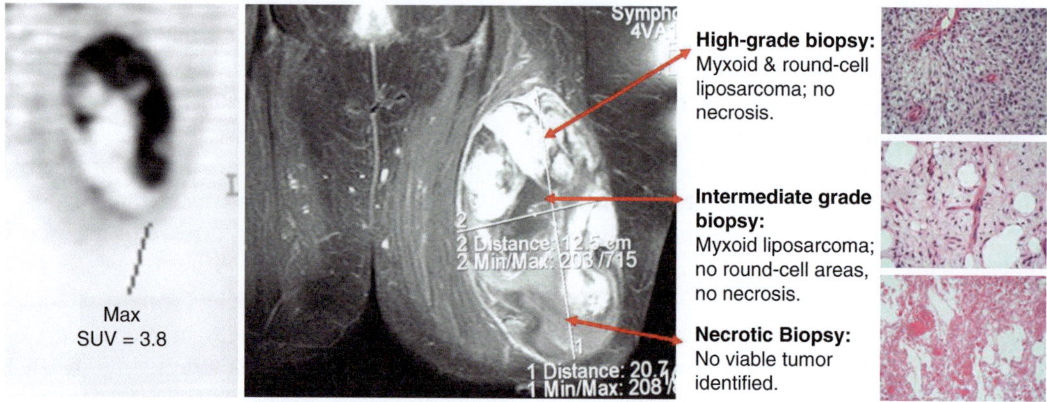

Fig. 8.2 Tumor heterogeneity and the challenges of sarcoma biopsy. Soft tissue sarcoma of the thigh in an adult patient. Sampling from three distinct areas of the tumor identified three distinct histopathologic subtypes. Due to the large size and heterogeneity of the tumor, errors in biopsy diagnosis, grade, and subtype may occur

targets develop with specificity to certain tumor subtypes, PET imaging should improve its accuracy and applications for monitoring the patient's response to adjuvant treatment.

The successful treatment of high-grade sarcomas relies on an accurate initial diagnosis, tumor grade, and the identification of the histologic response to adjuvant treatment, as well as appropriate surgical resection. Initial tumor imaging and accurate biopsy are critical first assessments for all neoplasms and a very challenging first step for many sarcoma patients (Fig. 8.2 Tumor heterogeneity and the challenges of sarcoma biopsy). The accurate biopsy of sarcomas includes the issues of tumor heterogeneity, the quantification of mitotic activity, and the challenges of sampling error for many types of sarcomas. PET scans assist in both the diagnostic and treatment challenges of sarcomas with their initial assessment of tumor grade, response to treatment, and the identification of local recurrence and metastasis [2].

Preoperative Imaging of Soft Tissue Sarcomas: The Neoadjuvant PET Sarcoma Treatment Model

The adequate treatment of soft tissue sarcomas requires multiple factors, beginning with the diagnosis and preoperative evaluation. An initial and accurate high-grade diagnosis from a biopsy,

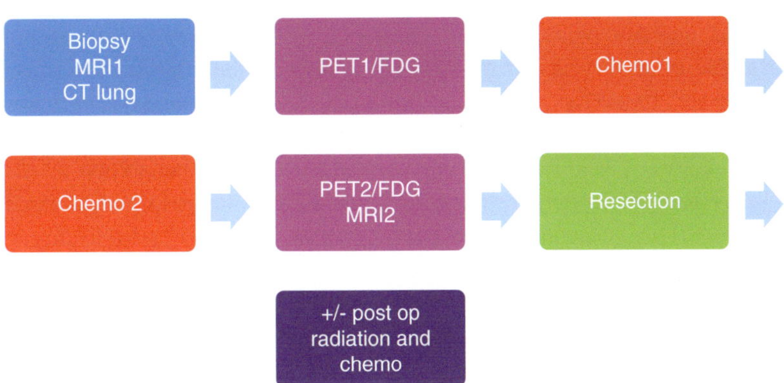

Fig. 8.3 Sarcoma PET neoadjuvant treatment model. Sequence of events following diagnosis of bone or soft tissue sarcoma. PET scans before and after neoadjuvant chemotherapy allow for monitoring and trending of SUVs

preoperative MRI, and PET imaging for all high-grade tumors is a crucial step in the patient's treatment algorithm (Fig. 8.3 Sarcoma PET "neoadjuvant" treatment model for sarcoma). The prognosis and risk of local tumor recurrence or metastasis following resection is mostly related to tumor grade, size, and anatomic location. High-grade sarcomas have a higher risk of local recurrence and metastasis compared to low-grade sarcomas, as do larger or axial tumors, occurring in the spine and pelvis. Those higher-risk tumors have a greater need for more careful imaging with PET imaging in a neoadjuvant model. That model in its initial description included repeat PET imaging after two cycles and four cycles of neoadjuvant chemotherapy with an identification of the greatest tumor response after the first two cycles of chemotherapy [4]. Low-grade sarcomas, with one exception, typically have a low (approximately 10%) risk of local recurrence and are usually associated with a lower risk of regional or distant (pulmonary) metastasis. Desmoid tumor is considered a low-grade soft tissue sarcoma which has a relatively high risk of tumor recurrence (30–50% depending on the size and location). Its confirmation as a low-grade tumor and issues of possible local recurrence represent reasonable indications for PET imaging.

The primary surgical goal for patients with soft tissue and osseous sarcomas is an adequate surgical resection with negative margins to minimize the risk of local tumor recurrence. Contemporary sarcoma surgical resection margins were described initially by Enneking and described the surgical goal to obtain a "wide"

margin of "normal tissue" surrounding the resected tumor [6]. In surgical practice today, the goal of a wide surgical margin of normal tissue of 5–10 mm is frequently compromised by several areas of "marginal" or "contaminated" surgical margins in at least one or two areas of the resected specimen. Those thinner margins may represent thinner margins secondary to an adjacent preserved anatomic structure (femur, artery, nerve) or an area lacking anatomic soft tissue coverage. The preoperative routine of planning surgical margins should consider tumor location, planned surgical margins or boundaries, grade, and the tumor response to neo-adjuvant chemotherapy or radiation therapy. Preoperative surgical planning for soft tissue or osseous sarcomas should carefully consider the identified surgical margins prior to resection and label those margins for subsequent postoperative pathological assessment. In the upper and lower extremity, preoperative planning includes identification of resection planes as well as anticipating the need for osseous and soft tissue reconstructions. Identifying tumor involvement of a major vessel (artery or vein) or a major peripheral nerve is critical to determining the resectability of the tumor as well as predicting functional outcomes and facilitating appropriate preoperative patient discussions.

A high-grade sarcoma typically deserves a wide rather than an intralesional or marginal margin. If, however, the patient has been treated with effective neoadjuvant chemotherapy (or radiation therapy), the resection may contain one to two areas of marginal margins (e.g., adjacent to a critical neurovascular structure) and have a successful outcome without local recurrence. An example of a 65-year-old patient with a large, 20 cm soft tissue sarcoma of the posteromedial mid-thigh that presented with pulmonary metastases and preop MRI of a axial and coronal MRI (T2/STIR 5 B&C) demonstrated an initial PET SUV of 10.6 at presentation and a very close surgical margin at the superficial femoral artery on preoperative MRI. The preoperative surgical margin was predicted to be at least microscopically contaminated. Preoperative chemotherapy and radiation therapy were given with a close, marginal surgical margin and no evidence of local recurrence at 2 years despite progression of her lung metastases (Fig. 8.4: MRI and PET imaging for a high-grade soft tissue sarcoma – (A) Preop PET with high SUV = 10.6. (B) Preop MRI showing a probable, very close marginal surgical margin at the superficial femoral artery, (C) coronal preop MRI of a 25 cm high grade sarcoma treated with preop chemo, radiation, and resection without local recurrence, MRI and PET preoperative imaging for adult soft tissue sarcoma).

A favorable histologic response to preoperative chemotherapy is more common in pediatric sarcomas (both osseous and soft tissue) relative to their adult counterparts. Because children, in general, have better histologic responses to high grade-sarcomas treated with preoperative chemotherapy, compared to adults, pediatric patients can be managed surgically with resections that have smaller, marginal margins, if those patients are followed carefully with serial MRI and PET scans to evaluate their response to preop chemotherapy [7] have PET imaging response has been best described by multiple studies in pediatric osteosarcoma, where a good response to preoperative chemo is defined as a 40–50% reduction in the PET SUV measurements following 8–10 weeks of preoperative chemotherapy [8]. Patients with a significant (>40%) reduction in SUV 2 compared to SUV 1 have a higher survival and a lower risk of local recurrence than those patients with a smaller (<40%) reduction in SUV [9].

Traditionally, response to neoadjuvant chemotherapy was determined by postoperative histologic analysis of tumor necrosis by a pathologist. PET tumor imaging in combination with MRI has the ability to identify histologic response after two to four cycles of neoadjuvant chemotherapy prior to surgery. Preoperative PET imaging after neoadjuvant chemotherapy may be a more accurate method of determining treatment response than the assessment of histologic response [10].

Routine preoperative sarcoma imaging should both MRI and PET imaging for all high grade tumors which can be obtained either before or after tumor biopsy but should be requested prior to the initiation of preoperative adjuvant chemotherapy or radiation therapy in order to assess treatment response and plan the details of surgical resection. The prediction of adequate surgical margins and the assessment of initial treatment response is a critical step in the successful treatment of high-grade and large (greater than 7–8 cm) sarcomas, in addition to the assessment of all recurrent sarcomas, regardless of tumor size [11–13].

For example, a 21-year-old female with thigh soft tissue sarcoma is treated with four cycles of neoadjuvant chemotherapy prior to resection in an initial neoadjuvant trial that was intended to compare the tumor response after two cycles (PET2) vs four cycles (PET3) of neoadjuvant chemotherapy (Fig. 8.5 – Neoadjuvant chemoresponse after two vs four cycles). This particular patient showed a greater SUV/PET response after the first 2 months of chemotherapy SUV (PET 2 vs PET1) compared to the PET SUV imaging after 4 cycles (PET 3 vs PET 1). That two- vs four-cycle chemotherapy comparison has been demonstrated in multiple patients, with serial preop PET scans after two vs four cycles. Comparing the initial chemotherapy response in PET 1-SUV1 (SUV = 14.3) with PET 2-SUV2 = 4.3 after two cycles vs PET 3-SUV3 (after 4 cycles), the first two cycles of chemotherapy in an adult soft tissue sarcoma population have demonstrated a greater tumor SUV response.

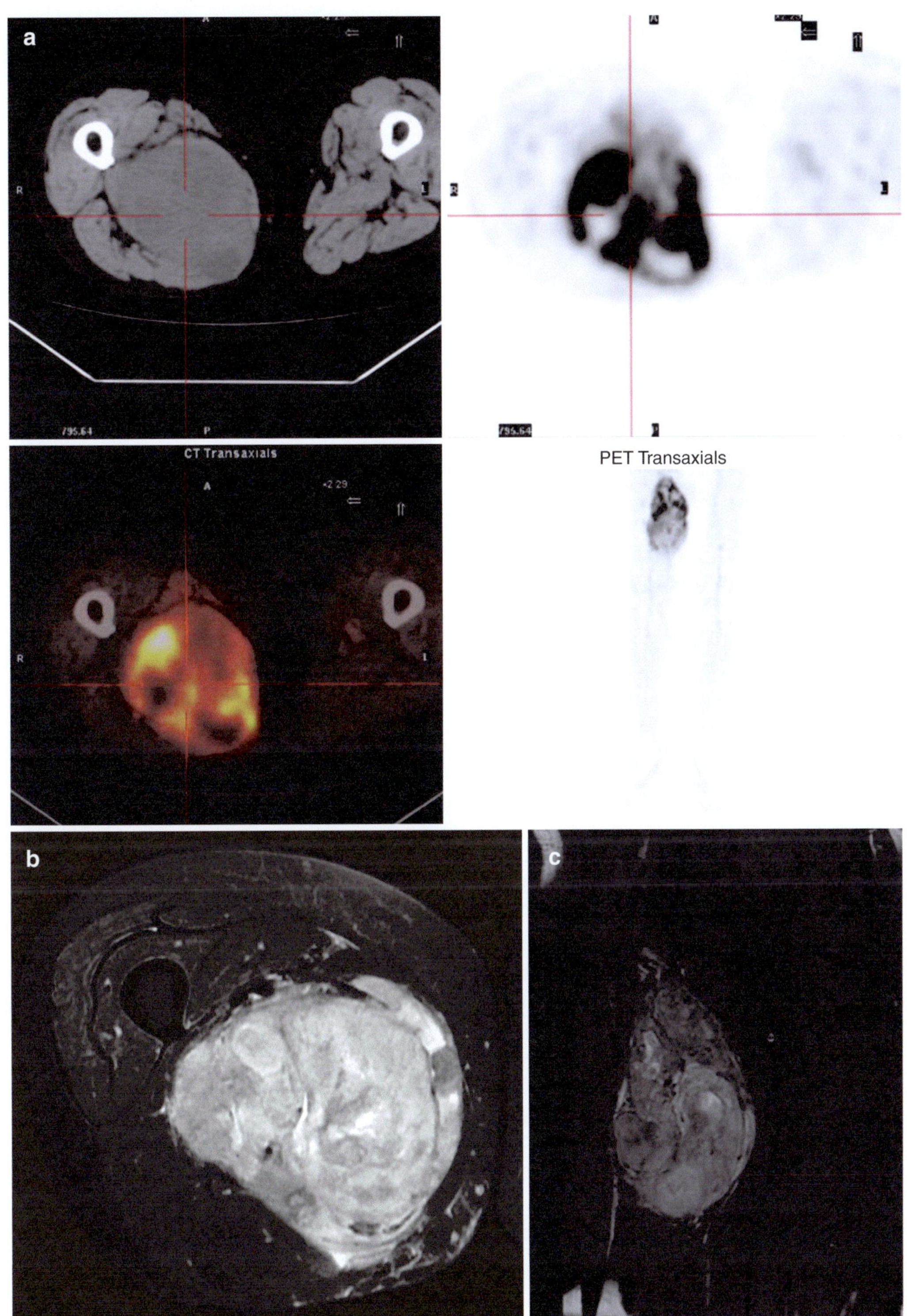

Fig. 8.4 MRI and PET imaging for high-grade soft tissue sarcoma. Imaging at initial presentation of a large, high-grade soft tissue sarcoma of the posteromedial thigh. Representative images of the lesion are (**a**) PET/CT with axial and coronal views, (**b**) axial, and (**c**) coronal fat-suppressed proton-density fast-spin-echo MRI. The maximum SUV of the mass was 10.6. This patient also had multiple pulmonary nodules found on PET/CT which were identified as metastases

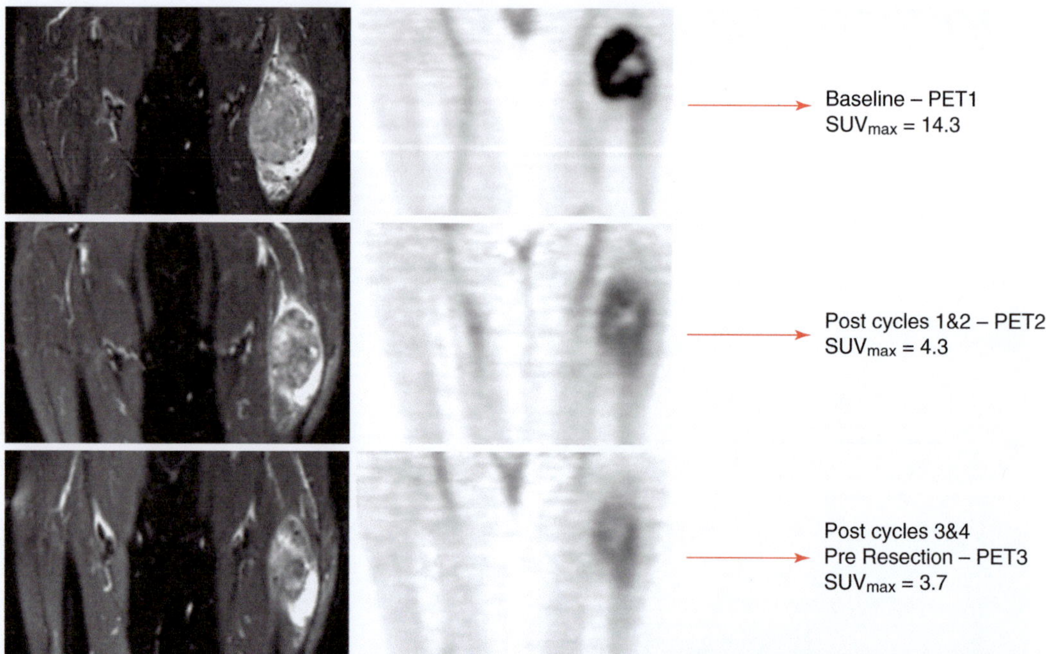

Fig. 8.5 Neoadjuvant chemotherapy response in a soft tissue sarcoma: Evaluating PET SUV after two vs four chemotherapy cycles. A 21-year-old female with a soft tissue sarcoma of the left thigh. Changes on MRI and PET scan in response to preoperative chemotherapy are seen sequentially. Decreasing SUVmax from prior to neoadjuvant chemotherapy (SUV1), following two cycles of neoadjuvant chemotherapy (SUV2) and following two additional cycles of neoadjuvant chemotherapy just prior to resection (SUV3). The biggest SUV changes occur between PET1 and PET2

Preoperative Assessment of Adult Osseous Sarcomas

Adult osseous tumors are comprised primarily of metastatic adenocarcinomas from primary tumors of the lung, breast, prostate, renal, or bone marrow (myeloma or lymphoma). A smaller number adult osseous sarcomas, including the diagnosis of chondrosarcoma or osteosarcomas. Metastatic adenocarcinomas to the skeleton comprise approximately 250,000 surgical orthopedic oncology patients per year in the United States [14]. These patients frequently require biopsy and skeletal stabilization or fixation, in addition to tumor staging and a diagnosis for what may be their presenting, initial diagnosis, requiring referral to medical oncology for systemic treatment of a new diagnosis.

Chondrosarcomas are the second most common primary malignant bone tumor, half of which are low grade or benign and are treated with marginal resection or intralesional surgical procedures [15]. The other half of adult chondrosarcomas are high grade and require careful wide resections. Chondrosarcoma carries a significant risk of local recurrence and pulmonary metastasis but has demonstrated only limited sensitivity to chemotherapy or radiation therapy. Consequently, there are currently limited indications for neoadjuvant treatment of high-grade chondrosarcomas. As a result, the surgical treatment for chondrosarcoma becomes more critical regarding control of both local recurrence and metastatic disease. As a general rule, chondrosarcomas do not occur in children unless they represent a variant of osteosarcoma (i.e., chondroblastic osteosarcoma), chondromyxoid fibroma (low-grade tumor), or "secondary" chondrosarcoma. Secondary pediatric chondrosarcomas occur following a transformation from a pre-existing pediatric dysplasia associated with multiple hereditary exostosis (MHE) or enchondromatosis (i.e., Ollier disease) and other similar diagnoses [16]. Many of these secondary chondrosarcomas will occur in adolescents or young adults and will require local resection [17].

Adult osteosarcoma occurs with an incidence of 1000 cases per year in the United States [15] compared to osteosarcoma in children which has an incidence of approximately 15,000 cases per year in the United States. These adult patients, like their pediatric counterparts, are treated with neoadjuvant chemotherapy and surgical resection, but have 50% survival compared to their pediatric counterparts. Adult osteosarcoma patients deserve careful assessment of their preoperative chemotherapy response with PET scans. Adult osteosarcoma patients deserve careful assessment of their preoperative chemotherapy response with PET scans, because of their poor response to chemotherapy and high risk of metastasis. Adult patients with osteosarcoma, who have a poor response to neoadjuvant chemotherapy, are at higher risk of local recurrence and distant metastasis than pediatric patients and deserve careful assessment of their response to treatment. The higher risk of relapse in adult osteosarcoma also unfortunately includes adolescents and young adults with osteosarcoma whose prognosis worsens in patients over the age of 18 years [9].

Figure 8.6 demonstrates conventional imaging and PET imaging for a 19-year-old with a large 20 cm distal femoral osteosarcoma who presented with metastatic disease after diaphyseal allograft reconstruction (Fig. 8.6a–d). He presented with a delayed diagnosis, metastatic disease, and a high initial PET SUV = 15.8. He had a poor response to preoperative chemotherapy. He was reconstructed with a cadaveric femoral allograft fixed with a femoral rod and fixation plates. Alternative osseous sarcoma reconstructions following resection of the knee joint for osseous sarcomas include oncologic total knee reconstructions for distal femoral or proximal tibial sarcomas (see Fig. 8.7: Oncologic total knee replacement for osseous sarcomas).

Surgical resection and reconstruction for osteosarcoma or chondrosarcoma usually requires a resection and reconstruction with a complex, oncologic endoprosthesis (i.e., megaprostheses). These patients usually require 3–6 months of orthopedic rehabilitation and continued oncologic follow-up to determine local recurrence or lung metastasis. Imaging follow-up for local control usually requires an MRI at 3–6-month intervals, but those MRI images are challenging to interpret for local recurrence because of the adjacent metal implant. PET scan imaging can assist with the assessment of those patients for the possible local recurrence because of the limitations of MRI assessment adjacent to a large metallic implant [18].

Assessing Tumor Response, Local Recurrence, and Metastatic Disease with Pelvic and Sacral Sarcomas

Overall treatment goals for sarcoma patients include the treatment of the primary tumor, and prevention of distant (most commonly pulmonary) metastases after a confident diagnosis has been achieved. Evaluation of the resected primary tumor site includes monitoring of the surgical site with radiographic follow-up, typically at three-month intervals. Chest CTs at routine 3-month intervals are most useful for screening for metastatic disease to the lungs. When a recurrence or metastasis is suspected, PET scanning may be key to confirming that development [19].

Some of the most challenging sarcoma patients are those with pelvic or sacral sarcomas, as recurrences are frequently difficult to diagnosis with MRI or CT alone. Pelvic sarcomas, whether they occur as osseous or soft tissue sarcomas, represent high-risk tumors for both local recurrence and metastatic disease. PET presents an opportunity to confirm the occurrence of an early tumor recurrence and, when paired with CT, can assist in diagnosing distant pulmonary metastases [16].

Pelvic sarcomas frequently present challenges with surgical resection and have significantly higher risks of local recurrence or surgical complications such as neurovascular injuries, bladder, bowel and ureter, massive blood loss, and intra-operative death (Fig. 8.8). Pelvic and sacral tumors have a higher risk of local recurrence (30–

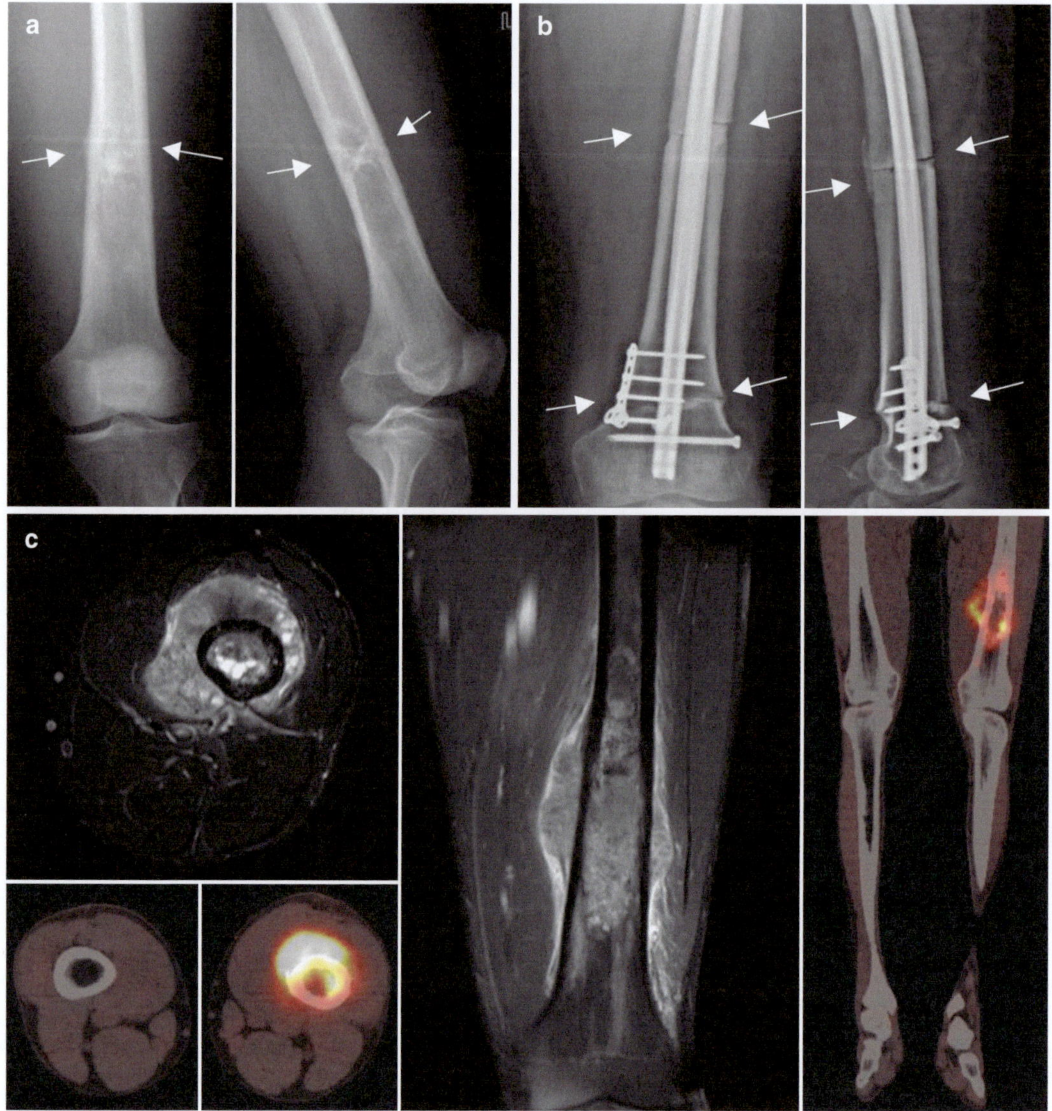

Fig. 8.6 Preop MRI and PET Imaging for a 19-year-old with femoral osteosarcoma. (**a**) Preop X-rays of femur, (**b**) postop cadaver femoral allograft reconstruction. (**c**) Pre-resection MRI. (**d**) Pre-resection PET. A 20-year-old male with a diaphyseal osteosarcoma. Preoperative (**a**) and postoperative (**b**) radiographs following a wide resection and reconstruction with an intercalary allograft fixed with an intramedullary rod as well as a unicortical plate and screws. (**b**) MRI and PET/CT scan of the same patient preoperatively. There is large, initial preoperative FDG uptake in his primary tumor site with SUV of 15.8. This patient also had multiple bilateral pulmonary metastases at presentation

50%), metastasis (30–50%), and death from their disease (10–20%) for high-grade sarcomas. Pelvic tumors also require careful preoperative imaging and surgical planning which includes both CT and MRI of the pelvis and abdomen as well as CT of the chest. Large, high-risk pelvic tumors can also be treated with neoadjuvant radiation therapy in addition to 2–3 months of neoadjuvant preop chemotherapy. In this situation, of both preop chemo and preop radiation, the surgical tumor resection will be delayed at least 12–18 weeks. Lastly, hemipelvic amputation is

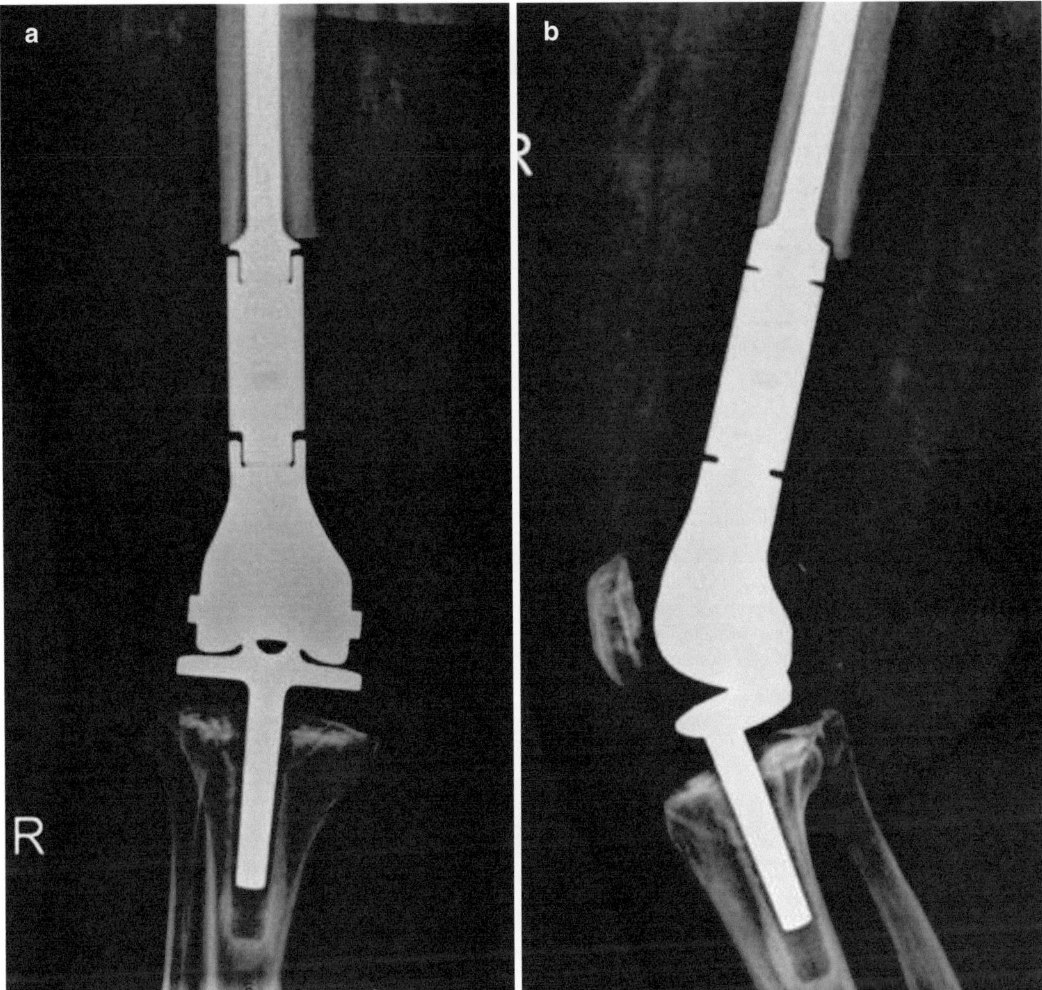

Fig. 8.7 Oncologic total knee – post 15 cm femoral resection. (**a**) Postop: Anterior view. (**b**) Postop: Lateral view

sometimes the best patient choice for resection but is also surgically challenging in obtaining adequate surgical margins at the pelvic and or sacral midline. Surgical resection for osseous pelvic tumors may also include intraoperative navigation to assist in resection accuracy which is more challenging in the pelvis than the extremities. Soft tissue sarcomas of the pelvis may present great challenges in histologic tumor response, especially as large pelvic or sacral sarcomas. Decisions regarding neoadjuvant chemotherapy and radiation therapy should be carefully planned for high-grade pelvic soft tissue sarcomas [20].

Osseous pelvic and sacral sarcomas, including osteosarcoma and osteosarcoma variants, are good candidates for preoperative chemotherapy, though they have a higher incidence of poor response to their preoperative treatment and much greater challenges with adequate surgical margins and local control after their resections. Large sacral tumors can present sarcoma imaging challenges because of PET "overlap" imaging with the bladder anteriorly, which will need resolution with both CT and MRI comparisons (Fig. 8.8: Sacral sarcoma preop imaging). Both preoperative and radiation therapy should be considered for pelvic sarcomas because of a greater challenge with local control and achieving a good response to chemo as seen with this 30-year-old male with a 14 cm syno-

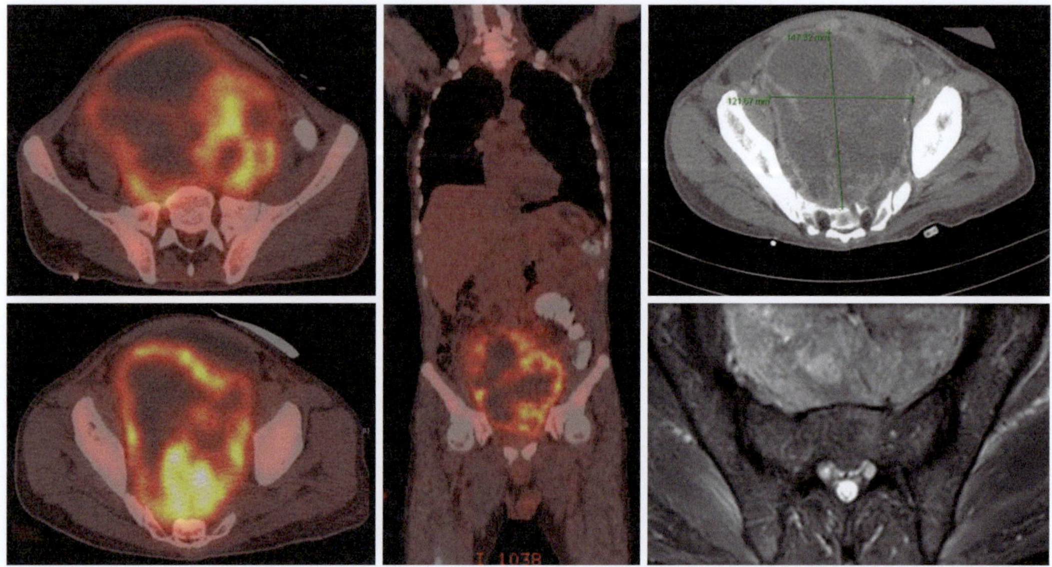

Fig. 8.8 MRI and PET Imaging for a large sacral sarcoma. Preoperative PET, CT, and MRI of a patient with a 17 cm sacral sarcoma. PET images demonstrated intense FDG activity peripherally (SUVmax = 12), with a central necrotic area. Needle biopsy demonstrated undifferentiated pleomorphic sarcoma

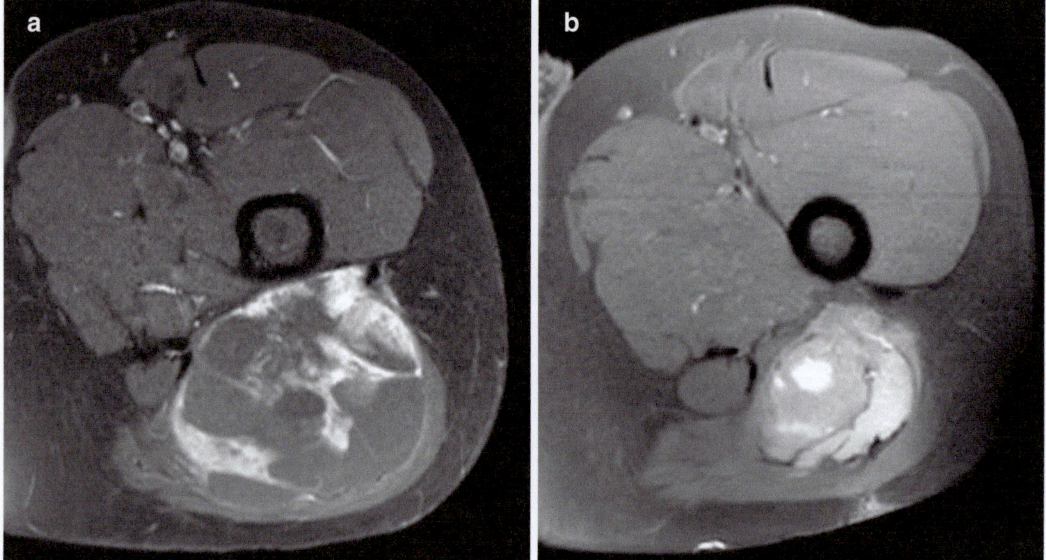

Fig. 8.9 A 30-year-old male with 15 cm posterior synovial sarcoma in the gluteus maximus – treated with preop chemotherapy and radiation therapy showing a decrease in size on pre-resection axial MRI (A pre-chemo vs B post-chemo) and a decrease in PET SUV1 (10.0) vs PET SUV2 (5.0). (**a**) Pre-chemo MRI. (**b**) Post-chemo MRI

vial sarcoma located in his gluteus maximus with a very close margin at the sciatic nerve. Figure 8.9 demonstrates a 30-year-old with a gluteal synovial sarcoma (A preop coronal FS T2 MRI) and Fig. 8.9b post-chemotherapy coronal MRI showing a decrease in tumor diameter following preop chemo therapy and radiation therapy. Preop-chemotherapy and radiation therapy allowed an uncontaminated marginal resection at the sciatic nerve after a good response to preoperative chemotherapy (preop SUV = 9.0 vs post SUV = 5.0).

After surgical resection, and after chemotherapy and radiation therapy, pelvic sarcoma patients should be followed with alternating pelvic CT and MRI at 3-month intervals for 2 years with consideration for PET scans at 6- or 12-month intervals postoperatively. As with all sarcoma patients, post-treatment follow-up should occur more frequently for the first 2 years followed by less frequent imaging for local recurrence and distant (lung) metastasis in years 3–5 [21].

Pediatric Sarcomas: The Best Indications for PET Imaging

The overall survival for pediatric patients following chemotherapy and resection is relatively high (60–70% 5-years survival) compared to their adult counterparts (40–50% 5-years survival) with a similar diagnosis. Pediatric patients with sarcomas are the optimal patients for PET imaging to assess response of neoadjuvant chemotherapy [22, 23]. Usually these patients have a better response to chemotherapy than their adult counterparts, which is usually predicted accurately by serial pre- and post-chemotherapy FDG-PET imaging. Multiple studies have corroborated the accuracy of PET in predicting chemotherapy response to pediatric osteosarcoma, Ewing sarcoma, and soft tissue sarcoma and the effectiveness of PET with pediatric staging [19, 24].

Predicting treatment response is particularly important for pediatric patients for several reasons. First, pediatric patients with a poor response to initial therapy, as measured by repeat PET/SUVs typically after 10–12 weeks of initial therapy, may receive a better and safer surgical resection or earlier modification in their systemic therapy if a poor response is appreciated on PET imaging. Second, surgical decisions and better surgical margins can be affected by the recognition of an initial positive or negative tumor response to chemotherapy is assessed. Patients with a good response are candidates for a smaller, more narrow surgical margins, potentially allowing the surgeon to spare an adjacent growth plate, knee joint, or leg with a more limited resection.

Lastly, both MRI and PET SUV have been demonstrated to have good accuracy in predicting surgical margins [7]. This approach for pediatric patients has been associated with good results with regard to local tumor control (90%) and may facilitate a more functional limb salvage procedure [25].

Osseous resections in pediatric sarcomas have the surgical options of amputation, rotation plasty (modified amputation, with transfer of the ankle to the knee), an oncologic total knee, or a joint sparing diaphyseal resection of the femur or tibia with a cadaveric allograft or fibular autograft reconstruction. Sparing the patients native, adjacent physis or growth plate is a major issue for surgical decisions, and osseous reconstructions sparing the physis are greatly facilitated by serial MRI and PET/SUV imaging. The prognosis for pediatric osteosarcoma or Ewings sarcoma worsens with patient age, tumor size, or the presence of metastatic disease at presentation, and higher-risk patients require careful observation at 3–6-month intervals for 3–5 years to exclude the risk local recurrence or pulmonary metastases. Surgical treatment for children under the age of 10–12 years is associated with a better response to initial chemotherapy, but surgical resections are more challenging decisions because of the desire to spare the adjacent growth plate (physis) and/or articular joint. As a result of growth issues and a better response to preoperative chemotherapy, surgery for younger pediatric patients involves more surgical options and more challenging surgical decisions.

References

1. Cates JMM. Simple staging system for osteosarcoma performs equivalently to the AJCC and MSTS systems. J Orthopeadic Res. 2018;36(10):2802–8. PMID: 29718558.
2. Guillou L, Coindre JM, Bonichon F, Nguyen BB, Terrier P, Collin F, Vilain MO, Mandard AM, Le Doussal V, Leroux A, Jacquemier J, Duplay H, Sastre-Garau X, Costa J. Comparative study of the National Cancer Institute and French Federation of Cancer Centers Sarcoma Group grading systems in a population of 410 adult patients with soft tissue sarcoma. J Clin Oncol. 1997;15(1):350–62.

3. Costelloe CM, Macapiniac HA, Madewell JE, et al. 18F-FDG PET/CT as an indicator of progression-free and overall survival in osteosarcoma. J Nucl Med. 2009;50(3):340–7. https://doi.org/10.2967/jnumed.108.058461.

4. Scheutze SM, Rubin BP, Vernon C, Hawkins DS, Bruckner JD, Conrad EU, Eary JF. Cancer. Use of positron emission tomography in localized, extremity soft tissue sarcoma treated with neoadjuvant chemotherapy. Cancer. 2005;103(2):339–48.

5. Conrad EU, Morgan HD, Vernon C, Schuetze SM, Eary JF. Fluorodeoxyglucose positron emission tomography scanning: basic principles and imaging of adult soft-tissue sarcomas. J Bone Joint Surg Am. 2004;86-A(Suppl 2):98–104.

6. Enneking WF, Spanier SS, Malawer MM. The effect of the Anatomic setting on the results of surgical procedures for soft parts sarcoma of the thigh. Cancer. 1981;47(5):1005–22.

7. Thompson MJ, Shapton JC, Punt SE, Johnson CN, Conrad EU. MRI identification of the osseous extent of pediatric bone sarcomas. Clin Orthop Relat Res. 2018;476(3):559–64. https://doi.org/10.1007/s11999.0000000000000068.

8. Hawkins DS, Rajendran JG, Conrad EU, Bruckner JD, Eary JF. Evaluation of chemotherapy response in pediatric bone sarcomas by [F-18]-fluorodeoxy-D-glucose positron emission tomography. Cancer. 2002;94(12):3277–84.

9. Byun BH, Kong CB, Park J, et al. Initial metabolic tumor volume measured by 18F-FDG PET/CT can predict outcome of osteosarcoma of the extremities. J Nucl Med. 2013;54(10):1725–32. https://doi.org/10.2967/jnumed.112.117697.

10. Folpe AL, Lyles RH, Sprouse JT, Conrad EU, Eary JF. (F-18) fluorodeoxyglucose positron emission tomography as a predictor of pathologic grade and other prognostic variables in bone and soft tissue sarcoma. Clin Cancer Res. 2000;6(4):1279–87.

11. Benz MR, Czernin J, Allen MS, et al. FDG-PET/CT imaging predicts histopathologic treatment responses after the initial cycle of neoadjuvant chemotherapy in high grade soft tissue sarcomas. Clin Cancer Res. 2009;15(8):2856–63. https://doi.org/10.1158/1078-0432.CCR-08-2537.

12. Evilevitch V, Weber WA, Tap WD, et al. Reduction of glucose metabolic activity is more accurate than change in size at predicting histopathologic response to neoadjuvant therapy in high-grade soft-tissue sarcomas. Clin Cancer Res. 2008;14(3):715–20. https://doi.org/10.1158/1078-0432.CCR-07-1762.

13. Palmerini E, Colangeli M, Nanni C, et al. The role of FDG PET/CT in patients treated with neoadjuvant chemotherapy for localized bone sarcomas. Eur J Nucl Med Mol Imaging. 2017;44(2):215–23. https://doi.org/10.1007/s00259-016-3509-z.

14. Hage WD, Aboulafia AJ, Aboulafia DM. Incidence, location, and diagnostic evaluation of metastatic bone disease. Orthop Clin North Am. 2000;31:515–28, vii.

15. Damron TA, Ward WG, Stewart A. Osteosarcoma, chondrosarcoma, and Ewing's sarcoma: National Cancer Data Base Report. Clin Orthop Relat Res. 2007;459:40–7.

16. Berrebi O, Steiner C, Keller A, Rougemont AL. Ratib O. F-18 Fluorodeoxyglucose (FDG) PET in the diagnosis of malignant transformation of fibrous dysplasia in the pelvic bones. Clin Nucl Med. 2008;33(7):469–71.

17. Brenner W, Conrad EU, Eary JF. FDG PET imaging for grading and prediction of outcome in Chondrosarcoma patients. European J Nuclear Med Mol Imaging. 2004;31(2):189–95.

18. Chang KJ, Kong CB, Choo WH, et al. Usefulness of increased 18 F-FDG uptake for detecting local recurrence in patients with extremity osteosarcoma treated with surgical resection and endoprosthetic replacement. Skelet Radiol. 2015;44(4):529–37. https://doi.org/10.1007/s00256-014-2063-7.

19. Francius C, Sciuk J, Daldrup-link HE, et al. PDG-PET for detection of osseous metastases from malignant primary bone tumours: comparison with bone scintigraphy. Eur J Nucl Med. 2000;27(9):1305–11.

20. Tregla G, Salsano M, Stefanelli A, et al. Diagnostic accuracy of 18F-FDG-PET and PET/CT in patients with Ewing sarcoma family tumours: a systematic review and a meta-analysis. Skelet Radiol. 2012;41(3):249–56. https://doi.org/10.1007/s00256-011-1298-9.

21. Meyer JS, Nadel HR, Marina N, et al. Imaging guidelines for children with Ewing sarcoma and osteosarcoma: a report from the Children's Oncology Group Bone tumor Committee. Pediatric Blood Cancer. 2008;51(2):163–70.

22. Denecke T, Hundsdorfer P, Misch D, et al. Assessment of histological response of paediatric bone sarcomas using FDG PET in comparison to morphological volume measurement and standardized MRI parameters. Eur J Nucl Med Mol Imaging. 2010;37(10):1842–53. https://doi.org/10.1007/s00259-010-1484-3.

23. Raciborska A, Bilska K, Drabko K, et al. Response to chemotherapy estimates by FDG PET is an important prognostic factor in patients with Ewing Sarcoma. Clin Transl Oncol. 2016;18(2):189–95. https://doi.org/10.1007/s12094-015-1351-6.

24. Volker T, Denecke T, Steffen I, et al. Positron emission tomography for staging of pediatric sarcoma patients: results of a prospective multicenter trial. J Clin Oncol. 2007;25(34):5435–41.

25. Agarwal M, Puri A, Gulia A, Reddy K. Joint-sparing or physeal-sparing diaphyseal resections: the challenge of holding small fragments. Clin Orthop Relat Res. 2010;468(11):2924–32.

FDG PET in the Diagnosis and Management of Pediatric and Adolescent Sarcomas

Andrew B. Smitherman, Stuart H. Gold, and Ian J. Davis

Introduction

Pediatric sarcomas are a heterogeneous group of cancers of likely mesenchymal cell origin that constitute approximately 14% of cancer diagnoses among children and adolescents, about 12 cases annually in the USA per one million children ages 0–19 years [66, 78]. Primitive mesenchymal cells differentiate into bone, cartilage, skeletal and smooth muscle, fat, and fibrous connective tissues, as such sarcomas may arise from any of these tissue types. The most common pediatric primary bone sarcomas are osteosarcomas (5.1 per million) and Ewing sarcomas (and associated Ewing family of tumors, 2.9 per million) [78]. Soft tissue sarcomas include rhabdomyosarcoma and rarer sarcomas often grouped as non-rhabdomyosarcoma soft tissue sarcomas (NRSTS) or adult-type soft tissue sarcomas which include fibrosarcomas, synovial sarcomas, and malignant peripheral nerve sheath tumors among others. Rhabdomyosarcoma is the most common pediatric soft tissue sarcoma with an annual US incidence of 4.7 per one million [78].

The treatment of pediatric sarcomas is typically multimodal, including systemic chemotherapy coupled with local control using surgery and/or radiation depending on the extent of tumor resection and the tumor type. Systemic chemotherapy is often administered neoadjuvantly followed by definitive tumor resection and radiation therapy if indicated. Subsequent adjuvant chemotherapy is then used to consolidate remission. The evaluation of tumor response to chemotherapy can be prognostic for some sarcomas such as osteosarcoma in which a pathological response has been evaluated as a guide for subsequent treatment.

Historically, survival outcomes for patients with a pediatric sarcoma were quite poor unless localized and resectable; however, incorporation of systemic chemotherapy for some diseases has significantly improved survival for non-localized and unresectable disease such that most children and adolescents with a sarcoma diagnosis will become long-term survivors [73, 75]. Nevertheless, improvements in survival outcomes for pediatric sarcomas have lagged behind those of many other pediatric cancers presenting opportunities for improvement in therapy. Due to clinical trials some great strides have been made in the treatment of some pediatric sarcomas such as Ewing sarcoma.

Survival outcomes are particularly poor among patients with pediatric sarcomas with metastatic disease. This fact highlights the

A. B. Smitherman (✉) · S. H. Gold · I. J. Davis
Department of Pediatrics, University of North Carolina School of Medicine, Chapel Hill, NC, USA

Lineberger Comprehensive Cancer Center, University of North Carolina School of Medicine, Chapel Hill, NC, USA
e-mail: andrew_smitherman@med.unc.edu; stuart_gold@med.unc.edu; ian_davis@med.unc.edu

© Springer Nature Switzerland AG 2021
A. H. Khandani (ed.), *PET/CT and PET/MR in Melanoma and Sarcoma*,
https://doi.org/10.1007/978-3-030-60429-5_9

importance of thorough staging at diagnosis in order to guide intensity and scope of treatment. Pediatric sarcomas commonly metastasize hematogenously to the lungs, liver, lymph nodes, bones, or bone marrow.

Imaging plays a major role in the diagnosis and staging of pediatric sarcomas. Imaging of the primary site is critical for planning local control options, including possibilities for complete resection. Since sarcomas frequently metastasize, traditional staging for many pediatric sarcomas has included radiologic evaluation of the primary tumor site with computed tomography (CT) or magnetic resonance imaging (MRI), CT of the lungs for pulmonary metastases, and a bone scan using ^{99m}technetium methylene diphosphate bone scintigraphy to evaluate for bone metastases. In addition, since rhabdomyosarcoma and Ewing sarcoma can involve the bone marrow, bilateral pelvic bone marrow aspirates and biopsies are recommended as part of the staging process. Evaluation of spinal fluid with lumbar puncture is recommended for some forms of rhabdomyosarcoma.

For some diseases such as alveolar rhabdomyosarcoma, metastatic spread to lymph nodes (both locoregionally and distant) is associated with poorer outcomes [74]. Lymph node involvement is common with soft tissue sarcomas such as rhabdomyosarcoma (up to 23% of cases), clear cell sarcoma, epithelioid sarcoma, and angiosarcoma [87]. In a cooperative group study of rhabdomyosarcoma, 17% of patients were determined to have regional lymph node involvement by biopsy despite these nodes having no clinically abnormal features [62]. This has led to the investigation of including metabolic imaging techniques in addition to traditional anatomic imaging to identify lymph node metastasis and guide effective nodal sampling and treatment.

Radiographic evaluation plays a central role in the staging workup and surveillance for disease recurrence following completion of therapy. Surveillance typically includes imaging of the primary tumor site to examine for local recurrence as well as imaging of sites of distant disease. In addition, chest imaging is routine for most pediatric sarcomas since pulmonary metastases are the most common site of distant recurrence. Imaging of additional sites has been guided by physical exam and symptoms. Surveillance regimens are generally more intensive in the early post-therapy period with a gradual reduction of frequency as the risk of recurrence decreases.

Positron emission tomography (PET) has become increasingly available for use in pediatric medical centers. PET utilizes positron-emitting radiopharmaceuticals and the subsequent detection of positron-electron annihilation which results in the generation of photons. For evaluation of pediatric sarcomas, fluorine-18 fluorodeoxyglucose (FDG) is the most commonly used radiotracer. FDG is a glucose analogue that accumulates in cancer cells as a result of increased glucose transport and metabolic activity in these cells.

Many potential roles exist for incorporating FDG PET in the care of childhood and adolescent patients with sarcoma. From diagnosis and accurate staging, through assessment of tumor response to therapy, evaluation for degeneration of benign to malignant tumors, and surveillance of recurrence, FDG PET has the potential to enhance the management of these cancers. However, the benefits of FDG PET must be balanced with the associated risks and potential healthcare costs related to false-positive results. FDG PET uptake is not specific to cancer cells, and nonmalignant conditions such as infection and inflammation also result in increased FDG PET uptake. Brown fat is a metabolically active tissue more widely present in children than in adults [35]. The higher amounts of brown fat in children and adolescents can be a particular challenge for using FDG PET during cold months which can lead to increased radiotracer uptake and may obscure sites of disease [56]. For this reason, researchers have examined the use of other radiotracers that may be more specifically taken up by cancer cells, such as carbon-11-methionine [50]. However, to date, no radiopharmaceuticals superior to FDG PET for evaluation of pediatric sarcomas have been identified. A recent study evaluated the uptake of gallium-68-fibroblast activation protein inhibitor (FAPI) PET in 28 various cancer types among adults. Uptake of FAPI was particularly high in the eight sarcomas evaluated though likely related to the high level of cancer-associated fibroblasts and fibrosis in these tumors [54]. However, further study is needed to determine if this tracer outperforms FDG PET in the assessment of pediatric sarcomas.

The coupling of functional imaging using FDG PET with anatomical imaging such as CT or MRI enables the association of hypermetabolic tissues with anatomical changes. FDG PET alone is limited by poor anatomical detail. The addition of CT serves to better differentiate normal from pathological metabolic tracer uptake [48] reducing the rate of false-positive studies. Another particular advantage of PET/CT is in the identification of small pulmonary metastases below the spatial resolution of PET alone. The addition of CT with breath-holding to FDG PET can improve sensitivity for detecting pulmonary nodules especially in the lung bases where respiratory excursion has its greatest impact on imaging [52].

FDG PET may also play an increasingly important role in early-phase clinical trials for assessing response to novel therapeutics where changes in tumor volume may be an inadequate biomarker of treatment response such as with osteosarcoma [86].

This chapter reviews several common pediatric sarcomas, describes key concepts related to their diagnosis and treatment, and illustrates the application of FDG PET in diagnosis, assessment of treatment response, and surveillance for cancer recurrence. Overall, FDG PET has proven to enhance identification of distant bone, soft tissue, and lymph node metastases among pediatric patients with sarcomas but has been inferior for identifying pulmonary metastases, especially smaller nodules. In addition to the higher sensitivity of FDG PET, the specificity in identifying metastases is similar to that of conventional imaging techniques. For these reasons, FDG PET has been incorporated into the diagnostic and surveillance regimens in recent Children's Oncology Group (COG) sarcoma clinical trials. Coupling FDG PET with conventional diagnostic imaging is increasingly employed. The role of FDG PET in guiding response-adapted or risk-adapted therapy, as has been firmly established in Hodgkin lymphoma, is unclear for pediatric sarcomas.

Osteosarcoma

Osteosarcoma is the most common pediatric primary bone cancer with an incidence of 5.1 per million per year [78]. Approximately 800 new cases of osteosarcoma are diagnosed in the USA annually [75] with half of these in patients less than 20 years old. This malignant neoplasm is histologically characterized by the production of osteoid or immature bone by the neoplastic cells. Often tumors arise at the metaphysis of long bones among adolescents suggesting an association with rapid bone growth [36]. Ten to 20% of patients will have detectable metastatic disease at presentation, most commonly in the lungs, distant bones, or noncontiguous regions of the bone involved with the primary tumor (skip lesion). Prior to the inclusion of chemotherapy, survival rates for osteosarcoma treated by surgical resection and/or radiation were between 15% and 20%. Distant recurrences, most commonly in the lungs, indicated that despite a lack of radiographic evidence, most patients had subclinical metastases at diagnosis. The addition of neoadjuvant and adjuvant chemotherapy has dramatically increased long-term survival to nearly 80% among patients with localized disease at diagnosis [1]. Comprehensive imaging is critical in determining the extent of disease for surgical planning, including resection of distant metastases, which has been shown to improve survival outcomes [36].

Historically, comprehensive staging for osteosarcoma included X-rays and MRI of the primary site, chest CT, and bone scan, such as (99 m) Tc-methylene diphosphonate [(99 m)Tc-MDP] bone scintigraphy. Functional imaging with FDG PET in addition to CT and MRI has become increasingly used in staging osteosarcoma and offers several advantages for its clinical management. FDG PET has been used to stage osteosarcoma to identify distant metastases at diagnosis (or restaging at disease progression/recurrence), to determine disease response to therapy, and to aid in surveillance for recurrence and has been studied as a potential tool to provide prognostic information to guide risk-based or response-adapted management.

FDG PET in Staging Osteosarcoma

The presence of metastatic disease is the strongest prognostic feature for patients with osteosarcoma. As compared to nearly 80% 5-year survival among patients with localized disease, patients with pulmonary metastases have an approximately 50% survival with complete resection [9] and 25% survival among patients with more extensive metastatic disease not amenable to complete resection. Pulmonary metastases are the most common form of distant disease with other osseous site being second most common. Accurate identification of metastasis, whether at diagnosis or at recurrence, carries significant prognostic and management implications. Multiple studies have demonstrated improved sensitivity for the detection of distant bony metastatic disease at diagnosis or recurrence among patients with osteosarcoma using FDG PET as compared to conventional imaging alone. The role of FDG PET in identifying pulmonary metastases is less certain.

Studies have compared the performance of FDG PET and conventional imaging modalities for the identification of metastatic pulmonary nodules in osteosarcoma. The sensitivity of FDG PET to detect pulmonary metastases was explored in 43 pediatric patients with sarcoma [85]. Among 9 patients (three with osteosarcoma), 28 pulmonary nodules were present, all identified by chest CT. Twenty-one lung metastases were not identified by FDG PET, 11 of these in patients with osteosarcoma (sensitivity of 25%). All lesions that were not detected by FDG PET were <7 mm in diameter demonstrating the insensitivity of FDG PET for smaller lesions. The authors conclude that chest CT cannot be replaced with FDG PET in evaluation for pulmonary metastases in pediatric sarcomas.

Several studies have compared the sensitivity of FDG PET coupled with low-resolution chest CT for attenuation correction versus dedicated chest CT for the detection of pulmonary metastases in pediatric patients with osteosarcoma. A study of 20 pediatric patients with recurrent osteosarcoma assessed 56 pulmonary lesions (32 malignant) by either dedicated chest CT or FDG PET [69]. Fewer false negatives were observed with dedicated CT (diameter 2 and 5 mm, sensi-

tivity 93.8%) as compared to FDG PET (diameter 2–7 mm, sensitivity 84.4%). Five false positives were seen with FDG PET (specificity 79.2%) compared to seven with CT alone (specificity 70.8%). Of note, four of the false positives on CT (4–11 mm in diameter) were correctly identified as benign on FDG PET. The lower sensitivity for FDG PET as compared to dedicated chest CT in this study was attributed to the lower resolution of FDG PET which is performed during shallow respiration as compared to with breath-holding in dedicated CTs. In a study of 41 pediatric bone sarcoma patients (20 with osteosarcoma and 21 with Ewing sarcoma), FDG PET was noted to have lower sensitivity for detecting malignant pulmonary nodules than conventional imaging (80% v. 93.3%) but higher specificity (95.8% v. 87.3%) and overall accuracy (93.0% v. 88.4%) [55]. This study did not classify outcomes by histology of the tumors or provide the diagnostic data for the various types of conventional imaging. Cistaro and colleagues evaluated 36 pulmonary nodules among 11 patients with osteosarcoma; FDG PET was shown to have a sensitivity of 90.3% which was not dependent on the cut-off criterion used – visual analysis, diameter >6 mm, or maximum standardized uptake value (SUV_{max}) >1.09 [17]. The authors suggest a lower limit of resolution for osteosarcoma pulmonary metastases on FDG PET of 6 mm. For pulmonary nodules greater than 6 mm, an SUV_{max} cutoff of >1.09 was shown to have the highest combined sensitivity (90.3%), specificity (93.8%), and accuracy (92.1%) [ROC AUC 0.92]. With the lower sensitivity of FDG PET for the identification of pulmonary metastasis osteosarcoma, especially smaller nodules <6 mm, there continues to be a benefit to dedicated chest CTs in the staging of osteosarcoma. The combination of FDG PET with a dedicated chest CT has become a widely adapted modality for pediatric osteosarcoma staging offering the high sensitivity of the conventional imaging coupled with the increased specificity from the functional imaging (Fig. 9.1).

In contrast to the evaluation of pulmonary metastases, FDG PET demonstrates superiority over conventional imaging to identify bony metastases. Traditionally, evaluation for distant

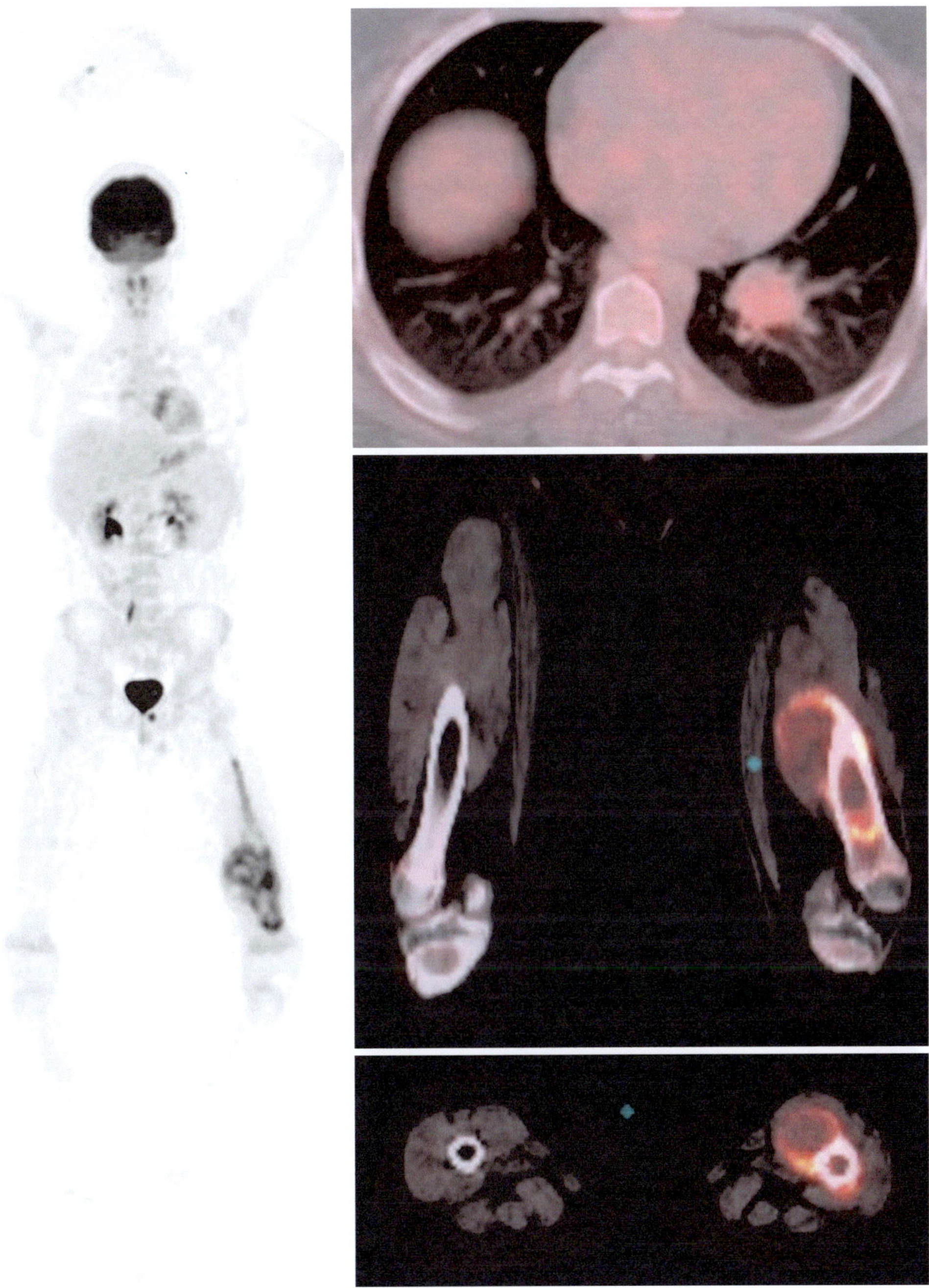

Fig. 9.1 12-year-old male with right distal femur osteosarcoma that also invades local musculature. The tumor extends proximally in the intramedullary space. Patient underwent left hip disarticulation and amputation. Eighteen months later the patient presented with hemoptysis. A 2.7 cm left lower lobe pulmonary nodule was found. The pulmonary recurrence was FDG avid with internal calcifications. No additional sites of recurrence were identified. Patient underwent left lower lobectomy

bony metastases in osteosarcoma relies on bone scintigraphy (bone scans) such as (99 m) Tc-methylene diphosphonate [(99 m)Tc-MDP]. Several studies have demonstrated higher sensitivity for identifying distant osseous metastases with FDG PET as compared with bone scintigraphy, particularly in areas around active growth plates. A study of 220 pediatric patients with osteosarcoma reviewed 833 FDG PET/bone scan pairs of which 84 studies identified potential bony metastases. As compared to bone scan, FDG PET had significantly higher sensitivity on both examination-based (95% v. 76%, $p = 0.015$) and lesion-based analysis (92% v. 74%, $p = 0.0013$) with comparable specificity (98% v. 97%) and diagnostic accuracy (98% v. 96%) [11]. A second study retrospectively examined paired FDG PET and bone scans in 39 patients (65 distant bone lesions evaluated). Lesion-based analysis of distant metastases revealed higher sensitivity with FDG PET compared to bone scan (79% v. 32%, $p = 0.035$) with similar specificity and diagnostic accuracy [46]. The combination of FDG PET with bone scan was found to have superior sensitivity in one study [11] but was not superior to FDG PET alone in the other [46]. Both studies observed significantly lower sensitivity for detection of metastases close to growth plates when using bone scan versus FDG PET. Two studies comparing FDG PET to bone scan for identification of bony metastases suggested that bone scans were equivalent or superior to FDG PET [32, 85]; however, these were small studies with limited number of identified metastatic lesions. Overall, FDG PET appears to have higher sensitivity than bone scan for identifying distant bony metastases in patients with osteosarcoma, particularly when the lesions are located close to an active growth plate and may replace bone scans in the evaluation for distant bony metastasis in osteosarcoma.

Surveillance for Local Recurrence

The identification of local recurrence of osteosarcoma can be very challenging due to postoperative changes and the frequent use of limb-sparing surgery with placement of metallic endoprostheses that complicate cross-sectional imaging. Studies have examined the use of FDG PET in diagnosing local recurrence of osteosarcoma comparing its performance to that of MRI or bone scan. Local recurrences have been reported more commonly in the soft tissues close to the area of the primary tumor and often are characterized by a peripheral and nodular uptake of the radiotracer. Multiple studies have shown that FDG PET is superior to conventional imaging such as MRI and bone scan in identifying local recurrences [2, 31, 77].

Evaluating Response to Therapy

Traditionally, response to therapy for osteosarcoma has been quantified by histological evaluation of the primary tumor resected at the time of local control (usually following two cycles of neoadjuvant chemotherapy). Following definitive local control with surgery, adjuvant chemotherapy is continued to address possible remaining micro-metastases. Greater than 90% necrosis noted on pathologic evaluation of the primary tumor after 10 weeks of therapy represents a good prognostic indicator for overall survival in osteosarcoma [58–60, 68]. Studies have evaluated the ability of FDG PET to predict both histological response and survival outcomes. The rationale for using interval FDG PET to evaluate tumor response in osteosarcoma is to guide possible changes in the therapeutic regimen (neoadjuvant chemotherapy, timing of surgery) in tumors demonstrating a suboptimal response to early treatment. FDG PET evaluation provides an earlier measure of response as opposed to waiting for histological evaluation following resection of the primary tumor at week 10 of therapy. A prospective study of 34 pediatric patients with osteosarcoma found that a lower SUV_{max} at week 5 (<4.04) and week 10 (<3.15) as well as a larger change in SUV_{max} from baseline (>60% decrease) to week 10 are predictive of a tumor histological response with greater than 90% necrosis [21]. In this study, changes in FDG PET intensity were not associated with event-free survival. Several additional studies have also observed an association between interim SUV measurements or changes in SUV and a good histological response [10, 22, 39, 53]. A meta-analysis of 8 studies that included 178 patients found that the pooled sensitivity and specificity of an interim FDG PET with an SUV <2.5 predicting a favorable histological response is 0.73 and 0.86, respectively [45]. All eight studies included adults in addition to pediatric patients. In a review article examining the results from 10 prospective and 12 retrospective studies, the authors concluded that significant evidence exists supporting the role of FDG PET in predicting histological response in osteosarcoma [13]. Not surprisingly, FDG PET serves as a superior biomarker as compared to change in tumor size for determining patient prognosis. To this point, FDG PET has not replaced the histological response noted following surgical local control. However, in the future it may provide additional information regarding early treatment response to help guide early modifications to therapy, although the role of additional chemotherapy has not been systematically evaluated.

As opposed to using FDG PET to predict another outcome proxy such as histological response to therapy, multiple studies have evaluated the ability of FDG PET to predict survival outcomes among patients with osteosarcoma. The results from these studies have been mixed. A higher SUV_{max} both at diagnosis (15 g/mL) and post-neoadjuvant chemotherapy at week 10 (5 g/mL) was associated with poorer event-free survival [19]. A higher SUV_{max} following neoadjuvant chemotherapy (3.3 g/mL) was also associated with poorer overall survival. High total lesion glycolysis (TLG) at diagnosis, a measure of average lesion SUV by tumor size, was also associated with poorer progression-free survival. Additional studies have reported similar findings of an association between tumor metabolic response to neoadjuvant therapy and progression-free survival [12, 41]. Further pediatric studies are needed to better understand the utility of FDG PET in predicting survival outcomes and whether this information could result in meaningful treatment modification. At this point, interim analysis of tumor metabolic response to initial therapy using FDG PET to guide risk-based, adaptive management, as in conditions such as Hodgkin lymphoma, has not been adopted for osteosarcoma.

Summary

The use of FDG PET has a growing role in staging newly diagnosed and recurrent osteosarcoma among pediatric patients. This is particularly true of identifying bony metastases where some have argued that it should replace bone scan. The role of FDG PET in identifying pulmonary metastases, particularly nodules <6 mm, is limited and does not eliminate the need for chest CT in the staging of osteosarcoma. Further studies are needed to determine the role of FDG PET in evaluating early response to therapy, predicting histological response, and gauging prognosis to guide risk-based, adaptive therapy.

Ewing Sarcoma

Ewing sarcoma (ES) is the second most common primary bone cancer in children, adolescents, and young adults following osteosarcoma with an annual incidence of approximately 2.9 per million per year [66] and represents approximately 3% of all pediatric cancers. Having both a male (1.2:1) and White predominance (6:1, White: Black), cases are most commonly diagnosed prior to the third decade. The Ewing family of tumors (EFTs) has been histologically characterized as small round cell sarcomas with some degree of neuroectodermal differentiation. Ewing sarcoma can develop in diverse sites, including common ES of the bone, extraosseous ES (eES), primary cutaneous ES (pcES), and Askin tumor (ES of the chest wall). Ewing family tumors are distinguished genetically by translocations between the *EWSR1* (and much less commonly *FUS*) and various partners in the ETS family of transcription factors. The most common of these translocations results in a fusion of the *EWSR1* and *FLI1* genes. In approximately 10% of cases of ES, *EWSR1* translocates next to other ETS family genes including *ERG*, *ETV1*, *ETV4*, or *FEV* [65].

The overwhelming majority of ES presents with a bony primary site most commonly in the pelvis or the diaphyseal region of appendicular long bones. The lesions are often associated with an area of local soft tissue extension. Detectable metastases are present in approximately 25% of cases at diagnosis with the most common metastatic sites being the lungs, bone marrow, or distant bones [66]. Treatment typically includes neoadjuvant chemotherapy with surgical or radiation-based local control following 12 weeks of therapy and subsequent adjuvant consolidation. Prior to the addition of chemotherapy to the treatment of ES, fewer than 10% of patients achieved long-term survival despite adequate local control with surgery, radiation, or a combination of these [66]. These outcomes indicated that micro-metastatic disease is commonly present at diagnosis and led to the inclusion of systemic therapy. The presence of detectable metastatic disease at diagnosis has proven to be the most important prognostic factor with survival rates of less than 20% for patients presenting with multiple sites of metastasis.

FDG PET in Staging Ewing Sarcoma

As with all pediatric cancers, due to the importance of staging to determine prognosis and inform local treatment approaches, the use of functional modalities such as FDG PET is increasingly common (Fig. 9.2). A meta-analysis combining data from 5 studies, 152 patients, and 279 FDG PET evaluations yielded a pooled sensitivity of 96% (95%CI: 91–99%) and specificity of 92% (95%CI: 87–96%) [82] for the detection of ES lesions on a per evaluation analysis. The area under the receiver operator curve for this analysis was 0.97. Among studies reporting per-lesion analysis, the sensitivity and specificity were lower primarily due to the inability for FDG PET to identify small lesions [38].

FDG PET performs well in identifying ES bone lesions. Several studies have reported higher sensitivity and specificity for the detection of bone metastases with FDG PET as compared to traditional imaging studies, particularly technetium-based radionuclide whole body bone scans [20, 32, 71, 85]. In a study directly comparing FDG PET and bone scintigraphy, the sensitivity and specificity for detection of bony metastases was higher for FDG PET (100% and 96%, respectively, for FDG PET versus 68% and 87% for bone scan) [32]. FDG PET is thought to be superior to bone scintigraphy since it reflects the increased glucose metabolism of the tumor rather than the secondarily increased osteoblastic activity detected by bone scan, better detects small epiphyseal lesions near growth plates which are active on bone scan, and identifies soft tissue lesions. However, FDG PET is less sensitive for ES lesions of the cranium due to the high glucose metabolism of the brain.

A prospective study of 46 pediatric and adolescent patients with sarcoma (23 with ES) demonstrated the superiority of FDG PET for identifying metastatic lesions at diagnosis over

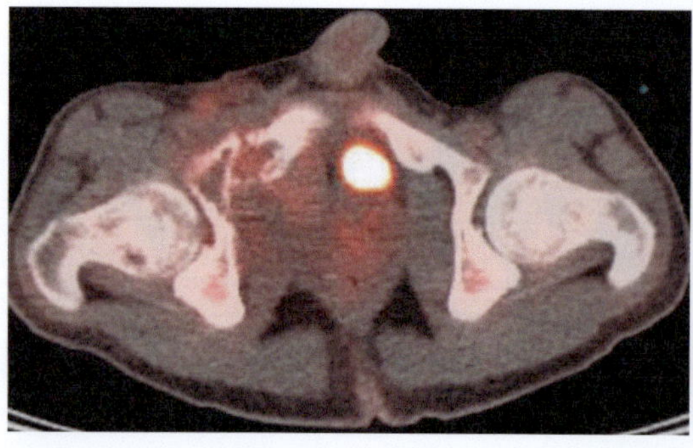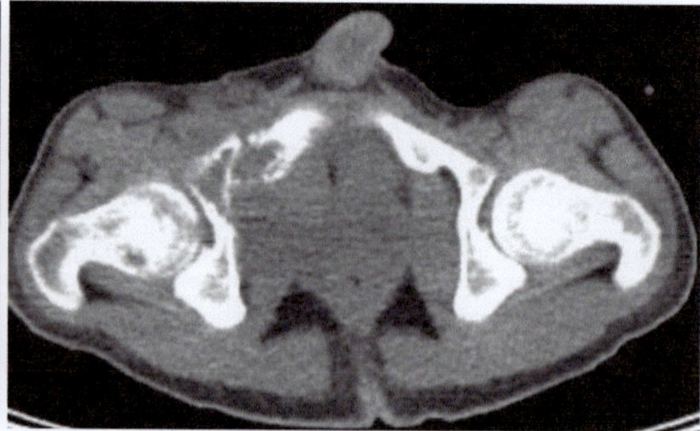

Fig. 9.2 14-year-old male with Ewing sarcoma (ES) of the right pubic ramus. An extraosseous component of the tumor is displacing the urinary bladder to the left. Asymmetric FDG avidity is noted in the subtrochanteric left femur marrow indicative of involvement with ES. Bone marrow biopsy at bilateral posterior superior iliac crests were negative

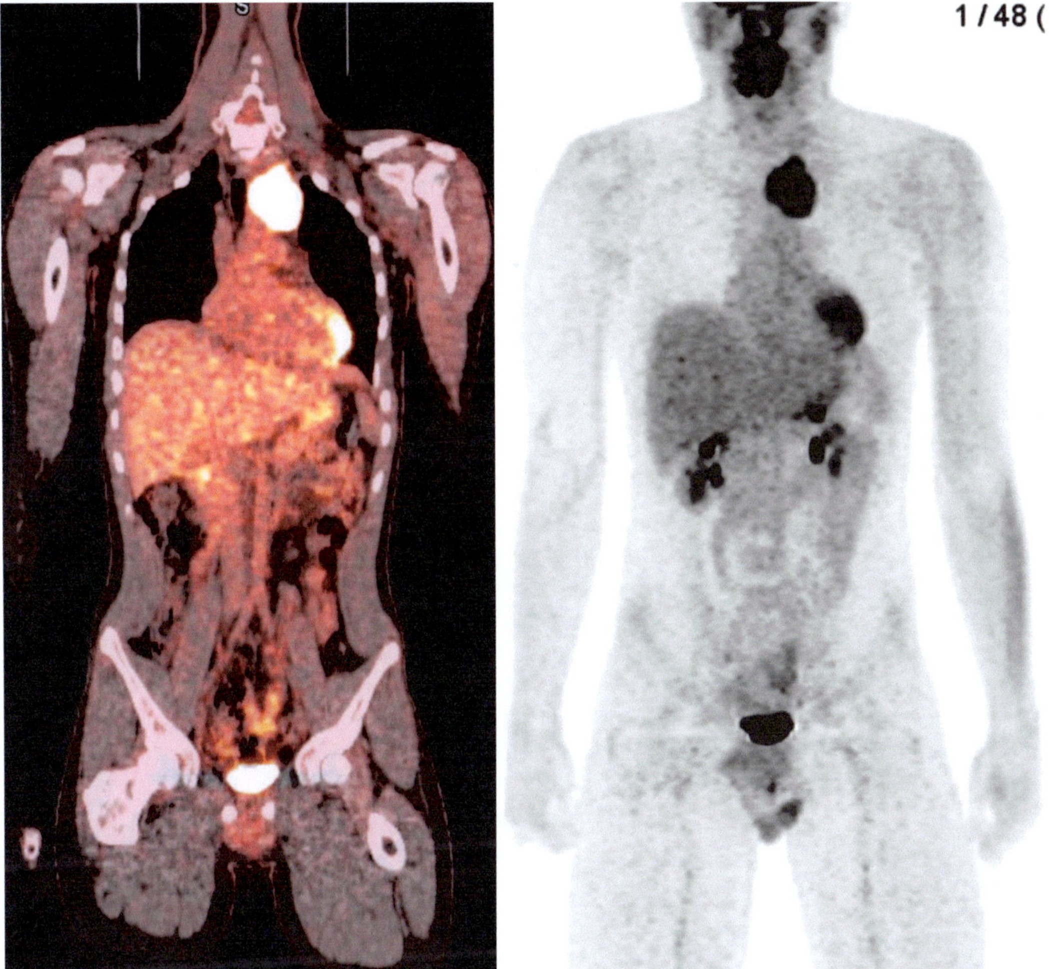

Fig. 9.3 17 year-old male with recurrent Ewing sarcoma. Initially diagnosed at the age of 14 with right lung extraosseous Ewing sarcoma that recurred in his left upper mediastinum

several forms of standard imaging including bone scintigraphy, MRI, ultrasound, and computed tomography [85]. In addition to higher sensitivity for identification of bony metastases compared to scintigraphy, FDG PET also better identified lymph node metastases among many of the cancers evaluated (sensitivity 95% for FDG PET versus 25% for other modalities); however, only one patient with ES was included in the lymph node analysis.

Regarding the detection of ES pulmonary metastases, FDG PET is inferior to standard imaging techniques. In the previously described study of 46 patients, conventional diagnostic CT had a higher sensitivity for detecting pulmonary metastases as compared to FDG PET (sensitivity of CT 100% versus 25% for FDG PET). Lesion size was the primary contributing factor for false negatives with FDG PET. Lesions smaller than 7 mm were not detected by the FDG PET with low-resolution CT. In a study of 39 patients with ES, FDG PET has a sensitivity for detecting pulmonary metastases of 56% and specificity of 91%, while CT had a sensitivity of 100% (using the criteria of any lesion larger than 5 mm or multiple lesions less than 5 mm to define a positive CT) and specificity of 78% [30]. Several studies have reported improved detection of local and distant ES lesions through the combination of FDG PET with conventional imaging such as diagnostic CT [16, 34, 57, 81, 85] (Fig. 9.3). With demonstrated superiority in identifying distant metastases, especially bony lesions and those that fall outside the field of conventional imaging, FDG PET has become incorporated into routine whole body diagnostic staging of pediatric bone sarcomas.

Multiple studies have also demonstrated that FDG PET has high sensitivity and specificity for detecting recurrent osseous ES [2, 16, 34, 57, 61, 76]. For several of its clinical trials, the Children's Oncology Group has recommended FDG PET for baseline and interim evaluation. FDG PET was a required evaluation on the latest ES study, AEWS1221. Combining FDG PET with the structural and anatomic evaluation of conventional imaging can provide highly sensitive and specific staging information to inform treatment decisions. One such algorithm was proposed by Newman et al. to evaluate bony ES lesions. If an initial FDG PET is negative, further imaging for bony metastases is likely unnecessary. With an initial positive FDG PET demonstrating distant bony lesions, further imaging with a bone scan may be beneficial in identifying additional areas of osseous metastasis [63].

Response to Therapy and Treatment Outcomes

Several studies have evaluated the ability of FDG PET to determine ES response to chemotherapy and to predict survival outcomes. Early PET response may be used to guide measures of local control and subsequent consolidative adjuvant therapy. Several studies have reported a correlation between histological response and FDG PET measures following neoadjuvant therapy [33, 37, 42, 43, 71]. In a study of 50 pediatric and adolescent patients with ES who received neoadjuvant chemotherapy and underwent local control with surgical resection, pretreatment and presurgery FDG PETs were obtained. In addition to the extent of necrosis, lower standard uptake values (SUVs) noted on FDG PET following neoadjuvant therapy were associated with improved event-free and overall 3-year survival outcomes [71]. Of note, the median follow-up time for this study was only 27 months despite the possibility

of late recurrence in Ewing sarcoma. A smaller study of 36 ES patients also demonstrated that decreased SUV on post-neoadjuvant FDG PET was significantly associated with improved 4-year progression-free survival. This demonstrates that PET-determined response to neoadjuvant chemotherapy is an indicator of outcome. While use of this information to guide response-adapted therapy in ES has yet to be adopted, such information may provide an additional data point to consider when planning local control and adjuvant consolidation.

Summary

Among pediatric and adolescent patients with ES family tumors, FDG PET can improve the detection of non-pulmonary metastatic disease both at diagnosis and at recurrence over conventional imaging modalities. FDG PET is particularly useful in identifying sites of bony metastasis and can be beneficial in identifying areas of soft tissue spread such as in lymph nodes. As a single modality, FDG PET is inferior to diagnostic CT for the detection of pulmonary ES metastases. The combination of FDG PET with conventional modalities such as a dedicated chest CT increases the sensitivity and specificity of the studies. FDG PET is increasingly being incorporated into pediatric cooperative group research trials as a recommended modality for staging. Although promising, the use of FDG PET for assessing response to treatment and predicting clinical outcomes remains under investigation and at this time is not routinely used to guide response-adapted treatment modifications.

Rhabdomyosarcoma

Rhabdomyosarcoma (RMS) is a tumor of mesenchymal cell origin that expresses immunohistochemical markers of skeletal muscle differentiation. RMS is the most common soft tissue sarcoma among pediatric patients, with an annual incidence of 4.7 cases per one million children and adolescents. The majority of cases occur in the first decade of life [78]. While these neoplasms can develop in most any anatomical location, common sites include the head and neck region (40%), genitourinary tract (25%), and extremities (20%). Several well-described factors are associated with prognosis for rhabdomyosarcoma including primary site, size of tumor, histology, regional lymph node involvement, extent of disease post local surgery, and presence of distant metastases. Approximately 20% of cases present with distant metastatic lesions. Although pulmonary metastases are most common, regional lymph nodes, bones, or bone marrow can be involved. Outcomes are considerably poorer among patients with metastatic disease at presentation compared to those with localized disease. As with other pediatric sarcomas, treatment generally consists of neoadjuvant chemotherapy followed by local control with surgery and/or radiation and subsequent adjuvant consolidation chemotherapy to eradicate micro-metastases.

The WHO Classification of Tumours of Soft Tissue and Bone classifies rhabdomyosarcoma into four histological subtypes: embryonal (ERMS), alveolar (ARMS), pleomorphic, and spindle cell/sclerosing. Pleomorphic and spindle cell are rare in children. Although histology has classically defined RMS subtypes, genomic studies of RMS now classify pediatric RMS into a low mutational burden tumor class characterized by chromosomal rearrangements that result in the fusion oncoproteins *PAX3-FOXO1* or *PAX7-FOXO1* (typically with alveolar histology) and those with a higher mutational burden but without *FOXO1* rearrangement (typically embryonal histology) [65]. These distinctions have prognostic and treatment implications.

FDG PET in Staging Rhabdomyosarcoma

Accurate staging of rhabdomyosarcoma is essential to guide appropriate surgery and radiation. Traditionally, staging of rhabdomyosarcoma included imaging of the primary tumor with MRI or CT, evaluation for pulmonary nodules with chest CT, bone scintigraphy, bone marrow evaluation, as well as lumbar puncture for patients with parameningeal disease. Since approximately 20% of cases present with metastases at diagnosis and are associated with significantly poorer outcomes, improved accuracy of staging could significantly impact the care of rhabdomyosarcoma. In a systematic review of 8 studies including 272 patients with rhabdomyosarcoma, researchers found that the sensitivity and specificity for identifying metastatic disease in lymph nodes was higher with FDG PET as compared to conventional imaging (MRI, CT, ultrasound) [64] (Figs. 9.4 and 9.5). Sensitivity for FDG PET ranged from 80% to 100% with specificity of 89–100%. Pooled estimates were not calculated due to the small number of combined observations. Overall identification of distant metastatic lesions was improved with FDG PET; however, the detection of pulmonary nodules was not better than conventional imaging, a finding similar to osteosarcoma and Ewing sarcoma [3, 30, 70]. Identification of bone and bone marrow metastases was higher using FDG PET as compared to traditional technetium bone scintigraphy (bone scan) [25, 26, 72, 80] leading some authors to suggest the replacement of bone scans with FDG PET in the staging assessment of patients with rhabdomyosarcoma [26]. However, there were small numbers of patients evaluated in these studies.

FDG PET for Predicting Outcomes in Rhabdomyosarcoma

The ability of FDG PET at diagnosis and during treatment to predict survival outcomes and success of local control has been studied. A retrospective study of 107 patients with rhabdomyosarcoma demonstrated that FDG PET intensity at diagnosis (SUV cutoff of 9.5), continued FDG PET positivity following induction chemotherapy, and residual positivity following local control were associated with poorer 3-year progression-free and overall survival [15]. Alveolar subtype and more advanced conditions were more highly represented in this study than

A. B. Smitherman et al.

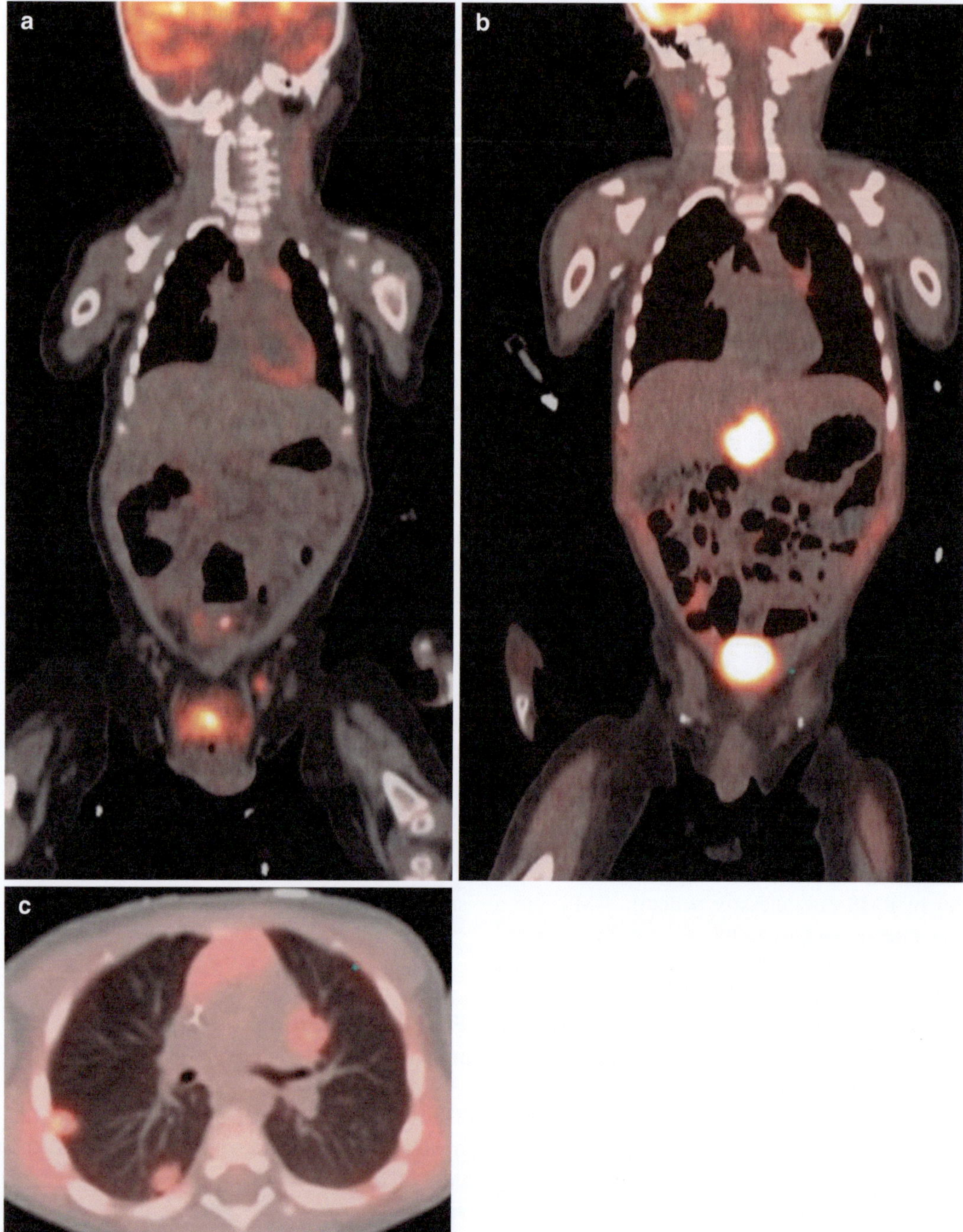

Fig. 9.4 Patient with FOXO-1 negative perineal rhabdo-myosarcoma. (**a**) was acquired at diagnosis (4 months old) demonstrating perineal primary at the base of the penis adjacent to the corpus spongiosum. FDG avid left inguinal lymph node determined to be involved with rhabdomyo-sarcoma following excision and histological evaluation. (**b**) and (**c**) acquired at completion of initial therapy demonstrating new metastatic lesions to the lungs and liver (segment III) confirmed by histological evaluation of pulmonary nodules

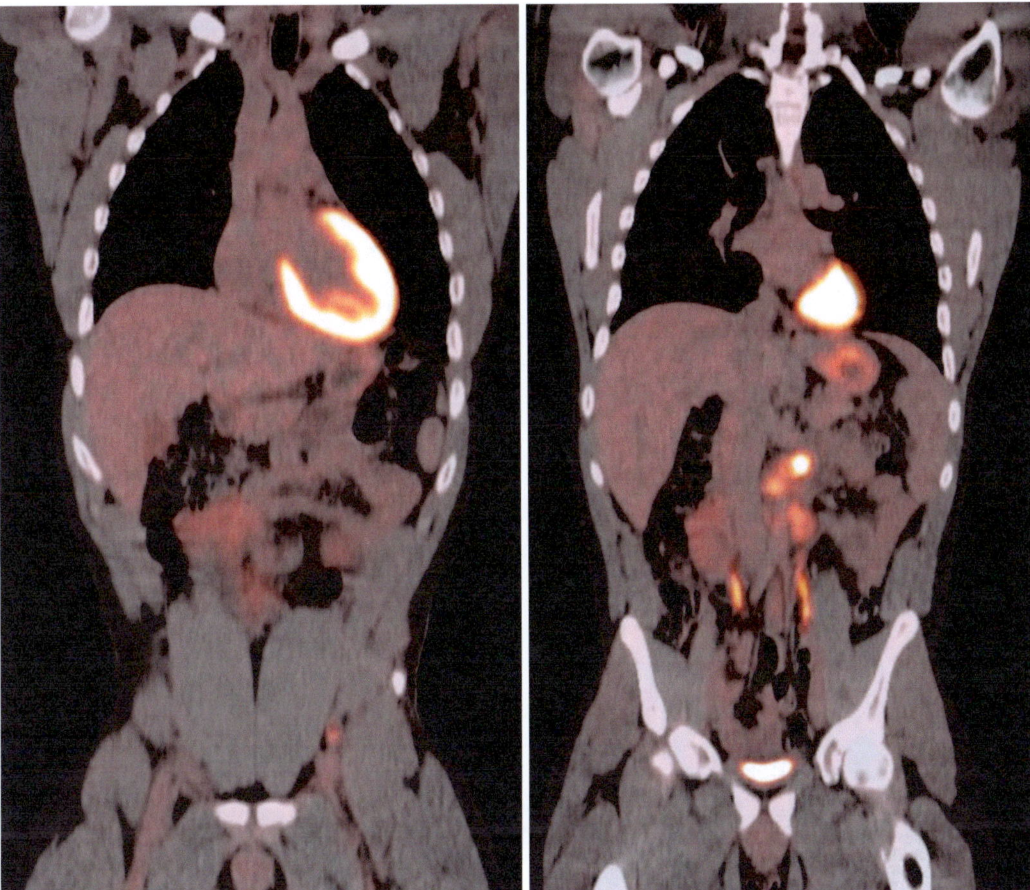

Fig. 9.5 19-year-old male with paratesticular FOXO-1 negative rhabdomyosarcoma. Patient was referred following left radical orchiectomy for further evaluation. Multiple strongly FDG avid para-aortic and infrarenal lymph nodes noted. A left iliac lymph node was also noted to be positive. Patient underwent retroperitoneal and left iliac lymph node dissection. Eight of nine para-aortic lymph nodes were involved with rhabdomyosarcoma, the largest 2.7 cm. No left iliac lymph nodes were involved with rhabdomyosarcoma. The FDG avidity seen in the left iliac nodes was likely related to prior orchiectomy

typically observed, suggesting that these findings may only be relevant for patients with poorer prognostic features. However, the authors suggest that this information may be used to modify both local control and consolidation therapy to improve outcomes in these high-risk populations. A more recent study combining results from two COG cooperative studies of intermediate- and high-risk RMS patients reported no difference in 3-year progression-free survival between patients with complete metabolic response versus those without a complete response on FDG PET either following induction chemotherapy or local con-trol with radiation [40]. Among patients without metastatic disease at diagnosis, a complete response after 4 weeks of adjuvant therapy was associated with improved 3-year EFS, although not statistically significant (67% with CR as compared to 52% with PR/SD/PD, $p = 0.65$). As only three patients experienced a CR, the study may have lacked the power necessary to confirm no difference in EFS between the groups. Further study is needed to determine the role of FDG PET in assessing response to therapy and for guiding modifications in treatment. The current COG intermediate-risk RMS study (ARST1431) evaluates this question and includes a secondary aim examining the association between interim FDG PET results after week 9 of induction and survival outcomes.

Summary

Among pediatric and adolescent patients with RMS, FDG PET appears to offer an advantage over conventional imaging for identifying distant sites of bone and soft tissue metastasis. This is particularly true for the identification of regional and distant lymph node involvement, more commonly seen with RMS as compared to other sarcomas. Research is ongoing to better understand the utility of interim FDG PET is predicting survival outcomes with the potential for guiding risk-adapted therapy.

Nonrhabdomyosarcoma Soft Tissue Sarcomas

Soft tissue sarcomas account for approximately 7% of cancers among children and adolescents [66]. Rhabdomyosarcoma constitutes one-half of the soft tissue sarcomas in children and adolescents. The other half are collectively known as nonrhabdomyosarcoma soft tissue sarcomas (NRSTS) or adult-type soft tissue sarcomas, a heterogeneous group of tumors that arise from various mesenchymal progenitor cells. NRSTS is more prevalent than rhabdomyosarcoma in infants and adolescents/young adults. NRSTS constitute a large number of rare tumors. Common histological subtypes of NRSTS among children and adolescents include synovial sarcoma, malignant peripheral nerve sheath tumors, fibrosarcoma, and leiomyosarcoma [67, 79]. Several NRSTS subtypes are associated with genetic predisposition conditions such as Li-Fraumeni syndrome (various mutations in the *TP-53* gene), mutations in the retinoblastoma gene, neurofibromatosis type 1, and familial adenomatous polyposis.

Accurate diagnosis of NRSTS is complex and requires integration of histological, immunohis-tochemical, molecular, cytogenetic, and clinical factors. Many of these tumors harbor characteristic genetic changes that are increasingly used for enhanced diagnostic precision. Mutations in gene coding for tumor suppressor proteins, growth factors, and signaling pathway elements are commonly associated with this family of tumors. For some NRSTS, localized and low-grade disease is treated with surgical resection alone. Treatment of high-grade and non-localized NRSTS generally includes chemotherapy such as ifosfamide and an anthracycline given in combination with local control measures. Radiation is used depending on the extent of resection and tumor margins.

Several prognostic factors are used to stratify NRSTS. Most importantly is the extent of disease (localized versus metastatic). Other prognostic factors include the histological grade, tumor size, and extent of surgical resection. Determining the extent of disease for NRSTS has historically been performed with CT or MRI. Because lymph node involvement is rare for most NRSTSs, lymph node evaluation is not routinely performed. However, some aggressive subtypes may have regional lymph node involvement in up to 15% of cases [24]. Subtypes associated with higher risk of lymph node involvement include clear cell sarcomas, epithelioid sarcomas, and angiosarcomas [47]. The addition of whole body metabolic imaging with FDG PET may help address the limitations of conventional cross-sectional imaging in the initial disease evaluation and accurate staging of pediatric patients with NRSTS.

FDG PET in Staging NRSTS

FDG PET is increasingly being used in the diagnostic evaluation and staging of NRSTS, the utility of which is a common object of study. A recently published study including 26 pediatric patients with either rhabdomyosarcoma or NRSTS (6 patients) reported increased identification of lymph node metastases with FDG PET [24]. Of 84 metastatic lesions identified in the study, 16 were identified by both FDG PET and conventional CT or MRI, 12 were identified by FDG PET alone (primarily in lymph nodes), and 56 were identified only with CT or MRI (lung metastases). This study supports many others that have demonstrated benefit for adding functional imaging with FDG PET to conventional anatomical imaging for the identification of soft tissue) metastases such as lymph node involvement while cautioning regarding the lack of sensitivity of FDG PET for identifying pulmonary metastases. The authors conclude that FDG PET is beneficial when added to conventional imaging for precise initial staging of pediatric soft tissue sarcomas and could be included in routine initial evaluation (Figs. 9.6 and 9.7).

Response to Treatment

FDG PET may also be useful in assessing early response to treatment or serving as a surrogate for early histological response to therapy in NRSTS. Multiple studies among adults with soft tissue sarcomas have reported an association between the reduction of FDG avidity and early histological response, response to therapy, and survival outcomes [5, 23, 44]. As studies of interim FDG PET for the assessment of response in pediatric soft tissue sarcomas are lacking, this question has been incorporated into the recent NRG and Children's Oncology Group NRSTS treatment study, ARST1321. The study aims to associate FDG PET findings following neoadjuvant therapy with pathological response and event-free survival. At this time the study has closed to enrollment, but data collection continues.

Malignant Transformation of Benign Neurogenic Tumors

In addition to improving the accuracy of diagnostic staging and providing a modality for the early assessment of therapy response among pediatric patients with soft tissue sarcomas, FDG PET may

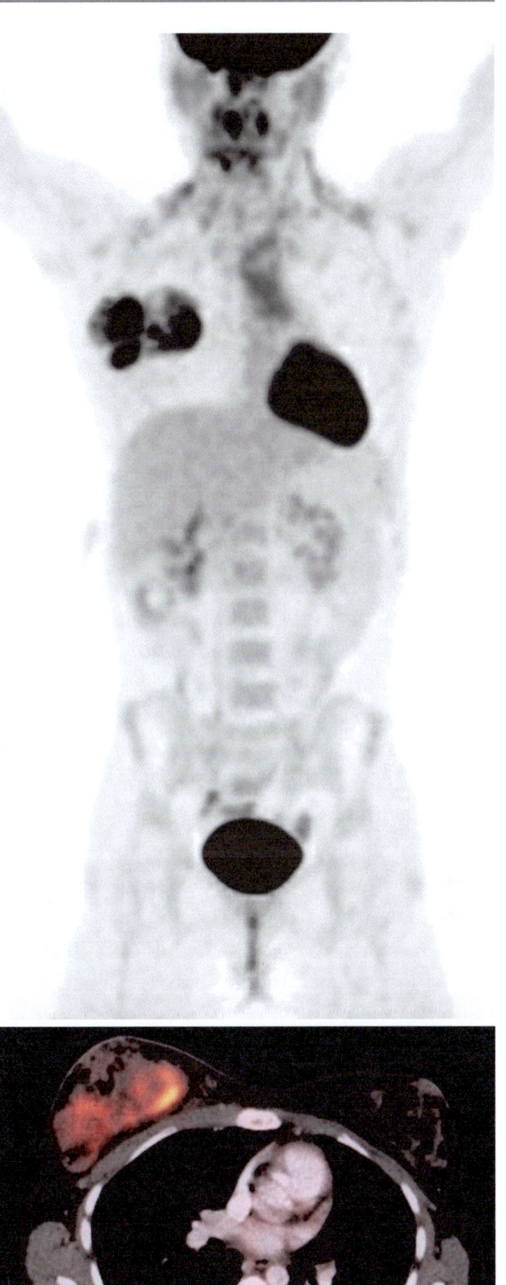

Fig. 9.6 17-year-old female with angiosarcoma localized to the right breast. Patient was treated with neoadjuvant chemotherapy and radiation followed by total resection and adjuvant consolidation chemotherapy

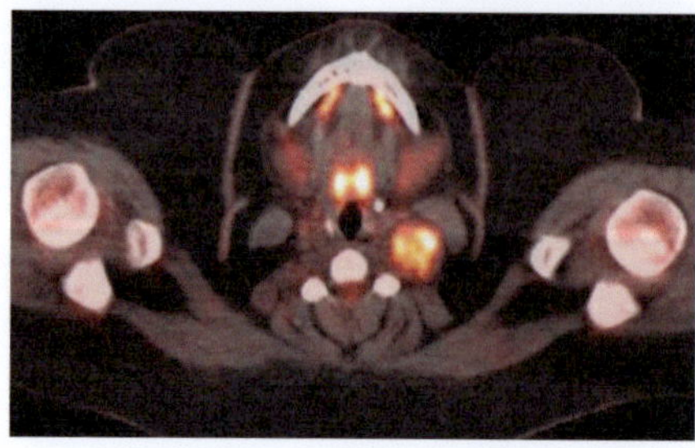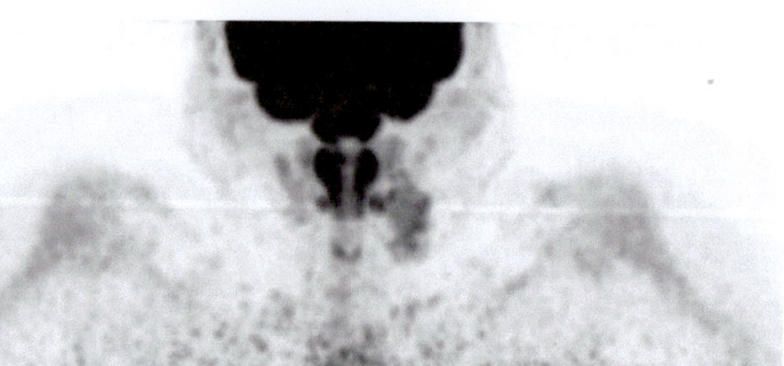

Fig. 9.7 14-year-old female with left neck mixed low-grade fibromyxoid sarcoma/sclerosing epithelioid fibrosarcoma. The lesion had slowly grown over the course of 12 months becoming increasingly painful prompting medical evaluation. She underwent gross total resection with residual microscopic margins. She was subsequently treated with radiation therapy as consolidation

have a role in the management of specific NRSTS subtypes. One such function may be to help identify the malignant transformation of benign neurogenic tumors in patients with neurofibromatosis type 1 (NF-1). Individuals with NF-1 often develop benign tumors (such as subcutaneous neurofibromas or plexiform neurofibromas) that can degenerate into malignant peripheral nerve sheath tumors (MPNST). Approximately 10% of patients with NF-1 will develop an MPNST over their lifetime, and MPNSTs represent the leading cause of mortality among these patients [84]. Numerous studies among adult patients with NF-1 have demonstrated the efficacy of using FDG PET to discriminate between benign and malignant neurogenic tumors [4, 6–8, 14, 18, 27, 28, 49, 51, 83]. Two studies that primarily included pediatric patients <18 years old also demonstrated that FDG PET can be used to detect the malignant transformation of benign neurogenic tumors into MPNST in this population helping to guide decisions regarding biopsy, excision, and further treatment [29, 84].

Summary

As with other pediatric sarcomas, FDG PET has proven to be beneficial when coupled with conventional imaging for the diagnostic staging of NRSTS. This is particularly true for the identification of regional lymph node and distant soft tissue metastases; however, the sensitivity of FDG PET for the identification of pulmonary metastasis is lower than that of CT highlighting the continued role of conventional imaging modalities for pediatric NRSTS staging. A growing body of evidence suggests that FDG PET may have a role in determining early response to therapy and guiding subsequent treatment, but further study to confirm this is required and currently underway. FDG PET appears beneficial in distinguishing benign from malignant neurogenic tumors among patients with NF-1 and can help guide the biopsy and excision decisions for these tumors.

References

1. American Cancer Society (ACS). Survival rates for osteosarcoma 2019. Retrieved from https://www.cancer.org/cancer/osteosarcoma/detection-diagnosis-staging/survival-rates.html
2. Arush MW, Israel O, Postovsky S, Militianu D, Meller I, Zaidman I, Bar-Shalom R. Positron emission tomography/computed tomography with 18fluoro-deoxyglucose in the detection of local recurrence and distant metastases of pediatric sarcoma. Pediatr Blood Cancer. 2007;49(7):901–5. https://doi.org/10.1002/pbc.21150.
3. Barger RL Jr, Nandalur KR. Diagnostic performance of dual-time 18F-FDG PET in the diagnosis of pulmonary nodules: a meta-analysis. Acad Radiol. 2012;19(2):153–8. https://doi.org/10.1016/j.acra.2011.10.009.
4. Bensaid B, Giammarile F, Mognetti T, Galoisy-Guibal L, Pinson S, Drouet A, Combemale P. Utility of 18 FDG positon emission tomography in detection of sarcomatous transformation in neurofibromatosis type 1. Ann Dermatol Venereol. 2007;134(10 Pt 1):735–41. https://doi.org/10.1016/s0151-9638(07)92528-4.

5. Benz MR, Czernin J, Allen-Auerbach MS, Tap WD, Dry SM, Elashoff D, Eilber FC. FDG-PET/CT imaging predicts histopathologic treatment responses after the initial cycle of neoadjuvant chemotherapy in high-grade soft-tissue sarcomas. Clin Cancer Res. 2009;15(8):2856–63. https://doi.org/10.1158/1078-0432.CCR-08-2537.

6. Benz MR, Czernin J, Dry SM, Tap WD, Allen-Auerbach MS, Elashoff D, Eilber FC. Quantitative F18-fluorodeoxyglucose positron emission tomography accurately characterizes peripheral nerve sheath tumors as malignant or benign. Cancer. 2010;116(2):451–8. https://doi.org/10.1002/cncr.24755.

7. Bredella MA, Torriani M, Hornicek F, Ouellette HA, Plamer WE, Williams Z, Plotkin SR. Value of PET in the assessment of patients with neurofibromatosis type 1. AJR Am J Roentgenol. 2007;189(4):928–35. https://doi.org/10.2214/AJR.07.2060.

8. Brenner W, Friedrich RE, Gawad KA, Hagel C, von Deimling A, de Wit M, Mautner VF. Prognostic relevance of FDG PET in patients with neurofibromatosis type-1 and malignant peripheral nerve sheath tumours. Eur J Nucl Med Mol Imaging. 2006;33(4):428–32. https://doi.org/10.1007/s00259-005-0030-1.

9. Briccoli A, Rocca M, Salone M, Bacci G, Ferrari S, Balladelli A, Mercuri M. Resection of recurrent pulmonary metastases in patients with osteosarcoma. Cancer. 2005;104(8):1721–5. https://doi.org/10.1002/cncr.21369.

10. Byun BH, Kong CB, Lim I, Choi CW, Song WS, Cho WH, Lim SM. Combination of 18F-FDG PET/CT and diffusion-weighted MR imaging as a predictor of histologic response to neoadjuvant chemotherapy: preliminary results in osteosarcoma. J Nucl Med. 2013a;54(7):1053–9. https://doi.org/10.2967/jnumed.112.115964.

11. Byun BH, Kong CB, Lim I, Kim BI, Choi CW, Song WS, Lim SM. Comparison of (18)F-FDG PET/CT and (99 m)Tc-MDP bone scintigraphy for detection of bone metastasis in osteosarcoma. Skelet Radiol. 2013b;42(12):1673–81. https://doi.org/10.1007/s00256-013-1714-4.

12. Byun BH, Kong CB, Park J, Seo Y, Lim I, Choi CW, Lim SM. Initial metabolic tumor volume measured by 18F-FDG PET/CT can predict the outcome of osteosarcoma of the extremities. J Nucl Med. 2013c;54(10):1725–32. https://doi.org/10.2967/jnumed.112.117697.

13. Caldarella C, Salsano M, Isgro MA, Treglia G. The role of Fluorine-18-fluorodeoxyglucose positron emission tomography in assessing the response to neoadjuvant treatment in patients with osteosarcoma. Int J Mol Imaging. 2012;2012:870301. https://doi.org/10.1155/2012/870301.

14. Cardona S, Schwarzbach M, Hinz U, Dimitrakopoulou-Strauss A, Attigah N, Mechtersheimer section sign G, Lehnert T. Evaluation of F18-deoxyglucose positron emission tomography (FDG-PET) to assess the nature of neurogenic tumours. Eur J Surg Oncol. 2003;29(6):536–41. https://doi.org/10.1016/s0748-7983(03)00055-6.

15. Casey DL, Wexler LH, Fox JJ, Dharmarajan KV, Schoder H, Price AN, Wolden SL. Predicting outcome in patients with rhabdomyosarcoma: role of [(18)f]fluorodeoxyglucose positron emission tomography. Int J Radiat Oncol Biol Phys. 2014;90(5):1136–42. https://doi.org/10.1016/j.ijrobp.2014.08.005.

16. Charest M, Hickeson M, Lisbona R, Novales-Diaz JA, Derbekyan V, Turcotte RE. FDG PET/CT imaging in primary osseous and soft tissue sarcomas: a retrospective review of 212 cases. Eur J Nucl Med Mol Imaging. 2009;36(12):1944–51. https://doi.org/10.1007/s00259-009-1203-0.

17. Cistaro A, Lopci E, Gastaldo L, Fania P, Brach Del Prever A, Fagioli F. The role of 18F-FDG PET/CT in the metabolic characterization of lung nodules in pediatric patients with bone sarcoma. Pediatr Blood Cancer. 2012;59(7):1206–10. https://doi.org/10.1002/pbc.24242.

18. Combemale P, Valeyrie-Allanore L, Giammarile F, Pinson S, Guillot B, Goulart DM, Mognetti T. Utility of 18F-FDG PET with a semi-quantitative index in the detection of sarcomatous transformation in patients with neurofibromatosis type 1. PLoS One. 2014;9(2):e85954. https://doi.org/10.1371/journal.pone.0085954.

19. Costelloe CM, Macapinlac HA, Madewell JE, Fitzgerald NE, Mawlawi OR, Rohren EM, Marom EM. 18F-FDG PET/CT as an indicator of progression-free and overall survival in osteosarcoma. J Nucl Med. 2009;50(3):340–7. https://doi.org/10.2967/jnumed.108.058461.

20. Daldrup-Link HE, Franzius C, Link TM, Laukamp D, Sciuk J, Jurgens H, Rummeny EJ. Whole-body MR imaging for detection of bone metastases in children and young adults: comparison with skeletal scintigraphy and FDG PET. AJR Am J Roentgenol. 2001;177(1):229–36. https://doi.org/10.2214/ajr.177.1.1770229.

21. Davis JC, Daw NC, Navid F, Billups CA, Wu J, Bahrami A, Shulkin BL. (18)F-FDG uptake during early adjuvant chemotherapy predicts histologic response in pediatric and young adult patients with osteosarcoma. J Nucl Med. 2018;59(1):25–30. https://doi.org/10.2967/jnumed.117.190595.

22. Denecke T, Hundsdorfer P, Misch D, Steffen IG, Schonberger S, Furth C, Amthauer H. Assessment of histological response of paediatric bone sarcomas using FDG PET in comparison to morphological volume measurement and standardized MRI parameters. Eur J Nucl Med Mol Imaging. 2010;37(10):1842–53. https://doi.org/10.1007/s00259-010-1484-3.

23. Dimitrakopoulou-Strauss A, Strauss LG, Egerer G, Vasamiliette J, Schmitt T, Haberkorn U, Kasper B. Prediction of chemotherapy outcome in patients with metastatic soft tissue sarcomas based on dynamic FDG PET (dPET) and a multiparameter analysis. Eur

J Nucl Med Mol Imaging. 2010;37(8):1481–9. https://doi.org/10.1007/s00259-010-1435-z.

24. Elmanzalawy A, Vali R, Chavhan GB, Gupta AA, Omarkhail Y, Amirabadi A, Shammas A. The impact of (18)F-FDG PET on initial staging and therapy planning of pediatric soft-tissue sarcoma patients. Pediatr Radiol. 2020;50(2):252–60. https://doi.org/10.1007/s00247-019-04530-1.

25. Eugene T, Corradini N, Carlier T, Dupas B, Leux C, Bodet-Milin C. (1)(8)F-FDG-PET/CT in initial staging and assessment of early response to chemotherapy of pediatric rhabdomyosarcomas. Nucl Med Commun. 2012;33(10):1089–95. https://doi.org/10.1097/MNM.0b013e328356741f.

26. Federico SM, Spunt SL, Krasin MJ, Billup CA, Wu J, Shulkin B, McCarville MB. Comparison of PET-CT and conventional imaging in staging pediatric rhabdomyosarcoma. Pediatr Blood Cancer. 2013;60(7):1128–34. https://doi.org/10.1002/pbc.24430.

27. Ferner RE, Golding JF, Smith M, Calonje E, Jan W, Sanjayanathan V, O'Doherty M. [18F]2-fluoro-2-deoxy-D-glucose positron emission tomography (FDG PET) as a diagnostic tool for neurofibromatosis 1 (NF1) associated malignant peripheral nerve sheath tumours (MPNSTs): a long-term clinical study. Ann Oncol. 2008;19(2):390–4. https://doi.org/10.1093/annonc/mdm450.

28. Ferner RE, Lucas JD, O'Doherty MJ, Hughes RA, Smith MA, Cronin BF, Bingham J. Evaluation of (18) fluorodeoxyglucose positron emission tomography ((18)FDG PET) in the detection of malignant peripheral nerve sheath tumours arising from within plexiform neurofibromas in neurofibromatosis 1. J Neurol Neurosurg Psychiatry. 2000;68(3):353–7. https://doi.org/10.1136/jnnp.68.3.353.

29. Fisher MJ, Basu S, Dombi E, Yu JQ, Widemann BC, Pollock AN, Alavi A. The role of [18F]-fluorodeoxyglucose positron emission tomography in predicting plexiform neurofibroma progression. J Neuro-Oncol. 2008;87(2):165–71. https://doi.org/10.1007/s11060-007-9501-5.

30. Franzius C, Daldrup-Link HE, Sciuk J, Rummeny EJ, Bielack S, Jurgens H, Schober O. FDG-PET for detection of pulmonary metastases from malignant primary bone tumors: comparison with spiral CT. Ann Oncol. 2001;12(4):479–86. https://doi.org/10.1023/a:1011111322376.

31. Franzius C, Daldrup-Link HE, Wagner-Bohn A, Sciuk J, Heindel WL, Jurgens H, Schober O. FDG-PET for detection of recurrences from malignant primary bone tumors: comparison with conventional imaging. Ann Oncol. 2002;13(1):157–60. https://doi.org/10.1093/annonc/mdf012.

32. Franzius C, Sciuk J, Daldrup-Link HE, Jurgens H, Schober O. FDG-PET for detection of osseous metastases from malignant primary bone tumours: comparison with bone scintigraphy. Eur J Nucl Med. 2000;27(9):1305–11. https://doi.org/10.1007/s002590000301.

33. Gaston LL, Di Bella C, Slavin J, Hicks RJ, Choong PF. 18F-FDG PET response to neoadjuvant chemotherapy for Ewing sarcoma and osteosarcoma are different. Skelet Radiol. 2011;40(8):1007–15. https://doi.org/10.1007/s00256-011-1096-4.

34. Gerth HU, Juergens KU, Dirksen U, Gerss J, Schober O, Franzius C. Significant benefit of multimodal imaging: PET/CT compared with PET alone in staging and follow-up of patients with Ewing tumors. J Nucl Med. 2007;48(12):1932–9. https://doi.org/10.2967/jnumed.107.045286.

35. Gilsanz V, Hu HH, Kajimura S. Relevance of brown adipose tissue in infancy and adolescence. Pediatr Res. 2013;73(1):3–9. https://doi.org/10.1038/pr.2012.141.

36. Gorlick R, Bielack S, Teot L, Meyer J, Randall RL, Marina N. Osteosarcoma: biology, diagnosis, treatment, and remaining challenges. In: Principles and practice of pediatric oncology. 6th ed. Philadelphia: Lippincott, Williams & Wilkins; 2011. p. 1015–44.

37. Gupta K, Pawaskar A, Basu S, Rajan MG, Asopa RV, Arora B, Banavali S. Potential role of FDG PET imaging in predicting metastatic potential and assessment of therapeutic response to neoadjuvant chemotherapy in Ewing sarcoma family of tumors. Clin Nucl Med. 2011;36(11):973–7. https://doi.org/10.1097/RLU.0b013e31822f684b.

38. Gyorke T, Zajic T, Lange A, Schafer O, Moser E, Mako E, Brink I. Impact of FDG PET for staging of Ewing sarcomas and primitive neuroectodermal tumours. Nucl Med Commun. 2006;27(1):17–24. https://doi.org/10.1097/01.mnm.0000186608.12895.69.

39. Hamada K, Tomita Y, Inoue A, Fujimoto T, Hashimoto N, Myoui A, Hatazawa J. Evaluation of chemotherapy response in osteosarcoma with FDG-PET. Ann Nucl Med. 2009;23(1):89–95. https://doi.org/10.1007/s12149-008-0213-5.

40. Harrison DJ, Parisi MT, Shulkin BL, et al. 18F-2Fluoro-2deoxy-d-glucose positron emission tomography (FDG-PET) response to predict event-free survival (EFS) in intermediate risk (IR) or high risk (HR) rhabdomyosarcoma (RMS): A report from the Soft Tissue Sarcoma Committee of the Children's Oncology Group (COG). Paper presented at the ASCO Annual Meeting, Chicago, IL 2016.

41. Hawkins DS, Conrad EU 3rd, Butrynski JE, Schuetze SM, Eary JF. [F-18]-fluorodeoxy-D-glucose-positron emission tomography response is associated with outcome for extremity osteosarcoma in children and young adults. Cancer. 2009;115(15):3519–25. https://doi.org/10.1002/cncr.24421.

42. Hawkins DS, Rajendran JG, Conrad EU 3rd, Bruckner JD, Eary JF. Evaluation of chemotherapy response in pediatric bone sarcomas by [F-18]-fluorodeoxy-D-glucose positron emission tomography. Cancer. 2002;94(12):3277–84. https://doi.org/10.1002/cncr.10599.

43. Hawkins DS, Schuetze SM, Butrynski JE, Rajendran JG, Vernon CB, Conrad EU, Eary JF. [18F] Fluorodeoxyglucose positron emission tomography predicts outcome for Ewing sarcoma family of

tumors. J Clin Oncol. 2005;23(34):8828–34. https://doi.org/10.1200/JCO.2005.01.7079.

44. Herrmann K, Benz MR, Czernin J, Allen-Auerbach MS, Tap WD, Dry SM, Eilber FC. 18F-FDG-PET/CT imaging as an early survival predictor in patients with primary high-grade soft tissue sarcomas undergoing neoadjuvant therapy. Clin Cancer Res. 2012;18(7):2024–31. https://doi.org/10.1158/1078-0432.CCR-11-2139.

45. Hongtao L, Hui Z, Bingshun W, Xiaojin W, Zhiyu W, Shuier Z, Yang Y. 18F-FDG positron emission tomography for the assessment of histological response to neoadjuvant chemotherapy in osteosarcomas: a meta-analysis. Surg Oncol. 2012;21(4):e165–70. https://doi.org/10.1016/j.suronc.2012.07.002.

46. Hurley C, McCarville MB, Shulkin BL, Mao S, Wu J, Navid F, Bishop MW. Comparison of (18)F-FDG-PET-CT and bone scintigraphy for evaluation of osseous metastases in newly diagnosed and recurrent osteosarcoma. Pediatr Blood Cancer. 2016;63(8):1381–6. https://doi.org/10.1002/pbc.26014.

47. Jacobs AJ, Morris CD, Levin AS. Synovial sarcoma is not associated with a higher risk of lymph node metastasis compared with other soft tissue sarcomas. Clin Orthop Relat Res. 2018;476(3):589–98. https://doi.org/10.1007/s11999.0000000000000057.

48. Kapoor V, McCook BM, Torok FS. An introduction to PET-CT imaging. Radiographics. 2004;24(2):523–43. https://doi.org/10.1148/rg.242025724.

49. Karabatsou K, Kiehl TR, Wilson DM, Hendler A, Guha A. Potential role of 18fluorodeoxyglucose-positron emission tomography/computed tomography in differentiating benign neurofibroma from malignant peripheral nerve sheath tumor associated with neurofibromatosis 1. Neurosurgery. 2009;65(4 Suppl):A160–70. https://doi.org/10.1227/01.NEU.0000337597.18599.D3.

50. Kaste SC, Snyder SE, Metzger ML, Sandlund JT, Howard SC, Krasin M, Shulkin BL. Comparison of (11)C-Methionine and (18)F-FDG PET/CT for staging and follow-up of pediatric lymphoma. J Nucl Med. 2017;58(3):419–24. https://doi.org/10.2967/jnumed.116.178640.

51. Khiewvan B, Macapinlac HA, Lev D, McCutcheon IE, Slopis JM, Al Sannaa G, Chuang HH. The value of (1)(8)F-FDG PET/CT in the management of malignant peripheral nerve sheath tumors. Eur J Nucl Med Mol Imaging. 2014;41(9):1756–66. https://doi.org/10.1007/s00259-014-2756-0.

52. Kiratli PO, Tuncel M, Bar-Sever Z. Nuclear medicine in pediatric and adolescent tumors. Semin Nucl Med. 2016;46(4):308–23. https://doi.org/10.1053/j.semnuclmed.2016.01.004.

53. Kong CB, Byun BH, Lim I, Choi CW, Lim SM, Song WS, Lee SY. (1)(8)F-FDG PET SUVmax as an indicator of histopathologic response after neoadjuvant chemotherapy in extremity osteosarcoma. Eur J Nucl Med Mol Imaging. 2013;40(5):728–36. https://doi.org/10.1007/s00259-013-2344-8.

54. Kratochwil C, Flechsig P, Lindner T, Abderrahim L, Altmann A, Mier W, Giesel FL. (68)Ga-FAPI PET/CT: tracer uptake in 28 different kinds of cancer. J Nucl Med. 2019;60(6):801–5. https://doi.org/10.2967/jnumed.119.227967.

55. London K, Stege C, Cross S, Onikul E, Graf N, Kaspers G, Howman-Giles R. 18F-FDG PET/CT compared to conventional imaging modalities in pediatric primary bone tumors. Pediatr Radiol. 2012;42(4):418–30. https://doi.org/10.1007/s00247-011-2278-x.

56. Long NM, Smith CS. Causes and imaging features of false positives and false negatives on F-PET/CT in oncologic imaging. Insights Imaging. 2011;2(6):679–98. https://doi.org/10.1007/s13244-010-0062-3.

57. McCarville MB, Christie R, Daw NC, Spunt SL, Kaste SC. PET/CT in the evaluation of childhood sarcomas. AJR Am J Roentgenol. 2005;184(4):1293–304. https://doi.org/10.2214/ajr.184.4.01841293.

58. Meyers PA, Gorlick R, Heller G, Casper E, Lane J, Huvos AG, Healey JH. Intensification of preoperative chemotherapy for osteogenic sarcoma: results of the Memorial Sloan-Kettering (T12) protocol. J Clin Oncol. 1998;16(7):2452–8. https://doi.org/10.1200/JCO.1998.16.7.2452.

59. Meyers PA, Heller G, Healey J, Huvos A, Lane J, Marcove R, Rosen G. Chemotherapy for nonmetastatic osteogenic sarcoma: the memorial Sloan-Kettering experience. J Clin Oncol. 1992;10(1):5–15. https://doi.org/10.1200/JCO.1992.10.1.5.

60. Meyers PA, Schwartz CL, Krailo M, Kleinerman ES, Betcher D, Bernstein ML, Grier H. Osteosarcoma: a randomized, prospective trial of the addition of ifosfamide and/or muramyl tripeptide to cisplatin, doxorubicin, and high-dose methotrexate. J Clin Oncol. 2005;23(9):2004–11. https://doi.org/10.1200/JCO.2005.06.031.

61. Mody RJ, Bui C, Hutchinson RJ, Yanik GA, Castle VP, Frey KA, Shulkin BL. FDG PET imaging of childhood sarcomas. Pediatr Blood Cancer. 2010;54(2):222–7. https://doi.org/10.1002/pbc.22307.

62. Neville HL, Andrassy RJ, Lobe TE, Bagwell CE, Anderson JR, Womer RB, Wiener ES. Preoperative staging, prognostic factors, and outcome for extremity rhabdomyosarcoma: a preliminary report from the Intergroup Rhabdomyosarcoma Study IV (1991–1997). J Pediatr Surg. 2000;35(2):317–21. https://doi.org/10.1016/s0022-3468(00)90031-9.

63. Newman EN, Jones RL, Hawkins DS. An evaluation of [F-18]-fluorodeoxy-D-glucose positron emission tomography, bone scan, and bone marrow aspiration/biopsy as staging investigations in Ewing sarcoma. Pediatr Blood Cancer. 2013;60(7):1113–7. https://doi.org/10.1002/pbc.24406.

64. Norman G, Fayter D, Lewis-Light K, Chisholm J, McHugh K, Levine D, Phillips B. An emerging evidence base for PET-CT in the management of childhood rhabdomyosarcoma: systematic review. BMJ Open. 2015;5(1):e006030. https://doi.org/10.1136/bmjopen-2014-006030.

65. Pappo AS, Dirksen U. Rhabdomyosarcoma, Ewing sarcoma, and other round cell sarcomas. J Clin Oncol. 2018;36(2):168–79. https://doi.org/10.1200/JCO.2017.74.7402.

66. Pizzo PA, Poplack DG. Principles and practice of pediatric oncology. 6th ed. Philadelphia: Wolters Kluwer Health/Lippincott Williams & Wilkins; 2011.

67. Pratt CB, Pappo AS, Gieser P, Jenkins JJ, Salzbergdagger A, Neff J, Maurer H. Role of adjuvant chemotherapy in the treatment of surgically resected pediatric nonrhabdomyosarcomatous soft tissue sarcomas: a Pediatric Oncology Group Study. J Clin Oncol. 1999;17(4):1219. https://doi.org/10.1200/JCO.1999.17.4.1219.

68. Provisor AJ, Ettinger LJ, Nachman JB, Krailo MD, Makley JT, Yunis EJ, Miser JS. Treatment of non-metastatic osteosarcoma of the extremity with preoperative and postoperative chemotherapy: a report from the Children's Cancer Group. J Clin Oncol. 1997;15(1):76–84. https://doi.org/10.1200/JCO.1997.15.1.76.

69. Quartuccio N, Fox J, Kuk D, Wexler LH, Baldari S, Cistaro A, Schoder H. Pediatric bone sarcoma: diagnostic performance of (1)(8)F-FDG PET/CT versus conventional imaging for initial staging and follow-up. AJR Am J Roentgenol. 2015;204(1):153–60. https://doi.org/10.2214/AJR.14.12932.

70. Quartuccio N, Treglia G, Salsano M, Mattoli MV, Muoio B, Piccardo A, Cistaro A. The role of Fluorine-18-Fluorodeoxyglucose positron emission tomography in staging and restaging of patients with osteosarcoma. Radiol Oncol. 2013;47(2):97–102. https://doi.org/10.2478/raon-2013-0017.

71. Raciborska A, Bilska K, Drabko K, Michalak E, Chaber R, Pogorzala M, Dziuk M. Response to chemotherapy estimates by FDG PET is an important prognostic factor in patients with Ewing sarcoma. Clin Transl Oncol. 2016;18(2):189–95. https://doi.org/10.1007/s12094-015-1351-6.

72. Ricard F, Cimarelli S, Deshayes E, Mognetti T, Thiesse P, Giammarile F. Additional benefit of F-18 FDG PET/CT in the staging and follow-up of pediatric rhabdomyosarcoma. Clin Nucl Med. 2011;36(8):672–7. https://doi.org/10.1097/RLU.0b013e318217ae2e.

73. Ries, L. A., Smith, M. A., Gurney, J. G., Linet, M., Tamra, T., Young, J. L., & Bunin, G. R.. Cancer incidence and survival among children and adolescents: United States SEER Program 1975–1995 1999. Retrieved from Bethesda.

74. Rodeberg DA, Garcia-Henriquez N, Lyden ER, Davicioni E, Parham DM, Skapek SX, Hawkins DS. Prognostic significance and tumor biology of regional lymph node disease in patients with rhabdomyosarcoma: a report from the Children's Oncology Group. J Clin Oncol. 2011;29(10):1304–11. https://doi.org/10.1200/JCO.2010.29.4611.

75. SEER Program (National Cancer Institute (U.S.)), & National Cancer Institute (U.S.). Cancer incidence and survival among children and adolescents: United States SEER Program, 1975–1995. Bethesda, MD: National Cancer Institute; 1999.

76. Sharma P, Khangembam BC, Suman KC, Singh H, Rastogi S, Khan SA, Kumar R. Diagnostic accuracy of 18F-FDG PET/CT for detecting recurrence in patients with primary skeletal Ewing sarcoma. Eur J Nucl Med Mol Imaging. 2013;40(7):1036–43. https://doi.org/10.1007/s00259-013-2388-9.

77. Sharp SE, Shulkin BL, Gelfand MJ, McCarville MB. FDG PET/CT appearance of local osteosarcoma recurrences in pediatric patients. Pediatr Radiol. 2017;47(13):1800–8. https://doi.org/10.1007/s00247-017-3963-1.

78. Siegel DA, King J, Tai E, Buchanan N, Ajani UA, Li J. Cancer incidence rates and trends among children and adolescents in the United States, 2001–2009. Pediatrics. 2014;134(4):e945–55. https://doi.org/10.1542/peds.2013-3926.

79. Spunt SL, Hill DA, Motosue AM, Billups CA, Cain AM, Rao BN, Pappo AS. Clinical features and outcome of initially unresected nonmetastatic pediatric nonrhabdomyosarcoma soft tissue sarcoma. J Clin Oncol. 2002;20(15):3225–35. https://doi.org/10.1200/JCO.2002.06.066.

80. Tateishi U, Hosono A, Makimoto A, Nakamoto Y, Kaneta T, Fukuda H, Kim EE. Comparative study of FDG PET/CT and conventional imaging in the staging of rhabdomyosarcoma. Ann Nucl Med. 2009;23(2):155–61. https://doi.org/10.1007/s12149-008-0219-z.

81. Tateishi U, Yamaguchi U, Seki K, Terauchi T, Arai Y, Kim EE. Bone and soft-tissue sarcoma: preoperative staging with fluorine 18 fluorodeoxyglucose PET/CT and conventional imaging. Radiology. 2007;245(3):839–47. https://doi.org/10.1148/radiol.2453061538.

82. Treglia G, Salsano M, Stefanelli A, Mattoli MV, Giordano A, Bonomo L. Diagnostic accuracy of (1)(8)F-FDG-PET and PET/CT in patients with Ewing sarcoma family tumours: a systematic review and a meta-analysis. Skelet Radiol. 2012a;41(3):249–56. https://doi.org/10.1007/s00256-011-1298-9.

83. Treglia G, Taralli S, Bertagna F, Salsano M, Muoio B, Novellis P, Giordano A. Usefulness of whole-body fluorine-18-fluorodeoxyglucose positron emission tomography in patients with neurofibromatosis type 1: a systematic review. Radiol Res Pract. 2012b;2012:431029. https://doi.org/10.1155/2012/431029.

84. Tsai LL, Drubach L, Fahey F, Irons M, Voss S, Ullrich NJ. [18F]-Fluorodeoxyglucose positron emission tomography in children with neurofibromatosis type 1 and plexiform neurofibromas: correlation with malignant transformation. J Neuro-Oncol. 2012;108(3):469–75. https://doi.org/10.1007/s11060-012-0840-5.

85. Volker T, Denecke T, Steffen I, Misch D, Schonberger S, Plotkin M, Amthauer H. Positron emission tomog-

raphy for staging of pediatric sarcoma patients: results of a prospective multicenter trial. J Clin Oncol. 2007;25(34):5435–41. https://doi.org/10.1200/JCO.2007.12.2473.

86. Voss SD. Functional and anatomical imaging in pediatric oncology: which is best for which tumors. Pediatr Radiol. 2019;49(11):1534–44. https://doi.org/10.1007/s00247-019-04489-z.

87. Wagner LM, Kremer N, Gelfand MJ, Sharp SE, Turpin BK, Nagarajan R, Dasgupta R. Detection of lymph node metastases in pediatric and adolescent/young adult sarcoma: sentinel lymph node biopsy versus fludeoxyglucose positron emission tomography imaging-A prospective trial. Cancer. 2017;123(1):155–60. https://doi.org/10.1002/cncr.30282.

Stephen M. Moerlein, Sally W. Schwarz,
and Farrokh Dehdashti

Positron emission tomography (PET) is a unique imaging modality, as it intrinsically depends on the administration of a radiopharmaceutical to derive the information used for disease management. The images thereby derived are dependent on the tracer kinetics of the labeled drug, which are in turn dependent on the molecular and localization characteristics of the radiopharmaceutical. For this reason, an examination of radiopharmaceuticals used for cancer imaging is relevant to the broad topic of PET studies of melanoma and sarcoma.

There are several radiopharmaceuticals that have evolved from benchtop research to routine clinical use [39]. Among PET radiopharmaceuticals, the metabolic radiopharmaceutical [^{18}F]fluorodeoxyglucose (FDG), a glucose analogue, has established preeminence for clinical applications in oncology, including melanoma [45] and sarcoma [6]. Despite this success, FDG has limitations as a PET radiopharmaceutical in that it traces tissue glucose metabolic activity that is not explicitly related to oncological processes, and the specificity of images may be blunted by other concomitant processes such as inflammation.

These limitations have generated interest in the nuclear medicine community for novel radiopharmaceuticals that can be used for PET imaging of melanoma and sarcoma. Such an expansion of PET for tumor evaluation draws upon the myriad of tumor targets created by tumor heterogeneity and alternative radiopharmaceuticals that can be employed as biomarkers for these new imaging targets. Instead of measurement of glucose metabolism only, novel PET radiopharmaceuticals may allow assessment of tumor parameters like proliferation, hypoxia, receptor expression, and apoptosis. Such refinements in PET images may promote diagnostic specificity and improve therapeutic decision-making and clinical outcomes for cancer patients.

This chapter will discuss PET radiopharmaceuticals other than FDG that have been used for studies of patients with melanoma and sarcoma. An overview of PET radiopharmaceutical production methods and quality control will be presented, along with regulatory requirements for transitioning new radiotracers from preclinical evaluation to use in human subject research. The mechanisms of localization for selected PET radiopharmaceuticals will be discussed, together with clinical findings in patients with melanoma and sarcoma. The reader will be given a perspective on how future development of novel radiopharmaceuticals may proceed to improve PET for melanoma and sarcoma.

S. M. Moerlein (✉) · S. W. Schwarz · F. Dehdashti
Edward Mallinckrodt Institute of Radiology,
Washington University in St. Louis,
St. Louis, MO, USA
e-mail: moerleins@wustl.edu; schwarzs@wustl.edu;
dehdashtif@wustl.edu

© Springer Nature Switzerland AG 2021
A. H. Khandani (ed.), *PET/CT and PET/MR in Melanoma and Sarcoma*,
https://doi.org/10.1007/978-3-030-60429-5_10

PET Radiopharmaceutical Production

Radionuclides

The methodology of PET is unique in nuclear medicine in that it is dependent on coincident detection of the annihilation radiation following positron emission from a radionuclide. The emitted positron will travel only a short distance before it encounters an orbital electron. The physics of annihilation dictate that the masses of the positron and electron are converted into two 511-keV photons, emitted at approximately 180° from one another to conserve momentum. The orientation of these photons has several advantages for nuclear medicine imaging. By engineering coincident detection circuits in a ring around the subject being images, lines of detection in which the initiating decay is located within the joint field of view of two opposing detectors can be measured. Computerized consolidation of these lines of detection results in a PET image in which the distribution of radionuclide is determined.

There are several advantages of PET over conventional nuclear medicine imaging such single-photon emission tomography (SPECT). Because lead collimation is not required for image reconstruction, the sensitivity of PET detection is much greater than with conventional nuclear medicine imaging. Moreover, extremely accurate attenuation correction of PET data is accomplished by performing transmission scans of image sections using an external X-ray source. This is often accomplished via computed tomog-raphy (CT) on PET-CT so that attenuation correction and anatomic coregistration of the emission data from PET and anatomic information from CT can be ascertained during the same imaging session. By use of PET scanners with multiple rings of detectors, large fields of view can be imaged simultaneously for comprehensive measurements of tracer disposition. Because of accurate attenuation correction, time-activity data from calibrated PET scanners yield valuable information that can be used for quantitative tracer kinetic modeling. This approach has also been adopted in SPECT-CT scanners.

A further advantage of PET over conventional nuclear medicine imaging concerns the choice of radionuclides that can be used for labeling the corresponding radiopharmaceuticals. Conventional radiopharmaceuticals are labeled primarily with metallic radionuclides like ^{99m}Tc, ^{111}In, and ^{67}Ga. In order to be attached to the labeling substrate, bulky bifunctional chelating groups are needed to attach the radiometal, which precludes labeling of low-molecular-weight drugs or biochemicals. By contrast, positron-emitting radionuclides are available from such elements as carbon (^{11}C) and fluorine (^{18}F). These radionuclides can be incorporated into molecular structures via covalent bonds, facilitating a great diversity in the types of radiopharmaceuticals that can be formulated. Note that many positron-emitting radionuclides are also metallic, but the availability of covalently bound radionuclides is a unique advantage to PET compared to conventional nuclear medicine imaging.

Table 10.1 gives relevant physical characteristics of radionuclides commonly used for labeling

Table 10.1 Radionuclides used in PET radiopharmaceuticals[a]

Nuclide	Half-life	β^+ Branching fraction (%)	$E_{\beta\,max}$ (MeV)
Cyclotron-produced			
Oxygen-15	122 s	1.00	1.73
Nitrogen-13	10.0 min	1.00	1.20
Carbon-11	20.4 min	1.00	0.96
Fluorine-18	110 min	0.97	0.63
Copper-64	12.7 h	0.29	0.65
Generator-available			
Gallium-68	68 min	0.89	1.89

[a]Data from [14]

PET radiopharmaceuticals [14]. Information is provided regarding radionuclide source, half-life, positron energy, and branching ratio. Missing from the table is generator-available rubidium-82 ($T_{1/2}$ = 1.27 min). Although ^{82}Rb is widely used for myocardial perfusion measurements, it has not been used for PET evaluation of sarcoma or melanoma.

The nuclides in Table 10.1 are divided into those that are cyclotron-produced and those that are available as the daughter of a generator system. This categorization has practical relevance in that it circumscribes the availability of the radionuclide, as well as the utility of the radionuclide as a label for radiopharmaceuticals. The advantage of generator-produced radionuclides is that they permit formulation of PET radiopharmaceuticals without the necessity of a costly medical cyclotron. The disadvantage of generator-available radionuclides is that (like ^{99m}Tc in conventional nuclear medicine) they are metallic and the type of radiopharmaceuticals developed using them is limited by the chelation chemistry required. In contrast, most of the cyclotron-produced radionuclides in the table can be incorporated into radiopharmaceutical structures via covalent bonds. This gives great versatility to the types of radiopharmaceuticals that can be synthesized, and the literature is correspondingly replete with different categories of PET tracers labeled with these cyclotron radionuclides.

Important characteristics of radionuclides to be used for PET include half-life, positron flux, and mean energy of the emitted positron. Half-life is clearly important for radiopharmaceuticals because it defines the time available for preparation, distribution, and image acquisition. For this reason, oxygen-15 (^{15}O), nitrogen-13 (^{13}N), (and ^{82}Rb) have found limited use for PET study of melanoma or sarcoma. Their short half-lives of these nuclides limit their utility to PET measurement of organ perfusion or other physiological processes with rapid kinetics. Note that excessively long half-lives are also suboptimal because it creates unnecessary radiation burden to the subject being imaged. For this reason, the most popular radionuclides in PET have half-lives that are less than 2 h long.

Positron flux and mean positron energy (E_β) are both important determinants of the usefulness of a radionuclide for PET imaging. Ideally, the positron flux should be close to 100% (branching fraction 1.00) to make the PET signal as robust as possible and to minimize patient-absorbed radiation dose. Decays that proceed without emission of a positron do not contribute to the PET signal but instead generate emissions that can be absorbed in the body of the subject being imaged and increase radiation burden. Practically speaking, such non-imaged decays should be minimized as much as possible. Note in Table 10.1 that for the common PET nuclides, the β^+ branching ratios are all close to unity, minimizing non-informational decay processes.

Positron energy (E_β) affects the image quality of PET, since it corresponds to the distance the positron travels prior to undergoing annihilation, and production of the coincidence radiation that is detected by PET scanners. Ideally, E_β should be as low as possible to maximize PET image resolution. From this perspective, image degradation is more of a concern with gallium-68 (^{68}Ga)- and ^{15}O (and ^{82}Rb)-labeled PET radiopharmaceuticals, since E_β is relatively high for these nuclides.

Carbon-11 This radionuclide can be used to substitute for a stable carbon atom in a biomolecule of interest to create a PET tracer with identical properties to the original stable carbon molecule. An important advantage of ^{11}C as a radiolabel is the large number of drug and biochemical structures that contain carbon in their molecular framework, sites that potentially can be substituted with ^{11}C. An additional beneficial characteristic of ^{11}C is that the 20-min half-life is short enough to permit repeated studies to be performed in the same subject within a relatively short time, as well as sufficiently long to be used in appropriately designed multistep synthetic procedures.

Fluorine-18 Fluorine-18 is a unique radionuclide due to the chemical properties of the element. The high electronegativity confers unusual properties on biomolecules, and fluorine is often found on drug structures for this reason. Indeed, the fortuitous character of metabolic trapping that is used to advantage with FDG-PET derives from the introduction of fluorine onto the naturally occurring glucose molecule. The half-life of almost 2 h is very convenient for radiosynthesis, purification, and distribution to remote imaging sites. Radiopharmaceutical batch yields can be very high, making multidose preparation of radiopharmaceuticals feasible.

Oxygen-15 and Nitrogen-13 Like ^{11}C, positron-emitting ^{15}O and ^{13}N are potential choices for labeling considering their stable isotopes are ubiquitous in biologically active organic molecules. However, unlike ^{11}C, their short half-lives of 2 min for ^{15}O and 10 min for ^{13}N create severe constraints on their utility as labels for PET radiopharmaceuticals. Not only are the radiosynthetic options limited, but the short time available for PET imaging limits the biological functions that can be studied with these nuclides. On the other hand, for the appropriate applications, the short half-lives of ^{15}O or ^{13}N make repeated studies during a single imaging session very convenient with these nuclides. Examples of this would be brain activation studies using [^{15}O]water or cardiac rest/stress protocols using [^{13}N]ammonia.

Copper-64 Copper-64 decays by β^+ (18%) and β^- emission (39%), as well as via electron capture (43%), making it suitable for PET imaging as well as radiotherapy. The disadvantage of low positron yield for ^{64}Cu is compensated by the relatively long half-life (12.7 h) of the nuclide, making it especially useful for imaging biological processes that are slow (such as antibody imaging), and for long-distance shipping from production centers to imaging sites. Although ^{64}Cu-labeled PET tracers have not yet been applied to study patients with melanoma or sarcoma, it has been used preclinically [4, 34]. Copper-64 has found widespread application for the study of other tumor types, and it is likely that over time, there will be extension to this oncology subspecialty as well. The radionuclide has metallic characteristics and is attached to molecular structures via bifunctional chelates.

Gallium-68 An alternative to cyclotron production of positron-emitting radionuclides is to extract a daughter radionuclide from a radionuclide generator system. Generators have the advantage of facilitating clinical studies at PET sites that lack an on-site cyclotron, or as a supplemental radionuclide source at busy cyclotron sites with insufficient beam time available to supply all radionuclide demands. In these situations, generators may provide daughter radionuclides and associated radiopharmaceuticals on demand, once adequate ingrowth has occurred since the last elution.

The ^{68}Ge/^{68}Ga system is perhaps the most important generator in PET nuclear medicine today. The parent nuclide germanium-68 has a half-life of 270.8 days, giving a practical shelf-life to the generator of 9–12 months. Daughter nuclide ^{68}Ga is valuable as a PET radiopharmaceutical label because its half-life of 68 min corresponds to the tracer kinetics of small-molecular-weight compounds such as peptides, antibody fragments, aptamers, oligonucleotides, and nanoparticles. In addition, local (ground) distribution of ^{68}Ga-labeled radiopharmaceuticals throughout a metropolitan area is feasible.

The coordination chemistry of Ga^{3+} is well established, and several bifunctional chelates that are resistant to in vivo transchelation are available for use in labeling radiopharmaceuticals. Although the positron energy is higher than other radionuclides listed in Table 10.1, potentially causing lower image resolution, this does not seriously limit the clinical utility of ^{68}Ga. The ^{68}Ge/^{68}Ga generator has potential to substantially increase accessibility of clinical PET procedures to the patient population [25, 43, 66].

Radiolabeling Techniques

An overarching requirement of all radiolabeling techniques used for PET radiopharmaceutical production is that chemical steps must be rapid and give high radiochemical yields. This requirement is essential because of the short half-lives of PET radionuclides, the limited amounts of starting activities that are available, and the need to do quality control on the finished drug product before use in human subjects.

With this understanding in mind, the following sections give an overview of radiolabeling methodologies for the different PET radionuclides, whose chemistries differ depending on the specific element.

Carbon-11 Carbon-11 is an important positron-emitting radionuclide for labeling biomolecules because of the ubiquitous presence of carbon in drug structures and biochemicals. The nuclide is produced with medical cyclotrons via proton irradiation of pure ^{14}N according to the nuclear reaction $^{14}N(p,\alpha)^{11}C$. Two major ^{11}C target products for radiosyntheses are [^{11}C]carbon dioxide (CO) and [^{11}C]methane (CH_4), which are formed when small amounts of oxygen or hydrogen, respectively, are present in the target. These labeling precursors can readily be converted to reactive compounds like [^{11}C]methyl iodide (CH_3I), hydrogen [^{11}C]cyanide (HCN), [^{11}C] cyanogen bromide (CNBr), and [^{11}C]phosgene (Cl_2CO) [5]. These labeling reagents are used to insert ^{11}C into specific molecular sites of the substrate dictated by the directionality of the organic reaction that is utilized. The reactions used with ^{11}C are rapid and completed within a few minutes of heating. Further molecular modification of labeled intermediates is accomplished by addition of nonradioactive synthetic reagents to accomplish the desired drug structure. Purification of the ^{11}C-radiopharmaceutical is achieved using high-performance liquid chromatography (HPLC). The drug substance is isolated from the appropriate chromatographic fraction using a solid-phase extraction cartridge and reformulated in a physiologically compatible solvent.

Fluorine-18 Fluorine-18 can be produced by medical cyclotrons in the ionic form [^{18}F]F^- (fluoride) or the gaseous form, [^{18}F]F_2 (fluorine), dependent on the cyclotron target and the particle used to irradiate the target. Radiopharmaceutical labeling with [^{18}F]F_2 is less desirable due to several practical disadvan-

tages [56]. Labeling precursor [^{18}F]F_2 is typically made by the $^{20}Ne(d,\alpha)^{18}F$ nuclear reaction, in which the target neon-20 gas is spiked with a few percent nonradioactive F_2 to facilitate transfer of ^{18}F activity from the target container to the reaction vessel. The result of this approach is that ^{18}F-labeled radiopharmaceuticals that are made from [^{18}F]F_2 are of low specific activity. This is suboptimal since the additional mass in the radiopharmaceutical can saturate low-capacity target sites like receptors. In addition, it increases the potential for toxicity or side effects to occur with radiopharmaceutical use, since it is not administered in tracer, sub-pharmacological dose amounts during imaging studies. Another consideration is that cyclotron target yields of [^{18}F]F_2 are relatively low, making radiopharmaceutical production batch yields correspondingly low. Typically radiopharmaceutical production using [^{18}F]F_2 is done on a single-subject basis, rather than multidose batches. For this reason, $^{18}F_2$ is generally only used only for electrophilic labeling strategies, when use of the preferred labeling precursor $^{18}F^-$ is not feasible.

In contrast to [^{18}F]F_2, cyclotron production of fluorine-18 in the ionic form [^{18}F]F^- is robust. Nucleophilic [^{18}F]F^- is routinely produced in multi-curie amounts using the $^{18}O(p,n)^{18}F$ nuclear reaction on isotopically enriched [^{18}O]water. Methodology has been developed for recovery and reuse of the expensive [^{18}O]water, and high radiochemical yields are achieved through optimized nucleophilic [^{18}F]fluorination reactions that insert the radionuclide into specific molecular sites on appropriately designed labeling substrates. Labeling strategies involve site-specific insertion of the radionuclide via nucleophilic displacement of leaving groups like aromatic nitro ($-NO_2$) triflate ($-OTf$) or tosylate ($-OTs$) [56].

Because these displacement reactions must occur under strictly anhydrous conditions and [^{18}F]F^- is delivered from the target in aqueous solution, a resolubilization step is needed prior to labeling. Resolubilization involves azeotropic removal of the water solvent and (assisted by a phase-transfer catalyst such as potassium 2.2.2.Kryptofix) redissolution in an organic reaction solvent. The nucleophilic substitution reaction proceeds with a few minutes of heating, protecting groups are hydrolytically removed, and purification is done very similar to the methods used for ^{11}C-labeled radiopharmaceuticals. The ^{18}F-labeled drug substance is chromatographically purified (often using HPLC), isolated from the appropriate chromatographic fraction using solid-phase extraction methods, and reformulated in a physiologically compatible solvent.

Oxygen-15 and Nitrogen-13 As mentioned above, radiosynthetic procedures are handicapped by the short half-lives of these nuclides [16]. Oxygen-15 is commonly produced in a cyclotron by the $^{14}N(d,n)^{15}O$ nuclear reaction on a target of naturally abundant nitrogen-14 gas. The target product [^{15}O]oxygen (O_2) can be chemically converted on-line into [^{15}O]carbon monoxide (CO) for blood volume measurements or [^{15}O]water (H_2O) for perfusion measurements by PET.

Nitrogen-13 can be produced by the nuclear reaction $^{16}O(p,\alpha)^{13}N$ on a target of naturally abundant [^{16}O]water. Since ^{13}N is produced in the chemical form of nitrate or nitrite in water ($^{13}NO_x$), subsequent reduction with Devarda's alloy yields commonly used [^{13}N]ammonia (NH_3). Direct in-target production of [^{13}N]NH_3 can be accomplished by addition of ethanol as a scavenger to the target water. As mentioned above, only early time points are available for PET imaging of ^{15}O or ^{13}N, making investigation of the several biological processes that occur over hours or days impossible.

Gallium-68 The long half-life of parent ^{68}Ge (270.8 d) coupled with the convenient half-life of ^{68}Ga (68 min) makes this pair an almost ideal generator strategy. There are challenges, however, in the practical application of this generator for radiopharmaceutical production. Unlike the popular $^{99}Mo/^{99m}Tc$ generator commonly used in conventional nuclear medicine, concentrated hydrochloric acid (HCl) is used as the generator eluent. Potential breakthrough of the long-lived parent nuclide could have consequences that are more serious if not rigorously controlled. Metallic impurities such as Zn^{2+} from the decay of ^{68}Ga or

Fe^{3+} and other column residuals may be present in the eluate and interfere with labeling procedures. To minimize impurities in the generator eluate, controls on radiopharmaceutical procedures are followed that include standardized generator elution volumes and maximum time limits allowed since previous elution. Such practices prevent buildup of chemical, radiochemical, and radionuclidic impurities.

The aqueous solution chemistry of gallium is very similar to that of iron, and the Ga^{3+} ion resembles Fe^{3+} with respect to coordination chemistry [46]. Both elements are 3+ charged and have similar ionic radii and major coordination number of six. Like Fe^{3+}, in aqueous solution free hydrated Ga^{3+} ion is stable only under acidic conditions. In the pH range of 3–7, gallium forms insoluble $Ga(OH)_3$, and at physiological pH, solubility is high due to formation of $[Ga(OH)_4]^-$ ions. In vivo, transchelation of Ga^{3+} to the iron transport protein transferrin may be problematic for ^{68}Ga-labeled radiopharmaceuticals.

The primary prerequisites for a successful $^{68}Ga^{3+}$ chelate used for radiopharmaceutical purposes are thermodynamic stability toward hydrolysis and resistance to ligand exchange with serum transferrin during the period of clinical use. Radiopharmaceutical complexes should be either more stable than the Ga-transferrin complex or kinetically inert to exchange with this protein. To prevent hydrolysis and formation of $^{68}Ga(OH)_3$ during radiopharmaceutical preparation, stabilizing weak ligands such as acetate, citrate, or HEPES can be used.

Several bifunctional chelates that have a functionality for covalent binding to a targeting vector in addition to binding the metal cation $^{68}Ga^{3+}$ have been proposed and coupled to biomolecules for gallium labeling [58]. These chelate $^{68}Ga^{3+}$ rapidly when linked to the macromolecule, and the resulting complexes are stable over a pH range of 4–8 and in the presence of other serum cations (Ca^{2+}, Zn^{2+}, Mg^{2+}).

The most common of these chelates in clinical use is the macrocyclic DOTA (1,4,7,10-tetraazacyclododecane-1,4,7,10-tetraacetic acid). DOTA has been shown to form stable complexes and avoid loss of the $^{68}Ga^{3+}$

core under physiological conditions. A potential limitation of DOTA is that chelation of $^{68}Ga^+$ requires moderately high temperature (80–100 °C) which may decompose heat-sensitive compounds like proteins and large-molecular-weight peptides. Another radiopharmaceutical chelator for ^{68}Ga is HBED-CC (N,N′-Bis[2-hydroxy-5-(carboxyethyl)-benzyl] ethylenediamine-N,N′-diacetic acid), which has fast complexing kinetics and high complex stability.

The typical labeling procedure for ^{68}Ga-radiopharmaceuticals is straightforward and is similar to the "kit" type ^{99m}Tc-radiopharmaceutical preparations commonly performed in conventional nuclear pharmacies. The ^{68}Ga is eluted from the generator in a small volume (5 mL or less) of concentrated HCl directly into a vial containing the labeling substrate (usually a peptide with attached bifunctional chelate). A buffer containing a stabilizing weak ligand for ^{68}Ga is added, and the solution is heated for a few minutes to affect complexation of the radiometal. This is followed by a cooling period and possible addition of excipients, and the labeling process is complete. Unlike the more complicated radiosynthetic schemes with ^{11}C or ^{18}F, purification with HPLC or reformulation into a different vehicle is not required prior to human administration.

Radiopharmaceutical Automation

PET radiopharmaceutical production is often accomplished using automated systems. This is especially true for cyclotron-produced radiopharmaceuticals, where starting radioactivities at curie levels are common. Automation of drug synthesis has the advantages of minimizing the radiation dose to production personnel, as well as (since they are microprocessor-controlled) standardizing production parameters within levels suitable for regulatory compliance [3, 9].

Automated systems are commercially available for commonly used PET radiopharmaceuticals and consist of sterile, pyrogen-free cassettes and reagents that are loaded into a module that is situated within a shielded hot cell. Radioactivity from the cyclotron target is delivered directly through a shielded line to the module, and the radiosynthetic pathway commences. Operation of the synthesis module is controlled by software loaded onto a microprocessor and sends signals to pneumatically open and shut valves, heat and cool mixtures, and move reaction mixtures according to a pre-programmed schedule. The operator is able to observe the functioning of the module in real time and (within limits) make minor interventions as needed. The reformulated radiopharmaceutical product is delivered through a sterilizing filter into a sterile pyrogen-free vial positioned in a lead shield. A small aliquot is then aseptically removed from this vial for quality control testing prior to release of the vial contents for human administration.

Quality Control of PET Radiopharmaceuticals

PET radiopharmaceuticals that are used for diagnostic imaging have short expiration dates and are manufactured in small quantities on a per-patient or limited-patient basis shortly before use. Nevertheless, radiopharmaceuticals, like all drugs, must be shown to be safe and effective prior to administration to human subjects.

Quality control of PET radiopharmaceuticals must evaluate both pharmaceutical and radioactive characteristics. Examination of pharmaceutical parameters ensures that no microbiological, pyrogenic, or particulate contamination is present in the final preparation. Examination of radioactive parameters ensures that the radiation exposure of patients is minimized by confirmation that there are no radiochemical or radionuclidic impurities in the product that may affect the biodistribution of the radiopharmaceutical and the associated radiation dose to the patient.

Because radiopharmaceutical syntheses involve complicated chemical reactions with various reagents, side products, and solvents, a comprehensive battery of quality control tests is required to prove drug identity and purity prior to administration. This pertains to all levels of regulation, from licensed radiopharmaceuticals to investigational tracers. The short half-life of PET radionuclides creates special challenges for the quality control of radiopharmaceuticals, and it is essential that analytical methods be rapid and give test results in a robust fashion to comply with regulatory requirements.

Quality control tests can be categorized as physicochemical tests or biological tests. Physicochemical tests include assessment of pH, visual inspection, and radiochemical, chemical, and radionuclidic purity. Biological tests evaluate product sterility and bacterial endotoxin content. The methodologies applied in these tests to assess the quality of PET radiopharmaceuticals are summarized in Table 10.2, and the sections below discuss these instrumental techniques. Note that these tests are performed using the same small aliquot withdrawn from the drug product specifically for quality control purposes.

Appearance The product is visually inspected for signs of color or particulate matter. A dark and light background is applied in this test for improved identification.

Acidity The pH is assessed to confirm the product acidity lies within the product specification.

Radiochemical Purity This test evaluates the fraction of total radioactivity in the product that is chemical form of the drug. Because the radiochemical form of the radioactivity determines its biodistribution, control of radiochemical impurities is important to avoid the patient unnecessary radiation exposure. Radiochemical impurities have a different biodistribution than the drug and may invalidate the clinical outcome of PET imaging studies.

Radiochemical impurities derive from several factors, including parameters of radionuclide production, radiochemical conditions during the production process, and impurities in starting materials. Radiochemical impurities may also derive from decomposition of the radiopharmaceutical during storage. Quantification of radiochemical purity requires analytical methods capable of separating the different radiochemicals that may be present in the drug product. Chromatographic methods are commonly used for determination of radiochemical purity because they have high resolution and effectively separate the different radiochemical species in the sample.

Chromatography is based on the separation of compounds by the distribution between two phases, a stationary and a mobile phase. The phases can be solid-liquid, liquid-liquid, or gas-liquid. Chromatographic methods are used to separate radioactive or nonradioactive species in the sample for determination of radiochemical, chemical, and enantiomeric purity. For PET radiopharmaceuticals, high-performance liquid

Table 10.2 Quality control testing of PET radiopharmaceuticals

Drug characteristic	Analytical method	Principle
Appearance	Visual inspection	Observation of color, clarity, particulates
Acidity	pH Paper	Colorimetric change with H^+ concentration
Radiochemical identity	Radio-TLC	Radiopharmaceutical R_f vs. standard R_f
	Radio-HPLC	Radiopharmaceutical R_t vs. standard R_t
Radiochemical purity	Radio-TLC	Fraction of total radioactivity as drug
	Radio-HPLC	Fraction of total radioactivity as drug
Chemical purity	Colorimetric	Color intensity of sample vs. standard
	HPLC	Radiopharmaceutical R_t vs. standard R_t
	GC	Radiopharmaceutical R_t vs. standard R_t
Enantiomeric purity	HPLC	Radiopharmaceutical R_t vs. standard R_t
Radionuclidic Identity	Dose calibrator	$T_{1/2}$ radiopharmaceutical vs. theoretical
Radionuclidic purity	Germanium Detector	Drug γ-spectrum vs. expected emissions
BET	Colorimetry	Compare LAL clotting by drug vs. standard
Sterility	Medium growth	Growth TSB or TG media over 14 days

chromatography (HPLC), thin-layer chromatography (TLC), and gas chromatography (GC) are frequently used.

High-Performance Liquid Chromatography HPLC is used to separate compounds within a solution. HPLC consists of a column of packing material (stationary phase), a pump to move the liquid mobile phase through the column, an injector to add the small-volume sample, and detectors that identify compound peaks that can be used to measure retention times for identification and quantification. The retention time of a compound depends on physicochemical interactions between the molecule, the stationary phase, and the solvent used as a mobile phase. There are three categories of HPLC systems generally used for quality control of PET radiopharmaceuticals: normal-phase, reversed-phase, and ionic-exchange.

Normal-phase HPLC uses a polar stationary phase and a nonpolar mobile phase. The polar compounds in the sample are retained by the polar stationary phase. Reversed-phase HPLC uses a nonpolar stationary phase and a moderately polar aqueous mobile phase. It involves hydrophobic interactions between the stationary phase and relatively nonpolar compounds in the sample. With ion-exchange chromatography, retention of compounds in the sample occurs due to attraction between charged sites bound to the stationary phase and ionic sample compounds. Ions with the same charge as the mobile phase are eluted with the mobile phase.

There are different types of detectors configured in HPLC systems. Theses detect the presence of a compound passing through and generate electronic signals for data acquisition. In HPLC analysis of radiochemical purity, radiation detectors such as NaI scintillators or BGO detectors are used on-line for determination of radiochemical purity. The radioactivity in product peaks is integrated, and the ratios of the areas under the peaks give the percentages of the total radioactivity corresponding to each radiochemical. In addition, the retention times of each peak facilitates identification of the radiochemical components in the sample by comparison with that of no-radioactive standards. The nonradioactive standards are quantified via detection of ultraviolet, electrochemical, conductivity, or refractive index (RI) detectors, like for the measurement of chemical purity of PET radiopharmaceuticals (see below).

Thin-Layer Chromatography TLC is also used for measurement of radiochemical purity. Like HPLC, TLC consists of a stationary phase and a mobile phase and can be used to determine the number of radiochemicals in a sample and to verify their identity. The stationary phase is typically a polar absorbent, such as finely ground alumina or silica particles that is layered onto a glass or plastic support. A wide variety of solvent mixtures can be used as the mobile phase.

The TLC plate is marked at the origin and the front distance before sample is applied. A few microliters of radiopharmaceutical sample are spotted onto the origin site, and the TLC plate is transferred to a development chamber containing a small amount of mobile phase. The mobile phase travels up the TLC plate by capillary action, passes over the sample spot, and carries the compounds in the sample up the plate at different rates. The sample compounds are separated on the plate due to differences in their relative affinity for the stationary phase and the mobile phase. When the mobile phase reaches the front mark, the plate is removed and dried, and the position of radioactive spots is determined by measuring the radioactivity distribution on the plate with a collimated radiation detector. Radioactive peak areas are integrated, and the ratios of the peak areas give the percentage of total radioactivity contributed by each peak and calculation of radiochemical purity.

TLC also determines the R_f values for sample components. The R_f value describes for each separated chemical the ratio-to-front value expressed as a decimal fraction and is calculated as the distance traveled by a compound computed to the distance from the origin to the solvent front. Like retention times in HPLC, R_f values from TLC allow chemical identification of radiochemical components in a sample by comparison to those of nonradioactive standard compounds.

Enantiomeric Purity Measurement of enantiomeric purity is a subcategory of radiochemical purity. Enantiomers are optical isomers in which the molecules are mirror images of each other. They exhibit stereoisomerism when there is at least one chiral center in the molecular structure of the drug. In the case of PET radiopharmaceuticals with a chiral center, high enantiomeric purity is important for clinical application since the biologically inactive enantiomer is a radiochemical contaminant that blunts the robustness of the PET signal from the active enantiomer. Where relevant, the enantiomeric purity of PET radiopharmaceuticals is measured using chromatographic methods.

Chemical Purity Whereas radiochemical purity affects patient dosimetry, chemical purity can affect pharmacological toxicity to the subject. Chemical purity testing evaluates the nonradioactive materials in the PET radiopharmaceutical and includes chemical byproducts, solvents, and other residual components from the production process. Product components such as stabilizers and excipients intentionally added to the radiopharmaceutical may also be assessed. Chemical impurities may include nonradioactive substances that affect radiolabeling or induce adverse biological effects in subjects. Similar to radiochemical impurities, chemical impurities are usually assessed chromatographically. Radiopharmaceutical release criteria ensure suitable chemical purity by defining limits on specific chemical impurities.

Like radiochemical purity, chemical purity of PET radiopharmaceuticals is routinely measured by HPLC. The same HPLC separations are used, but instead of online detection of radioactivity, measurement of nonradioactive components are quantified via detection of ultraviolet, electrochemical, conductivity, or refractive index (RI) detectors. Peak areas are integrated and compared to a mass detection signal calibration curve for conversion of HPLC detector measurement to mass concentration. As with radiochemical analysis, comparison of the retention times of mass peaks from HPLC with those of standard compounds facilitates identification of unknown components, as well as identity verification for the drug substance.

A subcategory of chemical purity testing is measurement of residual solvents in the PET radiopharmaceutical. These are defined as organic volatile chemicals that were used in the preparation of the drug product and were not entirely removed and are therefore present at trace levels in the radiopharmaceutical product. Residual solvents may have been introduced during radiopharmaceutical preparation or during packaging and storage and should be present only at low concentrations. Residual solvents fall into three classes based on their toxicity. Class 1 solvents should be avoided during manufacturing process because of unacceptable toxicity or negative environmental impact. Class 2 solvents may be present but at limited concentration because they are associated with less toxicity, although less severe than class 1. Class 3 solvents have low toxic potential and lower risk to human health, so can be present at higher concentrations than the other two categories. Because residual solvents are volatile, they are usually measured using gas chromatographic (GC) techniques.

Gas Chromatography In GC an injected sample is vaporized onto a chromatographic column and transported through the column by an inert gaseous mobile phase such as nitrogen, helium, or argon. GC columns are either packed or capillary in design. The components in the radiopharmaceutical sample are separated due to repeated distribution between the stationary and mobile phases; transport of the components occurs when in the gas phase, while separation takes place when it is in the stationary phase. The effectiveness of a GC separation is dependent on how long and how often the various components stay in the stationary phase, which is determined by its functional groups. The column temperature can be manipulated during a GC separation to optimize resolution.

Like HPLC, the time a compound travels through the column to the detector is its retention time. The components in a radiopharmaceutical sample can be detected using various types of detectors, with flame ionization detection (FID) being a popular method. Due to the volatility of organic solvents, GC is used to identify and quantify residual solvents in radiopharmaceutical preparations.

Radionuclidic Identity Radionuclidic identity confirms that the measured radioactive half-life of the PET radiopharmaceutical is close to the theoretical half-life of the expected radionuclide. This test is accomplished by taking serial measurements of a quality control sample held in a stationary position, usually using a scintillation counter. The sample activity must be of sufficient quantity to allow measurements detected within a suitable interval of time. This test is simple and robust and can be completed for most PET radiopharmaceuticals prior to administration for imaging.

Radionuclidic Purity The radionuclidic purity refers to the fraction of the total radioactivity in a sample that is due to the expected radionuclide in the radiopharmaceutical. Radionuclidic impurities can negatively affect the overall radiation dose to the patient, as well as corrupt the PET image quality. Radionuclidic impurities derive from secondary nuclear reactions during the target irradiation involving isotopic impurities present in the target material or the target body. Release specifications for radiopharmaceuticals may set limits for specific radionuclidic impurities that are considered to be likely candidates.

Radionuclidic purity testing is accomplished by gamma spectrometry. Using this methodology, the expected radionuclide is allowed to decay so that small levels of impurities will not be masked. In contrast to radionuclidic identity testing (which is done pre-release on every batch), radionuclidic purity testing is done on a post-release basis, usually once or twice a year (unless there is a change in target material). Gamma spectrometry is used to obtain the spectrum of gamma rays in a sample, and the energy of any unknown photopeaks can be compared to gamma spectrum libraries to determine the exact identity of the nuclear contaminants.

Gamma Spectrometers: Gamma ray spectrometers function due to the proportionality between the energy deposited into the detector (usually a germanium crystal) by a gamma and the pulse amplitude at the output of the detector. These pulse amplitudes are analyzed to generate an energy spectrum of detected radiation. Radionuclides emit specific gamma ray energies, so the gamma ray spectra provide qualitative analysis of the radionuclides in a radiopharmaceutical sample.

Operationally, the gamma detection system must be calibrated as a function of energy and correction of the various peak areas for detector efficiency. Energy and efficiency calibration should be done over the range of energies that is relevant to the specific energies of interest. For calibration, NIST-certified sources are used that have specified level of accuracy and are traceable to the international system of measurement.

Calibrated gamma spectrometry systems are used for several applications in the quality control of PET radiopharmaceuticals. These include identification of γ-emitting radionuclides, accurate radioactivity measurement, detection and quantification of γ-emitting radionuclidic impurities, and estimation of the upper limit of detection for potential impurities.

For analysis of PET radiopharmaceuticals, the energy distribution of gamma radiation absorbed by the detector crystal is examined. Peak energies are then determined using the energy calibration of the system. Radiopharmaceutical samples may demonstrate several peaks and low-concentration impurity peaks may not be obvious by visual inspection. For this reason, sophisticated software is often used for spectrum analysis.

In some cases there is more than one radionuclide emitting a specific gamma energy, like 511 keV for two positron emitters. In this situation, energy measurement is insufficient for radionuclide identification. Repetitive γ-spectrometer measurements of the decrease in peak area over time allow calculation of the nuclide's half-life, however, and thereby confirm its identification.

Bacterial Endoxins Test (BET) Bacterial endotoxins (pyrogens) are polysaccharides from bacterial gram-negative membranes. They are water-soluble, heat stable, and filterable, which means heat or membrane sterilization will not eliminate them from a radiopharmaceutical solution. Pyrogens in a parenteral drug solution can induce fever as well as leukopenia in immunosuppressed patients. Radiopharmaceuticals must be manufactured and dispensed under aseptic conditions to minimize the introduction of pyrogens. Endotoxins are quantified in a radiopharmaceutical preparation based on a blood-aggregating reaction initiated when pyrogens activate Limulus amebocyte lysate (LAL) derived from horseshoe crabs. Analytically, the BET may be accomplished using a gel-clot, turbidogenic, or chromogenic technique. Pyrogens must be measured before release of a PET radiopharmaceutical for human use.

The gel-clot technique detects clot formation induced by the reaction between endotoxins and LAL. A clotting protein is cleaved by an activated clotting enzyme and the insoluble cleavage products coalesce by ionic interaction to form a gel. The entire reaction sequence has not been identified, but it is known that the reaction leading to clot formation initiates a cascade of enzyme activation steps.

The turbidimetric technique observes the changes in turbidity that is associated with the clotting protein formed in the reaction between endotoxins and LAL. Endotoxin concentration is quantified by the quantitative relationship between endotoxin concentration and the turbidity (measured by absorbance or transmission) of the reaction mixture. The end-point version of the test measures turbidity at the end of the incubation period and the kinetic version of the test measures the time required for the reaction mixture to reach a predetermined absorbance or transmission level of turbidity.

The chromogenic technique uses a chromogenic peptide, which releases a chromophore (p-nitroaniline) from the reaction of endotoxins with LAL. Endotoxin activates the components of LAL in a proteolytic cascade that results in the cleavage of a colorless artificial peptide substrate.

Proteolytic cleavage of the substrate then liberates p-nitroaniline with an absorbance of 405 nm. Endotoxin concentration can be determined by the correlation between endotoxin concentration and the amount of chromophore released. As above, an end-point and kinetic version of the test can be used, dependent on when light absorption is measured.

Sterility Like all parenteral drugs, PET radiopharmaceuticals can be manufactured under conditions that promote sterile products by excluding microbial contamination. The USP test for sterility is performed under aseptic conditions by inoculating the sample into each of two culture media: soybean-casein digest (SCD) medium and fluid thioglycollate (FT) medium and rhen incubating for 14 days. SCD is a culture media for aerobic bacteria and fungi, while FT is primarily for the culture of anaerobic bacteria. Growth promotion tests should be performed as positive controls by incubating reference bacteria in the two media. Bacterial growth should be visible within the period of incubation to indicate that both SCD and FT capable of supporting bacterial growth and that results of the sterility test are valid. A system suitability test should also be performed to demonstrate that the product does not have intrinsic antimicrobial activity that would negate the validity of the test.

Because of the 14-day requirement for sterility measurement, these tests are performed on a post-release basis for PET radiopharmaceuticals, even though immediate inoculation of SCD and FT is done.

Validation of Analytical Procedures The above sections illustrate that several analytical techniques are used to assess the various quality aspects of PET radiopharmaceuticals. Each of these analytical procedures must be validated the different instruments to demonstrate that it is suitable for the intended purpose. The specific characteristics of quality control testing that must be addressed during method validation are listed in Table 10.3.

Table 10.3 Methods validation for analytical procedures

Parameter	Relevance
Specificity	Assess drug in presence of interfering substances
Precision	Variance in repeated measurements
Accuracy	Closeness of test results to reference
Linearity	Proportionality of measurements to concentration
Range	Interval between upper and lower limits for linearity
Limit of detection (LOD)	Lowest detectable level of substance
Limit of quantitation (LOQ)	Lowest quantifiable level of substance
Robustness	Resistance to small variations in parameters

Specificity Specificity may also be called selectivity and is the ability of the procedure to assess the test substance in the presence of other components that are present in the drug formulation. Interfering components may include impurities, degradation products, and constituents of the product matrix. If a technique is not specific as a stand-alone test, the deficiency may be compensated by supplemental analytical tests.

Precision The precision of a method is the degree of agreement among test results when the procedure is applied repeatedly to multiple analyses of a sample. Precision of an analytical procedure is usually expressed as the variance, standard deviation, or coefficient of variation of the series of measurements. Precision may also be used as a measure the robustness of the method (see below).

Accuracy The accuracy of an analytical procedure is the closeness of test results compared to the true or reference value and reflects the ability of the technique to provide the correct answer. It is determined by analysis of a reference standard and comparison of the measured value to the reference value. The accuracy of a procedure must be determined for the entire range of its application.

Linearity The linearity of an analytical procedure is its ability to give results that are directly proportional to the sample concentration within a specific range. The linearity of the relationship between actual concentration and measurement is sometimes achieved though mathematical transformation of one of the two sets of data. Such transformations to attain a model that faithfully describes the concentration-response relationship are considered acceptable.

Range The range of an analytical procedure is the interval between the upper and lower concentrations of test substance that has acceptable precision, accuracy, and linearity. Range is expressed in the same units as test results. The range of a radiopharmaceutical quality control method should cover the concentrations expected in routine measurements.

Detection Limit The limit of detection (LOD) is the lowest amount of test substance in a sample matrix that can be detected (but not necessarily quantified) under defined conditions. Signal-to-noise ratios between 2- or 3-to-1 are generally considered to be acceptable for estimating LOD. The LOD verifies that the amount of test substance is above or below a certain level and is typically is expressed as a concentration.

Quantitation Limit The limit of quantitation (LOQ) is a descriptor for quantitative assays of low levels of test compounds within sample matrices. The LOQ is the lowest amount of test substance in a sample matrix that can be quantified under defined conditions. Signal-to-noise ratios of 10-to-1 are generally considered to be acceptable for estimating LOQ. For PET radiopharmaceuticals, this would pertain not only to impurities or degradation products in the drug product but also to the high specific activity radiopharmaceutical as well.

Robustness The robustness of an analytical procedure measures its tendency to remain unaffected by small variations in procedural parameters and shows its suitability for normal usage. Examples of parameters that may change are mobile phase pH, variations of temperature, mobile phase composition, flow rate, and different columns (different lots and/or suppliers). The robustness of a method can be demonstrated during the development phase of the analytical procedure.

Subcategories of robustness are reproducibility and ruggedness. The reproducibility of an analytical procedure compares use of the method in different laboratories, as in a multicenter study. The ruggedness of a procedure describes the within-laboratory variation, as when the procedure is performed on different days, by different analysts or using different equipment.

PET Radiopharmaceutical Regulation

In the translation of new tracers from the bench-top to clinical application as PET radiopharmaceuticals, there are legal requirements that must be met. These requirements are designed to promote development of novel and effective PET radiopharmaceuticals of benefit to the public, while protecting the safety of test subjects and patients. Such issues of public well-being are the purview of government, and independent nations have designed different approaches whereby these goals can be accomplished. In particular, comparison of the laws regulating investigational radiopharmaceuticals in the United States (USA) (see below) and European Union (EU) [8, 19, 40, 67] shows that they are similar in spirit but differ greatly in the details. Likewise, regulations in Japan, India, and Canada have unique regulatory pathways that differ from both the United States and EU.

There have been attempts to harmonize regulations at the international level and create a standardized regulatory platform to improve the availability of new PET radiopharmaceuticals to the public at large, but the hurdles remain challenging [53, 54] and attempts to harmonize regulations appears to be a distant goal. Indeed, harmonization within the 27-member EU itself must precede harmonization with outside regulatory bodies.

Because of the diversity of regulatory approaches at the global level, we will focus here on the key points of PET radiopharmaceutical regulation within the United States. This will serve as a representative example of the regulatory complexities that are encountered when working with drugs that are both medicinal and radioactive. The emphasis here is on the regulatory requirements for first-in-human and early-phase studies, since these are the points where it is most likely that paradigm-shifting changes in clinical PET applications will initiate.

Regulation in the United States

PET radiopharmaceuticals are regulated in the United States by the Food and Drug Administration (FDA). In concert with the regulatory developments at the FDA, the US Pharmacopoeia (USP) sets legal, enforceable purity standards for drug products, including PET radiopharmaceuticals. The FDA Modernization Act (FDAMA) in 1997 directed that PET radiopharmaceuticals should be considered adulterated if not prepared according to USP standards and authorized FDA to establish its approval procedures and current good manufacturing practice (CGMP) requirements for PET radiopharmaceuticals. The Food and Drug Administration Amendments Act (FDAAA) in 2007 directed FDA to establish approval and review procedures, including the New Drug Application (NDA) and Abbreviated New Drug Application (ANDA) for radiopharmaceuticals. The FDA has published guidelines for CGMP for the manufacture of PET drugs and for the new drug application (NDA) and abbreviated new drug application (ANDA) process as it pertains to PET radiopharmaceuticals.

PET Radiopharmaceuticals Approved for NDA/ANDA

The current FDA-approved PET radiopharmaceuticals are listed in Table 10.4. Note that the majority of the new PET radiopharmaceuticals have been patented by and approved for commer-

Table 10.4 FDA-approved PET radiopharmaceuticals

[^{11}C]Choline
[^{18}F]Florbetaben (Neuraceq™)
[^{18}F]Florbetapir (Amyvid™)
[^{18}F]Fludeoxyglucose
[^{18}F]Fluciclovine (Auxumin™)
[^{18}F]Flutemetamol (Vizamyl™)
[^{18}F]Florbetapir (Amyvid™)
Sodium [^{18}F]fluoride
[^{68}Ga]DOTATATE (Netspot™)
[^{68}Ga]DOTATOC
[^{82}Rb]Rubidium chloride (Cardiogen-82™)

Table 10.5 Organization of the common technical document (CTD)

Module 1. Administrative information and prescribing information
Module 2. Overviews and summaries of modules
Module 3. Quality (pharmaceutical documentation)
Module 4. Non-clinical reports (pharmacology/toxicology)
Module 5. Clinical study reports (clinical trials)

cial pharmaceutical manufacturers. The PET radiopharmaceuticals listed in Table 10.4 are permitted to be used in clinical applications as well as for research purposes. For FDA approval of an NDA or ANDA, applications must be submitted to the FDA via electronic or paper format. Electronic submission using common technical document (CTD) is the current preferred method because it facilitates oversight of any critical information. The CTD format consists of five components, modules 1–5 (Table 10.5) [36].

Note that frequently PET radiopharmaceuticals may need to be used for clinical purposes even though an NDA or ANDA is lacking. For example, in rare diseases, it may be impractical to gain approval in the traditional NDA/ANDA route. In these circumstances the FDA may, in the interest of the patient, make an exception and permit use of the unapproved PET radiopharmaceutical. The mechanism for this special approval is the expanded access IND pathway, which is specifically designed for these relatively rare circumstances.

The list of FDA-approved PET radiopharmaceuticals in Table 10.4 is not insignificant but pales in comparison to the myriad of PET tracers that have proven worth in clinical research studies or have potential for translation from preclinical development to application in human subjects. The question then arises how to gain regulatory approval for human use of these valuable PET radiopharmaceuticals that lack an NDA or ANDA. The FDA permits this under one of two general approval pathways. These are FDA approval of an investigational new drug application (IND) [48] or approval by an in-house radioactive drug research committee (RDRC) [59].

Investigational New Drug (IND) Submission

The most comprehensive of these pathways is the submission of an IND according to 21 CFR 312. Note that this approach is the same as that followed by conventional drugs, of which the major phases are listed in Table 10.6. This table is more comprehensive than what is needed for initiation of a new PET radiopharmaceutical but is pre-

Table 10.6 Phases of clinical trials

Phase	Primary goal	Definition
Phase 0	Proof of concept	Enables further decision based on human data
		Healthy controls
Phase I	Safety	Adverse effects
		Tracer metabolism and excretion
		Healthy controls plus subjects with disease
		Dosimetry estimates
Phase II	Effectiveness	Demonstrate effectiveness of drug
		Healthy controls plus subjects with disease
Phase III	Commercialization	Demonstrate safety and efficacy in large samples
		Emphasis on patients with disease
		Compare to current gold standard
Phase IV	Post marketing	Monitor safety and efficacy post approval
		Identify potential new indications

Table 10.7 Major sections of an IND submission

I. FDA Form 1571
II. Table of Contents
III. Introductory Statement
IV. General Investigational Plan
V. Protocol
VI. Investigator's Brochure (multi-site studies)
VII. Chemistry, Manufacturing, and Controls (CMC)
VIII. Pharmacology and Toxicology
IX. Previous Human Experience
X. Additional Information
XI. Other Information

sented here to give the reader a sense of the evolution of an IND to the NDA and commercialization of a labeled drug. For investigation of a novel PET radiopharmaceutical for research, the focus is generally on Phase 0, which is also called an exploratory IND (eIND). The eIND is discussed in more detail below.

The major components of an IND submission are rigorously structured as outlined in Table 10.7. The sections are identified by roman numerals that are standardized for applications. Note that these major sections will differ according to the particular phase of the IND, becoming more comprehensive as the project evolves to include larger numbers of subjects ahead of NDA approval. For early-phase investigations at a single site, the application will not require an investigator's brochure, previous human experience, or case report forms. The IND application begins with a cover sheet and a cover letter from the principal investigator (PI), which is followed by Section I (FDA Form 1571). This form formats the name of the IND sponsor, sponsor address, name of PET radiopharmaceutical, proposed indication, specific contents of the IND application, and information regarding the principal contact individual. Section II (Table of Contents) precedes Section III (Introductory Statement) and presents the rationale for the study, a description of the PET radiopharmaceutical, and key references. Section IV is the general investigation plan, which gives an overview of the project in outline form. As mentioned above, Section V (Investigator's Brochure) is not required for studies performed at a single site. It is analogous to a package insert for the investigative PET radiopharmaceutical and is only required for multi-site clinical trials. Section VI (Protocol) is one of the most detailed parts of the IND. The protocol presents the background and rationale for the clinical research, objectives, methods (including research subjects, experimental design, expected results, experimental problems, and alternative approaches), data safety monitoring, and relevant references. The most comprehensive part of the IND is Section VII (Chemistry, Manufacturing, and Control Data (CMC). The CMC describes in great detail the raw materials, manufacture, environment, and quality control tests relevant to the investigational PET radiopharmaceutical. The CMC is discussed further below. Section VII (Pharmacology and Toxicology) focuses on the potential risk to human subjects based on preclinical findings in animals. Section VIII (Previous Human Experience) does not pertain to first-in-human applications, and Section IX (Additional Information) presents information about responsible individuals, radioassay equipment, and radiation dosimetry estimates. Section XI (Other Information) contains appendices with important supportive information. The appendices contain key information like the informed consent form, quality control (summary of quality control test results, stability testing results), preclinical pharmacology and toxicology results from animal studies, dosimetry estimates based on animal data, FDA Form 1572 and PI CV, and Form FDA 3674 (Certification of Compliance Clinical Trials).

CMC Section of the IND Submission

A goal of the IND is to foster clinical development of new PET radiopharmaceuticals while guarding subject and patient safety. A basic foundation of safety is manufacture of the radiolabeled drug with uncompromising control so that drug quality is rigidly maintained. The means whereby this goal is accomplished is the CMC section of the IND. The major components of the CMC section of an IND submission are summarized in Table 10.8, where key topics are arranged in the same order as they are presented in an IND.

The drug product is described by listing its components and quantitative composition.

Table 10.8 Key components of the CMC section of an IND

1. Drug product components and quantitative composition
2. Control for components/raw materials
3. Reference standard
4. Manufacturing and testing facilities
5. Manufacture of drug substance
6. Manufacture of drug product
7. Drug process evaluation
8. Controls for the finished dosage form
9. Stability testing
10. Environmental assessment

Control for components and raw materials (RM) is next, where each is listed individually with its supplier and certificate of analysis (COA). This section includes the target, other ingredients, reagents, solvents, gases, purification columns, and other auxiliary materials. Details for the reference standard are reported in the same fashion, with manufacturer and COA provided. The manufacturing and testing facility are described, including ISO class production environments.

The manufacture of the drug substance is described comprehensively. A batch formula lists each component used during the manufacturing process, including its function and the quantity used. Radionuclide production is explained, including particle accelerator, operating parameters, and description of the target body. Synthesis and purification of the drug substance is defined in terms of equipment used, operation, in-process controls, and post-synthesis procedures. Manufacture of the drug product is discussed with regard to production operation, reprocessing of PET drug product, packaging and labeling, and the container/closure that is used.

Drug/process evaluation is an important part of the CMC section. The various quality control tests that were discussed in general above are described in detail for the manufacturing site in the CMC, including details like specific equipment or techniques that will be used. These tests include membrane integrity testing, visual observation, pH, strength, radiochemical identity/purity, chemical purity (specific activity, residual solvents, reagents), radionuclidic identity/purity, BET testing, and sterility testing.

Controls for the finished dosage form are defined in the CMC. Sampling procedures and acceptance criteria are explained for the various QC tests. Regulatory specifications are defined, together with testing procedures (SOPs) and the testing schedule (pre-release, post-release, annually/biannually).

The CMC also reports results of stability testing, usually performed on three sequential batches to justify the expiration time that is defined.

The section concludes with an assessment of the environment for drug manufacturing. This environmental assessment involves both the general work area, as well as the critical ISO-5 manufacturing environment. Testing includes scheduled HEPA filtration certification, viable and nonviable particle counting, air settle and contact media plate testing, and personnel medial fill testing. All of these are to assure that the PET drug manufacturing process takes place in an environment that fosters patient safety.

USP Chapter 823

In addition to 21 CFR 312, the United States Pharmacopeia (USP) provides quality assurance standards for PET radiopharmaceuticals produced for compounding, investigational, or research purposes in the United States, and USP publishes monographs for FDA-approved PET radiopharmaceuticals. The Food Drug and Cosmetic Act states that any drug that has a monograph listed in the USP must meet this compendial standard for strength, quality, and purity.

Chapters in the USP are either enforceable by FDA or informational to serve as guidance to drug producers. Enforceable chapters are numbered below 1000, whereas informational chapters are numbered above 1000.

USP Chapter 823 (Positron Emission Tomography Drugs for Compounding, Investigational, and Research Purposes) is enforceable, and it is the position of FDA that (although less explicit than requirements of 21 CFR 212) are adequate for RDRC- and IND-approved PET radiopharmaceuticals. It is therefore acceptable to use the requirements of either of these regulatory documents to prepare PET radiopharmaceuticals. Table 10.9 gives the major subheadings of USP Chapter 823. Comparison of Table 10.9 with Table 10.8 shows a striking level of concurrence. The slight advantage of following USP Chapter 823 for PET drug manufacture is greater flexibility in microbiologic testing of aseptic workstations, more liberal verification of identities of components, containers and closures, and a less demanding schedule for sterility testing.

In addition to this enforceable chapter, the USP also published informational Chapter 1823 (Positron Emission Tomography Drugs). This chapter provides useful guidance on techniques for production and quality control, quality assurance, production, quality control, analytical methodologies, quality attributes, and sterility assurance. Guidance from this chapter is helpful for meeting regulatory requirements of either 21 CFR 212 or USP Chapter 823.

Alternatives to the IND: RDRC and eIND

To promote innovation in PET radiopharmaceutical development while simultaneously protecting subjects from harm, the FDA has developed alternative approval pathways to the traditional IND. These are the Radioactive Drug Research Committee (RDRC) programs and the exploratory IND (eIND; phase 0) application. Important differences between the RDRC, eIND, and IND processes are given in Table 10.10. The table illustrates that the requirements for the RDRC and eIND are much less restrictive than for the

Table 10.9 Sections of USP Chapter 823

Definitions
Personnel
Quality Assurance
Facilities and Equipment
Control of Components, Materials, and Supplies
Process and Operational Controls
Stability
Controls and Acceptance Criteria for Finished PET Drug Products
If a PET Drug Does Not Conform to Specifications
Reprocessing
Labeling

Table 10.10 Comparison of RDRC, eIND, and IND pathways for new PET radiopharmaceuticals

RDRC	eIND	IND
Purpose		
Basic research	Basic research	Clinical investigation of tracer
GRASE	Two to five tracers simultaneously	For diagnosis/therapy
NOAEL	Micro-dose studies	For safety/efficacy
Not for Dx/Tx	Must transition to IND	
Not for safety/efficacy	Not for diagnosis/therapy	
	Not for safety/efficacy	
Requirements		
Clinical protocol	Clinical Protocol	Clinical protocol
Manufacture per USP 823 or 21 CFR 212	Manufacture per USP 823 or 21 CFR 212	Manufacture per USP 823 or 21CFR 212
Dosimetry from rodents	Dosimetry from rodents	Dosimetry from rodents
	Toxicology in one species	Toxicology in two species
	No safety/pharmacology	Safety/pharmacology in two species
	No genotoxicity	Genotoxicity studies
Approval		
RDRC and IRB	FDA and IRB	FDA and IRB
Number of subjects		
<30	<30	No limit

traditional IND, but the scope of the research is correspondingly narrower. As points of concurrence, note that RDRC, eIND, and traditional IND all demand a clinical protocol, allow PET radiopharmaceutical manufacturing via USP Chapter 823 or 21 CFR 212, accept rodent data for estimation of human dosimetry, and stipulate approval from local IRB as part of the approval process.

Considering first the RDRC program, it is designed for studies with PET tracers that are generally recognized as safe and effective (GRASE). Institutional RDRC at are comprised of specialists with complementary expertise and basically function as an arm of the FDA in reviewing local research applications for safety and appropriateness. Under 21 CFR 36.1, the RDRC program permits human research using radioactive under certain conditions. An important requirement is that the investigation must be for basic research purposes only. Immediate therapeutic or diagnostic purposes are not permitted nor are studies to determine the safety or effectiveness of the tracer. These constraints are designed to thwart misuse of the RDRC for routine clinical applications or to acquire premarketing data that should instead be done under an IND. Another important restriction of the RDRC approval pathway is that the pharmacologic dose of the radioactive drug must not exceed the no-observed-adverse effect level (NOAEL). The NOAEL is the highest dose that under defined conditions of exposure causes no detectable adverse effect on morphology, functional capacity, development or life span. Because knowledge of the NOAEL in humans is needed beforehand, first-in-man studies are precluded for RDRC review. Also, RDRC-approved studies are limited to 30 subjects or less, since they are designed to show proof of concept. Despite these restrictions, the RDRC program provides a convenient means for initiation of research studies involving unapproved research PET radiopharmaceuticals in human subjects.

The eIND has several characteristics in common with the RDRC pathway for approval of new PET radiopharmaceuticals. Research plans are for basic research only, have no more than 30 subjects, and do not evaluate diagnostic/therapeutic information, nor radiopharmaceutical safety/efficacy. Major differences between the eIND and RDRC are that the eIND requires pre-clinical toxicology to be evaluated in one species. Whereas the RDRC relies on NOAEL, the eIND utilizes the concept of microdosing. A microdose is 1/100 of the dose calculated to cause a pharmacological effect. The eIND permits a mass dose of radiopharmaceutical ≤ 100 μg (or ≤ 30 nmol for protein products). Thus, for first-in-man studies, the eIND is far preferable to the RDRC approach. A further advantage of eIND submission is that two to five radiopharmaceuticals with similar molecular structures are permitted to be evaluated simultaneously to promote identification of the best derivative for further development as a labeled drug. These advantages of the eIND favor innovation and development of new radiopharmaceuticals for clinical PET. Note that following completion of an eIND, further development of a labeled drug must transition to the traditional IND pathway, with its more stringent safety requirements.

PET Imaging of Melanoma and Sarcoma

There have been several PET radiopharmaceuticals used to examine different aspects of melanoma and sarcoma. These are summarized in Table 10.11. In many cases, the studies involved multiple tracers, and tumor pathophysiology was examined from the perspective of different localization mechanisms. Also, in other situations, melanoma or sarcoma was just one of several cancers examined, and the different types of tumors were compared. The following is a summary of these studies, organized arbitrarily by radionuclide in the respective PET radiopharmaceutical.

[¹³N]Ammonia N-13 Ammonia is a perfusion tracer with widespread utility in cardiac blood flow studies with PET. The radiopharmaceutical was also found to be useful in asymptomatic early recurrence of fibrosarcoma, which is a rare

Table 10.11 Radiopharmaceuticals for PET imaging of patients with melanoma or sarcoma

Radiopharmaceutical	Localization mechanism
[^{13}N]Ammonia	Tumor vascularity
[^{11}C]Methionine (MET)	Amino acid transport
[^{11}C]Acetate (ACE)	Cell membrane constituent
[^{11}C]Choline (CH)	Cell membrane constituent
[^{18}F]Fluorocholine (FCH)	Cell membrane constituent
[^{18}F]Fluoroethyl-L-tyrosine (FET)	Amino acid transport
[^{18}F]Fluoroborono-L-phenylalanine (FBPA)	Amino acid transport
[^{18}F]FDOPA (Fluorodopa)	Amino acid transport
[^{18}F]Fluoroestradiol (FES)	Estrogen receptor
[^{18}F]Fluorothymidine (FLT)	DNA synthesis
[^{18}F]Mizonidazole (FMISO)	Hypoxia
Sodium [^{18}F]Fluoride (NaF)	Hydroxyapatite
[^{18}F]Fluciclatide (FC)	Integrin receptor
[^{18}F]Fluciclovine (FV)	Amino acid transport
[^{18}F]P3BZA	Melanin
[^{68}Ga]DOTATATE	Somatostatin receptor
[^{68}Ga]DOTANOC	Somatostatin receptor
[^{68}Ga]DOTATOC	Somatostatin receptor
[^{68}Ga]Pentixafor	Chemokine receptor type 4
[^{68}Ga]PSMA (prostate-specific membrane Antigen)	PSMA binding

tumor of the musculoskeletal system. These sarcomas are highly vascular, and imaging with the flow tracer allowed identification of early recurrence despite faint FDG avidity [29].

[^{11}C]Methionine (MET) Malignant transformation of cells increases utilization of amino acids (AA) for energy, protein synthesis, and cell division. There are approximately 20 AA transporter systems, and several are overexpressed in tumor cells. Expression of AA transporters in tumors varies widely, but in some cases represents proliferation speed and malignancy. Methionine is a precursor of S-adenosyl-L-methionine, which is a methyl group donor essential for cell growth. PET imaging of [^{11}C]methionine (MET) reflects methionine transport from plasma to tissues and has been used successfully for metabolic imaging of several types of cancer.

In a small study of malignant melanoma patients ($n = 10$), MET-PET detected primary and metastatic disease [standardized uptake values (SUV) of 1.8–12.7 [41]. The mean SUV of 6.3 was similar to that of non-Hodgkin's lymphoma, greater than that of non-small-cell lung cancer but less than that for breast cancer or head and neck cancer. Sensitivity of lesions >1.5 cm diameter was 100% and for lesions of any size 81%. MET-PET was effective for visualization of melanoma and may be useful for measurement of tumor metabolic activity in vivo.

Choroidal melanoma is the second most common intraocular malignant tumor after metastasis and is unique in that the tumors shrink slowly after radiotherapy and cannot be easily evaluated by histology. MET-PET was used to image 24 choroidal melanoma patients pre- and post- carbon ion beam therapy (CIBT) [60]. Tumor localization of MET was evaluated using a tumor-to-brain ratio (TBR) from the PET images. The mean TBR was 1.88 pre-therapy and decreased following therapy (1.73. 1.08. 0.67 and 0.65 at 1, 6, 12, and 24 months post CIBT, respectively). The imaging results at 1 month post-therapy were not useful due to increased activity secondary to inflammatory infiltration. MET-PET was effective at identification of choroidal melanoma and TBR after 6 months was a useful marker of therapeutic response.

A retrospective study of 85 patients with head and neck mucosal malignant melanoma evaluated whether MET-PET predicts outcomes from CIBT treatment [30]. The patients underwent MET-PET pre- and post-CIRT treatment, and image analysis involved calculation of the tumor-to-normal brain tissue ratio (TNR). Local recurrence, metastasis, and outcomes were studied in terms of the pre- and post-treatment TNR as well as the TNR change ratio. Kaplan-Meier curves demonstrated significant differences between higher and lower pre-CIRT TNR measurements with regard to local recurrences, metastasis, and outcome. The Cox proportional hazard model showed that pre-treatment TNR measurements are factors significantly influencing the risk of local recurrence, metastasis, and outcome, with hazard ratio HR = 19.0, 2.67, and 6.3, respectively.

A comparative study evaluated the uptake of MET versus FDG as predictive measures in nine patients with soft tissue sarcoma who underwent neoadjuvant radiotherapy [27] demonstrated that FDG-PET is superior to MET-PET discriminating between partial and complete responders. Pre-treatment mean MET SUV_{max} was 4.9 and 7.5 for complete and partial responders, respectively, whereas the mean FDG SUV_{max} was 7.1 and 13.2 for responders and nonresponders, respectively.

[¹¹C]Acetate (ACE) ACE is a metabolic tracer originally developed for cardiology applications of PET. Acetate is initially converted into acetyl-CoA by acetyl-CoA synthetase (EC 6.2.1.1), and its metabolic fate thereafter depends on the cell type and whether it follows a catabolic or anabolic pathway [28]. In myocytes, acetate is metabolized in mitochondria by the tricarboxylic acid cycle (TCA) to CO_2 and H_2O, which serves as the basis for use of ACE as a marker of myocardial viability. In contrast, tumor cells overexpress fatty acid synthetase (EC 2.3.1.85), which converts acetyl-CoA into fatty acids which then get incorporated into the phosphatidylcholine constituents of cell membranes of growing tumors. It is this latter anabolic pathway that engenders oncological utility to ACE. ACE has shown to have lower uptake than FDG in angiosarcoma and lung cancer [2].

[¹¹C]Choline (CH) As alluded above, choline is a key component of the phospholipids of cell membranes, and tissues with increased metabolism will have increased uptake of choline. Intracellular choline kinases phosphorylate choline, which is then incorporated into phospholipids after several biochemical steps. Since tumor cells have high metabolic rates, uptake of choline is high to meet the demands of phospholipid synthesis, and localization of CH at tumor sites can be detected by PET. CH may be useful to assess melanoma in sinuses due to its low background in comparison to FDG [49].

[¹⁸F]Choline (FCH) CH has major disadvantages in terms of the short half-life of the carbon-11 label, plus it localizes in healthy liver, kidney, and spleen and thereby generates unwanted background. FCH was developed as an alternative to CH with a longer physical half-life and with a potentially different biological fate. FCH-PET has demonstrated high tumor uptake in patients with cancer of the prostate, breast, brain, and melanoma [11]. FCH-PET may be useful in detecting metastatic melanoma [57] in patients with prostate cancer and, thus, may have significant impact in the therapeutic management of prostate cancer patients diagnosed with a second tumor, which may include melanoma.

O-(2-[¹⁸F]Fluoroethyl)-L-Tyrosine (FET) FET was originally developed as an F-18 labeled non-natural AA for detection of brain tumors based solely on L-AA transport (LAT). PET imaging of brain tumors has shown little difference between FET and MET, but there is improved discrimination between lesions and inflammation when FET is used compared to FDG. Several studies have demonstrated the utility of FET-PET to provide accurate identification of brain lesions, delineation of brain metastases, and detection of recurrent brain tumor.

Brain metastases occur in up to 17% of all cancer patients. In a study, the uptake characteristics of FET in newly diagnosed, untreated brain metastasis from a variety of primary tumors were evaluated. It was found that malignant melanoma had the highest variability in FET uptake, with TBR_{max} (1.25–9.47) [63]. Of all the patient subgroups studied by FET-PET, malignant melanoma had the highest individual TBR_{max} values. There was no significant correlation between TBR_{max} and lesion volume or diameter, and FET-PET may provide molecular biology information beyond simple morphologic tumor extent.

A novel therapeutic application of FET-PET is detection of checkpoint inhibitor-related pseudo-progression in patients with melanoma metastases at the early stages of increasing tumor burden [38]. Pseudoprogression presents as an initial increase in contrast-enhancing lesions that stabilize or resolve on follow-up in the absence of any treatment change. Exclusion of pseudoprogression is key to avoidance of inappropriate discontinuation of such checkpoint inhibitors as ipilimumab, nivolumab, or pembrolizumab. A retrospective study done on five patients that received FET-PET while on checkpoint-inhibitor therapy for melanoma brain metastases and demonstrated increased brain tumor burden according to contrast-enhanced MRI. The four patients diagnosed with tumor progression had significantly higher TBR_{max} (mean = 5.4) than the single pseudoprogression patient (TBR_{max} 2.5) [38]. Moreover, time-activity curves (TACs) from dynamic FET-PET demonstrated that the progression patients had much shorter time-to-peak (TP) values (mean 17 min) compared to the pseudoprogression case (45 min).

[¹⁸F]Fluorborono-L-Phenylalanine (FBPA) FBPA was developed as a PET theranostic agent for use in conjunction with boron neutron capture therapy (BNCT). The basis of BCNT is neutron capture by ^{10}B, followed by release of α particles and recoiling ^{7}Li in close proximity to the original boron atom. When the ^{10}B is delivered to the tumor in the chemical form of BPA, FBPA-PET can be employed to screen candidates that may benefit from BNCT. Dynamic FBPA-PET was performed as a BNCT screening test on 28 patients, 8 of which had malignant melanoma [47]. Malignant melanoma patients demonstrated a persistent pattern of FBPA localization, with insignificant changes in SUV_{max} or TNR over time. These data demonstrate the utility of FBPA-PET in patient selection for BNCT.

6-[¹⁸F]Fluoro-L-DOPA (FDOPA) Another synthetic amino acid used for PET imaging is FDOPA, which was originally developed for study of Parkinson disease and other movement disorders by virtue of its enzymatic concentration into dopaminergic neurons of the brain. Later, the utility of FDOPA for imaging brain tumors was identified, since it is transported into tumor cells by overexpressed AA transporters, and, unlike FDG, demonstrates relatively low background concentration in normal healthy brain tissue.

Tracer kinetic modeling of FDOPA, FDG, and the perfusion tracer [¹⁵O]water was performed to gain insight into the behavior of these radiopharmaceuticals in 11 pretreated melanoma patients [22]. FDG showed a 1.5-fold increase compared to surrounding tissue in 19/22 metastatic lesions, whereas FDOPA uptake was enhanced in 14/22 lesions. No correlation was noted between FDOPA transport constant K1 or SUV for FDOPA compared to FDG, nor between K1 for FDOPA and [¹⁵O]water. FDOPA uptake is therefore not perfusion dependent and provides different information than FDG, and patients with negative FDG findings may be helped by follow-up measurements with FDOPA-PET.

The adrenal gland is the fourth most common site of metastasis after the lungs, liver, and bone, and distinguishing between functioning adrenal and malignancy is challenging. This is particularly relevant to malignant melanoma, since the incidence of adrenal metastasis is approximately 50%. FDG detects metastasis from malignant melanoma but frequently demonstrates false positives. FDOPA-PET and FDG-PET were in concordance in a patient with metastatic melanoma to the adrenal glands, both demonstrating intense uptake in the adrenal masses. Final diagnosis was massive bilateral adrenal metastases from malignant melanoma [55].

As much as 20% of malignant melanoma patients develop brain metastasis, with poor prognosis and a mean survival of 2–5 months. FDOPA-PET has been shown to be useful to differentiate progression of metastatic melanoma from radionecrosis following radiosurgery (gamma knife) [31]. A study of 28 patients with brain tumors (19 gliomas, 9 brain metastases, 1 of which was melanoma) was investigated by FDOPA-PET prior to surgery and anti-LAT1 immunohistochemistry on surgical specimens to assess whether uptake of the tracer correlated with LAT1 expression [18], as FDOPA is believed to be taken up by tumors via the AA transporter LAT1. Significant association was observed between FDOPA uptake and LAT1 score, but there was no linear correlation. Parameters besides LAT1 must be involved in brain tumor enrichment by FDOPA. Additional studies investigated the utility of FDOPA-PET in comparison with FDG-PET in evaluating metastatic melanoma to the brain [13]. Both high-grade and low-grade tumors were identified by FDOPA-PET, and the sensitivity was substantially higher than for FDG. For the 81 brain tumor patients evaluated by FDOPA-PET, a sensitivity of 98% and specificity of 86% was attained. PET using FDOPA was found to be more accurate than FDG for evaluation of low-grade tumors and for distinguishing between tumor recurrence and radiation necrosis.

16α-$[^{18}F]Fluoro$-17β-$Estradiol$ (FES)

Estrogens are endogenous hormones that act primarily by regulating gene expression. Estrogen receptors (ER) are located in the cell nuclei within the female reproductive tract, breast, pituitary, hypothalamus, bone, liver, and other tissues. Estrogens passively diffuse through the cell membrane and bind to ER located in the nucleus.

ER are expressed by breast cancer and other types of cancers. Responsiveness to estrogen-receptor-targeted therapy is predicted by tumor ER content, but receptor binding assays suffer from inter-assay variability and intrinsic tumor ER heterogeneity. Unlike analysis of ER in tissue biopsies, ER imaging with FES can assess heterogeneity in ER expression. FES-PET has been shown to be valuable for in vivo evaluation of ER status and prognosis of therapy in breast cancer patients. ER are expressed in uterine leiomyomas in comparison to sarcomas. FES-PET and FDG-PET were performed in 38 patients with uterine tumors to examine the relationship between ER expression and glucose utilization [62]. Differences were noted between patients with endometrial carcinoma, endometrial hyperplasia, leiomyoma, and sarcoma. Uterine sarcoma ($n = 4$) showed the lowest uptake of FES and an insignificant difference between the SUV for FES and FDG, due to large variability of the latter. PET measurement of ER expression and glucose utilization may be a means for the differential diagnosis of uterine tumors. Another study examined 76 patients with suspected uterine sarcoma based on ultrasound, and MRI findings were studied using FDG-PET [70]. Of these, 24 patients also underwent FES-PET studies due to equivocal FDG-PET findings. Based on FES-PET, 11 patients were diagnosed as uterine sarcoma and 13 as leiomyoma, verified by histological examination. The addition of FES-PET in equivocal cases can decrease the number of false positive FDG findings and thereby improve diagnostic accuracy.

The pretreatment FDG/FES ratio was found to be a useful predictor of uterine sarcoma outcomes [69]. The SUV for FDG and FES and the FDG/FES ratio for a group of 18 patients with different histological subtypes of uterine cancer were examined for correlation with progression-free survival (PFS) and overall survival (OS). Patients with FDG SUV >5.5 had worse OS and patients with FES SUV ≤1.5 had worse PFS. For FDG/FES >2.6, both PFS and OS were worse. Measurement of the pretreatment FDG/FES ratio has predictive value for the prognosis of uterine sarcoma patients.

$3'$-$Deoxy$-$3'$-$[^{18}F]Fluorothymidine$ (FLT)

Unchecked proliferation is a common characteristic of tumor cells, and measurement of the proliferation rate of lesions helps to differentiate benign from malignant tumors and from normal tissues. Tumor metabolism, as measured with FDG, is often affected by inflammatory processes that may include necrotic cells. Thymidine (TdR) is a standard marker of DNA synthesis, and the TdR analog, FLT, has been developed for PET measurement of tumor proliferation. FLT is phosphorylated by thymidine kinase-1 (TK-1), an enzyme expressed in the cell cycle during the DNA synthesis phase. Intracellular FLT monophosphate does not permeate the cell membrane and remains metabolically trapped within cells. Most cancer cells have much greater TK-1 activity than normal cells, so uptake and accumulation of FLT is an index of cellular proliferation. FLT-PET has been successfully used for detection and monitoring of tumor proliferation, staging of tumors, and for detection of metastases.

FLT was evaluated in 16 patients with 18 untreated thoracic tumors (two of which were sarcoma) as a means for PET diagnosis and staging [23] and was compared with FDG. All tumors demonstrated significant FLT accumulation, although less than for FDG. FLT-PET accurately visualized tumors, but background accumulation in liver and bone marrow may hamper detection of nearby tumors. Another study examined the usefulness of FLT for staging metastatic melanoma [17]. Ten patients with Stage III melanoma metastatic to local LN underwent FLT-PET. Region-based sensitivity for detection of LN metastatic disease was 88%, with a specificity of 60%. The low specificity results may be due in part to the low number of false-positive and true-negative lesions in this patient population. FLT-PET is particularly useful in predicting/assessing response to therapy and, thus, discriminating responding and nonresponding melanoma patients early after anticancer therapy to aid in individualizing therapy. In one study, 14 melanoma patients with lymph node metastases were administered dendritic cell (DC) vaccine therapy via intranodal injection, and response was assessed by FLT-PET at various times afterward [1]. Immune response was readily visualized in treated lymph nodes and persisted for up to 3 weeks. FLT uptake in the LN significantly correlated to levels of circulating antigen-specific IgG antibodies and antigen-specific proliferation of T cells. Of note there was no such correlation with FDG uptake. FLT-PET is a sensitive method to assess kinetics, localization, and involvement of lymphocyte subsets in response to DC vaccination.

FLT-PET has also been used to predict therapeutic response of mucosal malignant melanoma patients to carbon ion radiotherapy (CIRT) treatment. FLT-PET was performed before and 1 month after CIRT in 13 patients with mucosal malignant melanoma [32]. Pre- and post-FLT SUV measures, reduction rate, and relevant clinical parameters were evaluated in relation to survival estimates. Pre-SUV_{max} $\geq$4.3, age $\geq$80 year, and tumor volume $\geq$39 mL were prognostic for better overall survival, whereas pre-SUV_{max} $\geq$5.0, age $\geq$80 year, sinusoidal cavity tumor location,

and absence of nodal involvement were prognostic for metastasis-free survival. Application of such data may lead to development of optimal treatment strategies based on prognostic factors for individual patients.

FLT-PET also has been used in soft tissue sarcoma. Twenty patients with resectable, high-grade soft tissue sarcoma were examined by FLT-PET before and after neoadjuvant therapy to evaluate tumor viability and proliferation [7]. Baseline tumor SUV_{peak} averaged 7.1 and decreased to 2.7 on follow-up, but reductions were not specific for histopathological response. Marked reductions were not noted in most patients with sarcoma, and, thus, FLT-PET does not appear to be promising for the reliable prediction of response to neoadjuvant treatment of patients with soft tissue sarcoma.

[^{18}F]Fluoromisonidazole (FMISO) Hypoxia is an important aspect of tumors to assess because it can affect the outcome of anticancer treatment. Tumors can become relatively resistant to therapy because of lack of oxygen, which is a potent radiosensitizer. For this reason, substantial effort has been dedicated to the development of methods and imaging techniques for measuring oxygen in tissues. Positron-emitting tracers have been developed to measure tumor hypoxia, offering a less invasive and less technically demanding alternative to the Eppendorf (oxygen) electrode method. Such an imaging technique also avoids sampling bias.

[^{18}F]Fluoromisonidazole (FMISO) has become the most widely used nitroimidazole derivative for this technique. FMISO selectively accumulates in hypoxic cells and has been used to quantitatively assess tumor hypoxia in the lung, brain, and head and neck cancer and in myocardial ischemia. The mechanism for FMISO accumulation is chemical reduction and binding to macromolecules within hypoxic cells. FMISO is relatively lipophilic and passively diffuses across cell membranes. Because of the slow reaction mechanisms and passive diffusion of FMISO, its application for quantification of hypoxic tumor areas requires long examination protocols. Another limitation of FMISO-PET is that severe cases of tissue hypoxia are underestimated, possibly due to a threshold below which bioreduction and sequestration of FMISO stops increasing.

To examine the relationship between tumor hypoxia and metabolism, 19 patients (10 male, nine female) with soft tissue sarcoma underwent FMISO-PET and FDG-PET prior to neoadjuvant chemotherapy or surgery [51]. Ten of the patients were also studied by both radiotracers after their third cycle of chemotherapy. Significant hypoxia was found in 76% of tumors before therapy, and there was no correlation between hypoxic volume and tumor grade or volume. The correlation between FMISO and FDG uptake was only 0.49, and most tumors demonstrated reduced uptake of both FMISO and FDG after therapy. FMISO-PET revealed areas of significant and heterogeneous hypoxia in soft tissue sarcoma, and the discrepancy between FDG and FMISO uptake indicated that regional metabolism and hypoxia do not always correlate. In another study the correlation coefficient between FDG and FMISO uptake was 0.32 in patients with soft tissue sarcoma [50]. There were highly significant difference among the different tumor types, and whereas hypoxia can affect glucose metabolism, some hypoxic tumors can have modest glucose metabolism, and some highly metabolic tumors are not hypoxic. This discordance in tracer uptake may be tumor type specific.

Patients with soft tissue sarcoma were evaluated with [^{11}C]thymidine, FMISO, and [^{11}C]verapamil in a single PET session to assess cellular proliferation, hypoxia, and P-glycoprotein activity, respectively [24]. [^{15}O]Water and [^{15}O]carbon monoxide measurements of perfusion and tissue pH were also done by PET. Tumor uptake parameters varied between the patients, and specific characteristics suggest that each patient tumor has a unique biological profile. Multi-agent PET may be valuable tool for assessing individual tumor characteristics and personalized therapeutic decision-making.

Sodium [^{18}F]Fluoride (NaF) NaF is chemically the simplest ^{18}F radiopharmaceutical to prepare (it is essentially a cyclotron target product or

labeling precursor), but it nevertheless has useful clinical applications due to the behavior of the ion in vivo. [^{18}F]Fluoride anions localize to bone via exchange with hydroxyl ions on the surface of hydroxyapatite crystals, which has led its use in PET imaging of bone lesions, benign and malignant, and vulnerable atherosclerotic plaque. Besides bone, NaF can also localize to extraosseous calcifying lesions in non-boney tissues.

Both NaF-PET and FDG-PET are individually informative imaging procedures that provide complementary information to the clinician. FDG is recommended for evaluation of both soft tissue sarcoma and bone sarcoma, whereas NaF is preferred for evaluation of bone sarcomas only. A novel approach is to combine the two radiopharmaceuticals and scan both tracers simultaneously during the same imaging session. A retrospective review of 21 patients with biopsy-proved sarcoma [33] demonstrated an overall sensitivity of 82% for NaF-PET/FDG-PET, but the overall specificity was relatively low 60%. NaF-PET also has been shown to be superior to FDG in detection of hepatic metastasis from osteosarcoma [12]. There are several examples where NaF-PET has been shown to be clinically valuable in patient assessment and treatment planning. This is especially true in evaluation for metastasis, where new tumor seeding can appear in unexpected locations [35] such as osteosarcoma with metastasis to right ventricule [15] or abdominal muscles [64]. However, extraosseous findings (vascular uptake) on NaF-PET can be important by unmasking clinically relevant non-malignant findings that influence clinical decision-making [68].

[^{18}F]Fluciclatide (FC) FC is a small synthetic cyclic peptide that contains an RGD-sequence (Arg-Gly-Asp) labeled with ^{18}F for PET imaging of tumors. The RGD architecture of FC binds to $\alpha_V\beta_3$ and $\alpha_V\beta_5$ integrin receptors, which are frequently upregulated on tumor cell surfaces and endothelial cells in the tumor vasculature. The labeled peptide may be of use in PET measurements of changes in tumor vascularity that occur in response to antiangiogenic agents. Limited clinical studies have shown 100% visualization of malignant melanoma lesions by FC-PET [44]. There was variable tumor uptake of FC; however, a good correlation between PET-derived Patlak influx rate constant (K_i) and $\alpha_V\beta_5$ optical density (OD) was observed (correlation coefficient of $r = 0.83$).

[^{18}F]Fluciclovine (FV) FV is a synthetic AA analogue of L-leucine radiolabeled with fluorine-18. Like AA, FV appears to enter cells through the energy-independent LAT system. Because it is an AA analogue, FV is preferentially accumulated in tumor cells due to their increased metabolic requirements. However, since FV is a synthetic nonnatural AA, it is not metabolized. Such a metabolic trapping mechanism leads to cellular enrichment by FV and potential tumor visualization using PET. FV has been used in a patient with recurrent melanoma [61].

N-(2-(diethylamino)-ethyl)-5-[^{18}F]fluoropico-linamide ([^{18}F]P3BZA; FP3BZA) A recent approach for detection of malignant melanoma is to target melanin pigment itself, since only 2–8% of melanomas are amelanotic. FP3BZA is a ^{18}F labeled benzamide with affinity for binding to melanin. In a small study of five patients with multiple melanomas, FP3BZA-PET and FDG-PET detected the primary tumors, two lymph node metastases, and one bone metastasis [42]. Tumoral FP3BZA uptake was higher than that of FDG (the average SUV_{max} was 19.7 ± 5.3 for FP3BZA and 10.8 ± 2.7 for FDG, and 18.2 ± 3.7 and 6.3 ± 2.2, respectively, for metastases). The higher uptake by FP3BZA has potential of increasing the accuracy of diagnosis and treatment monitoring compared to FDG-PET in patients with malignant melanoma.

^{68}Ga-Labeled Octreotide Analogs Somatostatin is a 28 amino acid peptide with a plasma half-life of approximately 3 minutes, so it is not appropriate for radiolabeling. Instead, eight amino acid analogs like octreotide (OC) have been developed for therapeutic and imaging purposes. SSTR ligands labeled with ^{68}Ga have had the most success, and their development has evolved over several years based on earlier work done

with ^{99m}Tc- and ^{111}In-labeled SPECT radiopharmaceuticals based on OC.

For PET, ^{68}Ga is bound to the chelating group 1,4,7,10-tetraazacyclodecane-N,N′,N″,N‴-tetraacetic acid (DOTA) which is covalently linked to the peptide. There have been several octreotide analogs labeled with ^{68}Ga in this fashion. Octreotide itself is inadequate because it binds mainly to SSTR2 with moderate affinity. The major ^{68}Ga-labeled SSTR-binding radiopharmaceuticals are metal complexes of DOTANOC ([DOTA0, 1-Nal3]octreotide), DOTATATE ([DOTA0, Tyr3, Thr8]octreotide), and DOTATOC ([DOTA0, Tyr3]octreotide). This class of PET drugs represents the most clinically applied of all ^{68}Ga-labeled pharmaceuticals in nuclear medicine.

Imaging of SSTR-expressing tumors with ^{68}Ga-labeled peptides has been applied for tumor detection and staging, prediction of the response to therapeutic somatostatin, and treatment planning for SSTR-directed radionuclide therapy. The most clinically accepted indication is tumor localization and staging, for which SSTR imaging has become part of the clinical routine for carcinoids and other neuroendocrine tumors. These tumors, frequently arising from the gut or other abdominal structures, can be challenging to identify by conventional anatomic imaging; such well-differentiated neuroendocrine tumors have limited FDG uptake and modest effectiveness of FDG-PET in neuroendocrine tumor staging.

[^{68}Ga](DOTA)-1-Nal3-octreotide([^{68}Ga]-DOTA-NOC; Ga-DOTANOC) Malignant melanoma can undergo neuroendocrine differentiation. Ga-DOTANOC-PET has been shown to be useful in identifying metastatic lesions from melanoma and alveolar rhabdomyosarcoma [37, 71]. However, preliminary results for Ga-DOTATOC-PET in patients with metastatic malignant melanoma were disappointing [10]. Ga-DOTATOC-PET detected metastatic lesions in 11 of the 18 patients (61%), but only 59 of 263 lesions (22%) on a lesion-by-lesion basis. FDG-avid lesions were missed by Ga-DOTATOC, and the mean SUV_{max} was only 3.1 for Ga-DOTATOC-PET

compared to 28.2 for FDG-PET. This is likely due to low levels of SSTR in the lesions.

[⁶⁸Ga](DOTA)-Tyr(3)-Thr(8)-Octreotide ([⁶⁸Ga]-DOTA-TATE; Ga-DOTATATE) Carney triad is a rare syndrome characterized by the synchronous occurrence of gastrointestinal stromal tumors, pulmonary chondroma, and extrarenal paraganglioma. Ga-DOTATATE-PET has been successfully used for restaging of extra-adrenal metastasizing paraganglioma and determined eligibility of the patient for targeted radionuclide therapy [20]. Similarly, Ga-DOTATATE-PET demonstrated high uptake in an epithelioid hemangioendothelioma, which is a rare tumor derived from vascular endothelial cells with potential for metastasis [21]. The uptake of Ga-DOTATATE was greater than that of FDG (SUV_{max} 10.7 and 3.7, respectively) and demonstrated patient eligibility for targeted radionuclide therapy (TRT).

[⁶⁸Ga]Pentixafor (Ga-PEN) Ga-PEN is a radioconjugate comprised of a synthetic, cyclic pentapeptide analog of stromal cell-derived factor-1 (SDF-1), which is a ligand for chemokine receptor C-X-C chemokine receptor type 4 (CXCR4). The chelating moiety for binding ⁶⁸Ga is DOTA, as in the above OC derivatives. CXCR4 can be expressed by cancer cells and is a marker of poorly differentiated cells. It plays a key role in tumor growth progression, invasiveness, and metastasis. The studies in malignant melanoma and soft tissue sarcoma with Ga-PEN have been disappointing, as the Ga-PEN uptake was much less than the FDG uptake in these lesions [65]. Thus, FDG-PET seems to be a more suitable general clinical diagnostic method, although Ga-PEN-PET may have merit in specialized applications such as stratification for targeted radionuclide therapy (TRT) with ⁹⁰Y- or ¹⁷⁷Lu-pentixafor or monitoring chemokine CXCR4-directed pharmacotherapy.

[⁶⁸Ga]HBED-CC-PSMA-11 (Ga-PSMA) Ga-PSMA is a ⁶⁸Ga-labeled PET radiopharmaceutical that targets the human prostate membrane antigen (PSMA). The PSMA-targeting peptide is Glu-urea-Lys(Ahx), and the ⁶⁸Ga is coordination by the bifunctional chelate N,N′-bis [2-hydroxy-5-(carboxyethyl)benzyl] ethylenediamine-N,N′-diacetic acid (HBED-CC). PSMA is a tumor-associated antigen and type II transmembrane protein expressed on the membrane of prostatic epithelial cells and overexpressed on prostate tumor cells. Ga-PSMA binds to the overexpressed PSMA via the Glu-urea-Lys(Ahx) moiety, is internalized, and thereby concentrates in tumor cells for detection by PET imaging. Due to the relatively small size of Ga-PSMA, unbound radio ligand is rapidly excreted resulting in high tumor to background ratios. Ga-PSMA-PET has been used to image all stages of prostate cancer. It has high sensitivity and specificity for localization of primary tumors and has been applied for image-guided biopsy. The technique may also have utility for lymph node staging, although this is controversial. Ga-PSMA-PET has also been used to evaluate local, nodal, and distant recurrence of prostate cancer. It has been shown that Ga-PSMA may be useful to differentiate rare histologic subtype, partially differentiated sarcomatoid metastasis, of prostate cancer from adenocarcinoma of the prostate [26]. In addition, Ga-PSMA-PET has shown promise in detecting osteosarcoma arising from fibrous dysplasia [52], which highlights the ability of Ga-PSMA-PET to detect neoangiogenesis in osteosarcoma and may have implications for assessing antiangiogenesis-based therapeutic options.

Future Perspective

There is great potential for the development of novel PET radiopharmaceuticals that enhance understanding of the pathophysiology of melanoma and sarcoma, with improvements for both diagnosis and monitoring of therapeutic approaches to these conditions. With the availability of several positron-emitting radionuclides and established radiolabeling techniques for each, there is great capability for the preparation of a wide variety of molecular structures as PET tracers. Innovative PET radiopharmaceuticals can thus be prepared that are based upon new tumor biomarkers discovered in preclinical or clinical research. Quality control methodology has been standardized and can readily be applied to new molecular structures. Regulatory approval via eIND or RDRC facilitates rapid translation of new radiopharmaceuticals to human studies in a safe manner.

Several PET studies of melanoma or sarcoma involving numerous PET radiopharmaceuticals with different localization mechanisms, while limited in scope, have demonstrated promising findings. Differences between these results and those from FDG-PET encourage further research and development of new PET biomarkers that map unique tumor targets. Such novel PET radiopharmaceuticals could be used in concert with traditional FDG imaging to give improved understanding of an individual patient's tumor pathophysiology. The improved clinical information gained from such new PET biomarkers for melanoma and sarcoma would translate to improved, personalized care of patients suffering from these afflictions.

References

1. Aarntzen EH, Srinivas M, De Wilt JH, Jacobs JF, Lesterhuis WJ, Windhorst AD, de Vries IJ. Early identification of antigen-specific immune responses in vivo by [18F]-labeled 3′-fluoro-3′-deoxy-thymidine ([18F]FLT) PET imaging. Proc Natl Acad Sci U S A. 2011;108(45):18396–9. https://doi.org/10.1073/pnas.1113045108.
2. Abiko T, Koizumi S, Takanami I. Dual primary subclavicular angiosarcoma and lung cancer imaging with C-11 acetate PET and FDG PET. Clin Nucl Med. 2009;34(5):302–4. https://doi.org/10.1097/RLU.0b013e31819e5242.
3. Alexoff DL. Automation for the radiosynthesis and application of PET radiopharmaceuticals. In: Welch MJ, Redvanly CS, editors. Radiopharmaceutical handbook. Radiochemistry and applications. Chichester: Wiley; 2004. p. 283–306.
4. Anderson CJ, Ferdani R. Copper-64 radiopharmaceuticals for PET imaging of cancer: advances in preclinical and clinical research. Cancer Biother Radiopharm. 2009;24(4):379–93. https://doi.org/10.1089/cbr.2009.0674.
5. Antoni GKT, Langstrom B. Aspects on the synthesis of 11C-labelled compounds. In: Welch MJ, Redvanly CS, editors. Handbook of radiopharmaceuticals. Radiochemistry and applications. Chichester: Wiley; 2003. p. 141–94.
6. Becher S, Oskouei S. PET imaging in sarcoma. Orthop Clin North Am. 2015;46(3):409–415, xi. https://doi.org/10.1016/j.ocl.2015.03.001.
7. Benz MR, Czernin J, Allen-Auerbach MS, Dry SM, Sutthiruangwong P, Spick C, Radu C, Weber WA, Tap WD, Eilber FC. 3′-deoxy-3′-[18F]fluorothymidine positron emission tomography for response assessment in soft tissue sarcoma: a pilot study to correlate imaging findings with tissue thymidine kinase 1 and Ki-67 activity and histopathologic response. Cancer. 2012;118(12):3135–44. https://doi.org/10.1002/cncr.26630.
8. Bormans G, Buck A, Chiti A, Cooper M, Croasdale J, Desruet M, Windhorst AD. Position statement on radiopharmaceutical production for clinical trials. EJNMMI Radiopharm Chem. 2017;2(1):12. https://doi.org/10.1186/s41181-017-0031-y.
9. Boschi S, Malizia C, Lodi F. Overview and perspectives on automation strategies in (68) Ga radiopharmaceutical preparations. Recent Results Cancer Res. 2013;194:17–31. https://doi.org/10.1007/978-3-642-27994-2_2.
10. Brogsitter C, Zophel K, Wunderlich G, Kammerer E, Stein A, Kotzerke J. Comparison between F-18 fluorodeoxyglucose and Ga-68 DOTATOC in metastasized melanoma. Nucl Med Commun. 2013;34(1):47–9. https://doi.org/10.1097/MNM.0b013e32835ae4ed.
11. Burgers AMG, Wondergem M, van der Zant FM, Knol RJJ. Incidental detection of a melanoma by 18F-Fluorocholine PET/CT performed for evaluation of primary hyperparathyroidism. Clin Nucl Med. 2018;43(4):265–6. https://doi.org/10.1097/RLU.0000000000001972.
12. Cai L, Chen Y, Huang Z, Wu J. Incidental detection of solitary hepatic metastasis by 99mTc-MDP and 18F-NaF PET/CT in a patient with osteosarcoma of the tibia. Clin Nucl Med. 2015;40(9):759–61. https://doi.org/10.1097/RLU.0000000000000769.
13. Chen W, Silverman DH, Delaloye S, Czernin J, Kamdar N, Pope W, Cloughesy T. 18F-FDOPA PET imaging of brain tumors: comparison study with 18F-FDG PET and evaluation of diagnostic accuracy. J Nucl Med. 2006;47(6):904–11. Retrieved from http://www.ncbi.nlm.nih.gov/entrez/query.fcgi?cmd=Retrieve&db=PubMed&dopt=Citation&list_uids=16741298.
14. Cherry SR, Dahlbom M. PET: physics, instrumentation, and scanners. In: Phelps ME, editor. PET. Molecular imaging and its biological applications. New York: Springer; 2004. p. 1–124.
15. Chou YH, Ko KY, Cheng MF, Chen WW, Yen RF. 18F-NaF PET/CT images of cardiac metastasis from osteosarcoma. Clin Nucl Med. 2016;41(9):708–9. https://doi.org/10.1097/RLU.0000000000001289.
16. Clark JCA. Chemistry of Nitrogen-13 and Oxygen-15. In: Welch MJRCS, editor. Handbook of radiopharmaceuticals. Radiochemistry and applications. Chichester: Wiley; 2004. p. 119–40.

17. Cobben DC, Jager PL, Elsinga PH, Maas B, Suurmeijer AJ, Hoekstra HJ. 3′-18F-fluoro-3′-deoxy-L-thymidine: a new tracer for staging metastatic melanoma? J Nucl Med. 2003;44(12):1927–32.

18. Dadone-Montaudie B, Ambrosetti D, Dufour M, Darcourt J, Almairac F, Coyne J, Burel-Vandenbos F. [^{18}F] FDOPA standardized uptake values of brain tumors are not exclusively dependent on LAT1 expression. PLoS One. 2017;12(9):e0184625. https://doi.org/10.1371/journal.pone.0184625.

19. Decristoforo C, Penuelas I, Patt M, Todde S. European regulations for the introduction of novel radiopharmaceuticals in the clinical setting. Q J Nucl Med Mol Imaging. 2017;61(2):135–44. https://doi.org/10.23736/S1824-4785.17.02965-X.

20. Derlin T, Hartung D, Hueper K. 68Ga-DOTA-TATE PET/CT for molecular imaging of somatostatin receptor expression in extra-adrenal paraganglioma in a case of complete carney triad. Clin Nucl Med. 2017a;42(12):e527–8. https://doi.org/10.1097/RLU.0000000000001864.

21. Derlin T, Hueper K, Soudah B. 68Ga-DOTA-TATE PET/CT for molecular imaging of somatostatin receptor expression in metastasizing epithelioid hemangioendothelioma: comparison with 18F-FDG. Clin Nucl Med. 2017b;42(11):e478–9. https://doi.org/10.1097/RLU.0000000000001814.

22. Dimitrakopoulou-Strauss A, Strauss LG, Burger C. Quantitative PET studies in pretreated melanoma patients: a comparison of 6-[^{18}F]fluoro-L-dopa with 18F-FDG and (15)O-water using compartment and noncompartment analysis. J Nucl Med. 2001;42(2):248–56. Retrieved from https://www.ncbi.nlm.nih.gov/pubmed/11216523.

23. Dittmann H, Dohmen BM, Paulsen F, Eichhorn K, Eschmann SM, Horger M, Bares R. [^{18}F]FLT PET for diagnosis and staging of thoracic tumours. Eur J Nucl Med Mol Imaging. 2003;30(10):1407–12. https://doi.org/10.1007/s00259-003-1257-3.

24. Eary JF, Link JM, Muzi M, Conrad EU, Mankoff DA, White JK, Krohn KA. Multiagent PET for risk characterization in sarcoma. J Nucl Med. 2011;52(4):541–6. https://doi.org/10.2967/jnumed.110.083717.

25. Fani M, Andre JP, Maecke HR. 68Ga-PET: a powerful generator-based alternative to cyclotron-based PET radiopharmaceuticals. Contrast Media Mol Imaging. 2008;3(2):67–77. https://doi.org/10.1002/cmmi.232.

26. Geraldo L, Ceci F, Uprimny C, Kendler D, Virgolini I. Detection of sarcomatoid lung metastasis with 68GA-PSMA PET/CT in a patient with prostate cancer. Clin Nucl Med. 2016;41(5):421–2. https://doi.org/10.1097/RLU.0000000000001157.

27. Ghigi G, Micera R, Maffione AM, Castellucci P, Cammelli S, Ammendolia I, Rubello D. 11C-methionine vs. 18F-FDG PET in soft tissue sarcoma patients treated with neoadjuvant therapy: preliminary results. In Vivo. 2009;23(1):105–10. Retrieved from https://www.ncbi.nlm.nih.gov/pubmed/19368133.

28. Grassi I, Nanni C, Allegri V, Morigi JJ, Montini GC, Castellucci P, Fanti S. The clinical use of PET with (11)C-acetate. Am J Nucl Med Mol Imaging. 2012;2(1):33–47. Retrieved from http://www.ncbi.nlm.nih.gov/pubmed/23133801.

29. Harisankar CN, Mittal BR, Watts A, Bhattacharya A, Sen R. Utility of dynamic perfusion PET using (1)(3)N-ammonia in diagnosis of asymptomatic recurrence of fibrosarcoma. Clin Nucl Med. 2011;36(2):150–1. https://doi.org/10.1097/RLU.0b013e318203be6c.

30. Hasebe M, Yoshikawa K, Nishii R, Kawaguchi K, Kamada T, Hamada Y. Usefulness of (11)C-methionine-PET for predicting the efficacy of carbon ion radiation therapy for head and neck mucosal malignant melanoma. Int J Oral Maxillofac Surg. 2017;46(10):1220–8. https://doi.org/10.1016/j.ijom.2017.04.019.

31. Hernandez Pinzon J, Mena D, Aguilar M, Biafore F, Recondo G, Bastianello M. Radionecrosis versus disease progression in brain metastasis. Value of (18)F-DOPA PET/CT/MRI. Rev Esp Med Nucl Imagen Mol. 2016;35(5):332–5. https://doi.org/10.1016/j.remn.2016.03.002.

32. Inubushi M, Saga T, Koizumi M, Takagi R, Hasegawa A, Koto M, Kamada T. Predictive value of 3′-deoxy-3′-[^{18}F]fluorothymidine positron emission tomography/computed tomography for outcome of carbon ion radiotherapy in patients with head and neck mucosal malignant melanoma. Ann Nucl Med. 2013;27(1):1–10. https://doi.org/10.1007/s12149-012-0652-x.

33. Jackson T, Mosci C, von Eyben R, Mittra E, Ganjoo K, Biswal S, Iagaru A. Combined 18F-NaF and 18F-FDG PET/CT in the evaluation of sarcoma patients. Clin Nucl Med. 2015;40(9):720–4. https://doi.org/10.1097/RLU.0000000000000845.

34. Jiang L, Wang D, Zhang Y, Li J, Wu Z, Wang Z, Wang D. Investigation of the pro-apoptotic effects of arbutin and its acetylated derivative on murine melanoma cells. Int J Mol Med. 2018;41(2):1048–54. https://doi.org/10.3892/ijmm.2017.3256.

35. Jones RP, Iagaru A. 18F NaF brain metastasis uptake in a patient with melanoma. Clin Nucl Med. 2014;39(10):e448–50. https://doi.org/10.1097/RLU.0000000000000371.

36. Jordan D. An overview of the ommon technical dossier (CTD) regulatory dossier. Med Writing. 2014;23(2):101–5.

37. Jung RS, Mittal BR, Bal A, Dey P, Shukla J, Kapoor R. Metastatic melanoma to the thyroid gland expressing somatostatin receptors-imaging with 68Ga-DOTANOC PET/CT. Clin Nucl Med. 2015;40(2):175–6. https://doi.org/10.1097/RLU.0000000000000636.

38. Kebir S, Rauschenbach L, Galldiks N, Schlaak M, Hattingen E, Landsberg J, Glas M. Dynamic O-(2-[^{18}F]fluoroethyl)-L-tyrosine PET imaging for the detection of checkpoint inhibitor-related pseudoprogression in melanoma brain metastases. Neuro-Oncology.

2016;18(10):1462–4. https://doi.org/10.1093/neuonc/now154.

39. Kowalsky RJF, Falen SW, editors. Radiopharmaceuticals in nuclear pharmacy and nuclear medicine. 3rd ed. Washington DC: American Pharmacists Association; 2011.

40. Lange R, ter Heine R, Decristoforo C, Penuelas I, Elsinga PH, van der Westerlaken MM, Hendrikse NH. Untangling the web of European regulations for the preparation of unlicensed radiopharmaceuticals: a concise overview and practical guidance for a risk-based approach. Nucl Med Commun. 2015;36(5):414–22. https://doi.org/10.1097/MNM.0000000000000276.

41. Lindholm P, Leskinen S, Nagren K, Lehikoinen P, Ruotsalainen U, Teras M, Joensuu H. Carbon-11-methionine PET imaging of malignant melanoma. J Nucl Med. 1995;36(10):1806–10. Retrieved from https://www.ncbi.nlm.nih.gov/pubmed/7562047.

42. Ma X, Wang S, Wang S, Liu D, Zhao X, Chen H, Cheng Z. Biodistribution, radiation dosimetry, and clinical application of a melanin-targeted PET probe, (18) F-P3BZA, in patients. J Nucl Med. 2019;60(1):16–22. https://doi.org/10.2967/jnumed.118.209643.

43. Maecke HR, Andre JP. 68Ga-PET radiopharmacy: a generator-based alternative to 18F-radiopharmacy. Ernst Schering Res Found Workshop. 2007;62:215–42. https://doi.org/10.1007/978-3-540-49527-7_8.

44. Mena E, Owenius R, Turkbey B, Sherry R, Bratslavsky G, Macholl S, Kurdziel K. [(1)(8)F]fluciclatide in the in vivo evaluation of human melanoma and renal tumors expressing alphavbeta 3 and alpha vbeta 5 integrins. Eur J Nucl Med Mol Imaging. 2014;41(10):1879–88. https://doi.org/10.1007/s00259-014-2791-x.

45. Mena E, Sanli Y, Marcus C, Subramaniam RM. Precision medicine and PET/computed tomography in melanoma. PET Clin. 2017;12(4):449–58. https://doi.org/10.1016/j.cpet.2017.05.002.

46. Moerlein SM, Welch MJ. The chemistry of gallium and indium as related to radiopharmaceutical production. Int J Nucl Med Biol. 1981;8(4):277–87. https://doi.org/10.1016/0047-0740(81)90034-6.

47. Morita T, Kurihara H, Hiroi K, Honda N, Igaki H, Hatazawa J, Itami J. Dynamic changes in (18) F-borono-L-phenylalanine uptake in unresectable, advanced, or recurrent squamous cell carcinoma of the head and neck and malignant melanoma during boron neutron capture therapy patient selection. Radiat Oncol. 2018;13(1):4. https://doi.org/10.1186/s13014-017-0949-y.

48. Mosessian S, Duarte-Vogel SM, Stout DB, Roos KP, Lawson GW, Jordan MC, Phelps ME. INDs for PET molecular imaging probes-approach by an academic institution. Mol Imaging Biol. 2014;16(4):441–8. https://doi.org/10.1007/s11307-014-0735-2.

49. Qin C, Hu F, Arnous MMR, Lan X. Detection of non-FDG-avid residual sinonasal malignant melanoma in the skull base with 11C-choline PET and contrast-enhanced MRI. Clin Nucl Med. 2017;42(11):885–6. https://doi.org/10.1097/RLU.0000000000001836.

50. Rajendran JG, Mankoff DA, O'Sullivan F, Peterson LM, Schwartz DL, Conrad EU, Krohn KA. Hypoxia and glucose metabolism in malignant tumors: evaluation by [¹⁸F]fluoromisonidazole and [¹⁸F]fluorodeoxyglucose positron emission tomography imaging. Clin Cancer Res. 2004;10(7):2245–52.

51. Rajendran JG, Wilson DC, Conrad EU, Peterson LM, Bruckner JD, Rasey JS, Krohn KA. [(18)F]FMISO and [(18)F]FDG PET imaging in soft tissue sarcomas: correlation of hypoxia, metabolism and VEGF expression. Eur J Nucl Med Mol Imaging. 2003;30(5):695–704. Retrieved from http://www.ncbi.nlm.nih.gov/entrez/query.fcgi?cmd=Retrieve&db=PubMed&dopt=Citation&list_uids=12632200.

52. Sasikumar A, Joy A, Pillai MRA, Alex TM, Narayanan G. 68Ga-PSMA PET/CT in osteosarcoma in fibrous dysplasia. Clin Nucl Med. 2017;42(6):446–7. https://doi.org/10.1097/RLU.0000000000001646.

53. Schwarz SW, Decristoforo C. US and EU radiopharmaceutical diagnostic and therapeutic nonclinical study requirements for clinical trials authorizations and marketing authorizations. EJNMMI Radiopharm Chem. 2019;4(1):10. https://doi.org/10.1186/s41181-019-0059-2.

54. Schwarz SW, Decristoforo C, Goodbody AE, Singhal N, Saliba S, Ruddock P, Ross AA. Harmonization of United States, European Union and Canadian first-in-human regulatory requirements for radiopharmaceuticals-is this possible? J Nucl Med. 2018;60(2):158–66. https://doi.org/10.2967/jnumed.118.209460.

55. Seshadri N, Wat J, Balan K. Bilateral adrenal metastases from malignant melanoma: concordant findings on (18)F-FDG and (18)F-FDOPA PET. Eur J Nucl Med Mol Imaging. 2006;33(7):854–5. https://doi.org/10.1007/s00259-006-0101-y.

56. Snyder SEK. Chemistry of Fluorine-18 radiopharmaceuticals. In: Welch MJ, Redvanly CS, editors. Handbook of radiopharmaceuticals. Radiochemistry and applications. Chichester: Wiley; 2004. p. 195–228.

57. Sollini M, Pasqualetti F, Perri M, Coraggio G, Castellucci P, Roncali M, Erba PA. Detection of a second malignancy in prostate cancer patients by using [(18)F]Choline PET/CT: a case series. Cancer Imaging. 2016;16(1):27. https://doi.org/10.1186/s40644-016-0085-1.

58. Spang P, Herrmann C, Roesch F. Bifunctional Gallium-68 Chelators: past, present, and future. Semin Nucl Med. 2016;46(5):373–94. https://doi.org/10.1053/j.semnuclmed.2016.04.003.

59. Suleiman OH, Fejka R, Houn F, Walsh M. The radioactive drug research committee: background and retrospective study of reported research data (1975-2004). J Nucl Med. 2006;47(7):1220–6. Retrieved from https://www.ncbi.nlm.nih.gov/pubmed/16818959.

60. Tamura K, Yoshikawa K, Ishikawa H, Hasebe M, Tsuji H, Yanagi T, Tsujii H. Carbon-11-methionine PET imaging of choroidal melanoma and the time course after carbon ion beam radiotherapy. Anticancer

Res. 2009;29(5):1507–14. Retrieved from https://www.ncbi.nlm.nih.gov/pubmed/19443358.

61. Teoh EJ, Tsakok MT, Bradley KM, Hyde K, Subesinghe M, Gleeson FV. Recurrent malignant melanoma detected on 18F-Fluciclovine PET/CT imaging for prostate cancer. Clin Nucl Med. 2017;42(10):803–4. https://doi.org/10.1097/RLU.0000000000001789.

62. Tsujikawa T, Yoshida Y, Mori T, Kurokawa T, Fujibayashi Y, Kotsuji F, Okazawa H. Uterine tumors: pathophysiologic imaging with 16alpha-[^{18}F]fluoro-17beta-estradiol and 18F fluorodeoxyglucose PET--initial experience. Radiology. 2008;248(2):599–605. https://doi.org/10.1148/radiol.2482071379.

63. Unterrainer M, Galldiks N, Suchorska B, Kowalew LC, Wenter V, Schmid-Tannwald C, Albert NL. (18)F-FET PET uptake characteristics in patients with newly diagnosed and untreated brain metastasis. J Nucl Med. 2017;58(4):584–9. https://doi.org/10.2967/jnumed.116.180075.

64. Usmani S, Marafi F, Rasheed R, Bakiratharajan D, Al Maraghy M, Al Kandari F. Unsuspected metastases to muscles in osteosarcoma detected on 18F-sodium fluoride PET-CT. Clin Nucl Med. 2018;43(9):e343–5. https://doi.org/10.1097/RLU.0000000000002191.

65. Vag T, Gerngross C, Herhaus P, Eiber M, Philipp-Abbrederis K, Graner FP, Schwaiger M. First experience with chemokine receptor CXCR4-targeted PET imaging of patients with solid cancers. J Nucl Med. 2016;57(5):741–6. https://doi.org/10.2967/jnumed.115.161034.

66. Velikyan I. Prospective of (6)(8) Ga-radiopharmaceutical development. Theranostics. 2013;4(1):47–80. https://doi.org/10.7150/thno.7447.

67. Verbruggen A, Coenen HH, Deverre JR, Guilloteau D, Langstrom B, Salvadori PA, Halldin C. Guideline to regulations for radiopharmaceuticals in early phase clinical trials in the EU. Eur J Nucl Med Mol Imaging. 2008;35(11):2144–51. https://doi.org/10.1007/s00259-008-0853-7.

68. Verma P, Purandare N, Agrawal A, Shah S, Rangarajan V. Unusual finding of a tumor thrombus arising from osteosarcoma detected on 18F-NaF PET/CT. Clin Nucl Med. 2016;41(6):e304–6. https://doi.org/10.1097/RLU.0000000000001174.

69. Yamamoto M, Tsujikawa T, Yamada S, Kurokawa T, Shinagawa A, Chino Y, Yoshida Y. 18F-FDG/18F-FES standardized uptake value ratio determined using PET predicts prognosis in uterine sarcoma. Oncotarget. 2017;8(14):22581–9. https://doi.org/10.18632/oncotarget.15127.

70. Yoshida Y, Kiyono Y, Tsujikawa T, Kurokawa T, Okazawa H, Kotsuji F. Additional value of 16alpha-[^{18}F]fluoro-17beta-oestradiol PET for differential diagnosis between uterine sarcoma and leiomyoma in patients with positive or equivocal findings on [^{18}F]fluorodeoxyglucose PET. Eur J Nucl Med Mol Imaging. 2011;38(10):1824–31. https://doi.org/10.1007/s00259-011-1851-8.

71. Zanoni L, Lopci E, Ambrosini V, Boschi S, Fanti S. Alveolar rhabdomyosarcoma with neuroendocrine differentiation detected by Ga-68 DOTA-NOC PET/CT: a case report. Clin Nucl Med. 2011;36(10):915–8. https://doi.org/10.1097/RLU.0b013e31821a2691.

Future Directions of PET and Molecular Imaging and Therapy with an Emphasis on Melanoma and Sarcoma

Arif Sheikh

Introduction to the Future of Molecular Imaging and Radiotheragnostics

The concepts for molecular imaging have been around for several decades and have come into clearer focus as pathology of disease has been better understood. In essence, the objective is to target a cell receptor, protein, antigen or a unique metabolic process with a radiolabelled tracer that yields information about the pathology and prognostic information about the disease, especially if it can predict response to disease. Radiolabelled antibodies have been available for animal imaging from almost the beginning of nuclear medicine. Clinical imaging started off with elemental or simple tracers, such as iodine-131 (I-131), gallium-67 citrate (Ga-67), thallium-201 chloride (Tl-201) and even F-18 sodium fluoride (NaF), which were found to be useful for evaluating malignant processes. The development of technetium-99m (Tc-99m) allowed radiolabelling of a wide variety of pharmaceuticals, revolutionizing the field. Later, more sophisticated peptide tracers such as In-111 octreotide and I-131 metaiodobenzylguanidine (I-131 mIBG) were developed for the evaluation of various neuroendocrine tumours. There was also subsequent work to develop tracers to evaluate specific tumours, but with limited success. Clinical use of radiolabelled monoclonal antibodies (mAb) fragments saw a brief period of use with the advent of Tc-99m anti-CEA mAb tracer to image colorectal carcinomas. The subsequent clinical introduction of F-18 flurodeoxyglucose (FDG) PET in the late 1990s and early 2000s was a paradigm shift, providing the needed aspects of pathology identification, prognostic information and therapeutic response for oncologic imaging, as well as a significant improvement in resolution compared to SPECT, and the ability to quantify uptake accurately. It also showed the potential of developing specific probes that could further answer clinical questions about the behaviour of disease; however, the astronomical success of FDG PET also had the effect that additional probes that were previously being developed became less relevant. Nevertheless, there was renewed interest in the field as limitations to FDG PET arose. Additionally, more sophisticated knowledge about pathologic metabolic processes, receptors, etc. along with advancements in radiochemistry, and mechanisms of antibody and ligand targeting, allowed development of more innovative approaches to evaluating disease.

Although FDG PET has been successfully used in both melanoma and sarcoma, some important limitations remain. Both diseases have variable FDG uptake in different types of tumour. Whereas just that property has inherent prognostic

A. Sheikh (✉)
Icahn School of Medicine, The Mount Sinai Hospital, New York, NY, USA
e-mail: arif.sheikh@mountsinai.org

© Springer Nature Switzerland AG 2021
A. H. Khandani (ed.), *PET/CT and PET/MR in Melanoma and Sarcoma*,
https://doi.org/10.1007/978-3-030-60429-5_11

information in the diseases, it nevertheless limits the ability to properly stage patients. Given this variability, small tumour deposits, especially in lymph nodes, are underestimated, and clinically important disease could be missed. There is also known limitations of finding brain or liver metastases due to physiologic FDG activity in those organs, all of which has led to interest in finding newer tracers that could improve imaging in these diseases. Yet, the task is not that easy in these processes. There are few targets that are specific to these diseases, or not abundant enough that they can be exploited for imaging. As a result, many of the strategies involve targeting metabolic processes, ligands or receptors which although overexpressed in melanomas and/or sarcomas, are also found in other diseases. Hence, there is great overlap with how these diseases are evaluated, similar to other malignancies.

The concept of targeted radionuclide therapies has been around since around World War II. With the early successes seen in using iodine-131 in benign and malignant thyroid diseases, and phosphorous-32 (P-32) for myelo dyscrasias, research has pursued the idea of being able to specifically deliver radionuclide-labelled vectors to target tissue, thereby delivering high radiation doses while minimizing non-target tissue radiation exposure. There were not many successes until the understanding of various disciplines were advanced, such as tumour biology, immunology as well as radiochemistry and radiobiology, amongst others. There were developments for cavitary ablation for malignant effusions using P-32 and radiosynovectomy for inflammatory arthritides, and the 1990s saw the rise of bone pain palliation treatments. The early 2000s introduced mAbs for the treatment of low-grade, follicular B-cell non-Hodgkin's lymphoma into clinical practice; however, these therapies were unutilized despite their clear benefit compared to other analogous treatments, partly due to financial incentives of the referring physicians.

The introduction of radium-223 dichloride (Ra-223) saw a shift in this attitude as the ALSYMPCA (ALpharadin in SYMPtomatic Prostate CAncer) trial showed a clear survival benefit in the appropriately selected prostate cancer patients with primarily metastatic bone disease [1]. The next major therapies were introduced just within the last 5 years for low-grade neuroendocrine tumours, using [^{177}Lu-DOTA0, Tyr3] octreotate (lutetium-177 DOTATATE) and norepinephrine (I-131 mIBG) analogues. These therapies had been used by many groups for over 30 years prior to that but were not studied in a formal clinical trial until recently and again show evidence of improved clinical outcomes [2]. There is now mounting evidence that newer upcoming therapies with radiolabelled prostate-specific membrane antigen (PSMA) may have a major impact in patients with prostate cancer as well and are thus a part of an upswing of interest in this modality of therapy for other diseases.

The renewed interest in therapy is also being driven by development in molecular imaging. As increasingly sophisticated methods are being found to target specific tumour processes and receptors for imaging, there is a growing realization that some of those targets are specific enough and have sufficiently high target to non-target count ratios that the relevant ligands could be radiolabelled with therapeutic radionuclides. Many of these agents in both the imaging and therapeutic versions are imaged with SPECT. Although there has been great interest in developing tracers for PET imaging due to its greater sensitivity and inherent capability of quantitative analysis over that of SPECT, the latter may be more practical in some cases and is a clear companion diagnostic agent to the PET agent, as the post-therapy scans can be imaged with SPECT, which allows correlation of response during the time of therapy with the initial diagnostic PET scan. Therefore, when molecular imaging and radionuclide therapeutics are intimately tied together, this is referred to as radiotheragnostics. Like molecular imaging, advances in radiochemistry, immunology and molecular biochemistry have significantly improved the understanding of targeting disease mechanisms for radiotheragnostics. Hence, PET and SPECT imaging should be viewed as complementary rather than competing modalities in molecular imaging that form the basis of clinical decisions and follow-up needed for radiotheragnostics.

In melanoma and sarcoma, there are some target mechanisms which can be exploited for therapy. Their embryological origins trace to ectoderm and mesodermal regions but share lineages with neural crest cells, amongst others. Thus, some specific targets are also shared by other tumours of those origins. There are more specific targets in melanoma than sarcomas. A part of the reason for this is that sarcomas represent a more heterogeneous set of tumours and so have different approaches for the various entities, whereas melanomas are derived from melanocytes and have a more direct embryological lineage. Still, some malignancies such as osteosarcoma have properties that can be utilized to deliver therapies despite having targets that are otherwise less specific. Nevertheless, molecular imaging and radiotheragnostics show great promise in the next generation of development of imaging and therapeutic modalities in the management of melanomas and sarcomas.

Evolving Applications in Sarcomas

Sarcoma imaging has been available from the earliest days of metabolic and targeted imaging in nuclear medicine. One of the earliest experiments around 70 years ago utilized murine anti-osteosarcoma antibodies against tumours in rabbits which was radioiodinated with I-131 [3]. Since sarcomas for the most part have few targets specific for it that can be utilized for imaging and therapy, advanced imaging approaches subsequently involve metabolic targets that are present in many cancers.

Several different imaging strategies have been developed in sarcomas. In the earlier days of nuclear medicine, sarcomas were imaged using Ga-67 imaging until the advent of FDG PET. Some entities like osteosarcoma could be evaluated with strategies that were clinically useful. Chemotherapy response in osteosarcoma has been studied with tracers such as Tl-201 and Tc-99m sestamibi imaging. Tl-201 is a marker of tumour viability, and loss of uptake in sites of disease after chemotherapy is considered a marker of positive response [4]. Conversely residual uptake on the Tl-201 scan is suggestive of residual viable tumour after treatment. Another important tool is the use of Tc-99m sestamibi scan imaging for the use of predicting chemotherapy response, since it is a marker of chemotherapy multidrug resistance (MDR) due to its clearance from cells with P-glycoprotein (Pgp). If significant washout was then seen during imaging, this would suggest active clearance of tracer from the tumour by Pgp and thus a marker of MDR, warranting an alternative therapeutic approach [5]. These strategies are not specific for osteosarcoma but were considered clinically useful in the disease, although these have now largely been replaced by FDG PET imaging. Additionally, osteosarcoma stands out from other sarcomas in its ability to be staged by bone scans, not only for extent of bone involvement, but also since metastatic soft tissue disease is frequently detected using Tc-99m phosphonate tracers with SPECT imaging. More recently, NaF PET scanning has shown to be quite useful for imaging osteosarcoma and can have a different pattern of uptake as compared to FDG [6]. This would suggest that NaF could be used as an additional prognostic biomarker along with FDG.

Another approach that has been used in the past has been with the differentiation of Kaposi's sarcoma from lymphoma in patients with acquired immunodeficiency syndrome (AIDS). Ga-67 has uptake in lymphomas, whereas Tl-201 has uptake in both entities [7]. This strategy was also used to help differentiate between infectious and granulomatous entities from malignant ones, although with limited accuracy, and is still occasionally used when FDG PET may not be readily available.

Finally, tracers for somatostatin (SSTR) imaging also demonstrate uptake in some cases of sarcomas and were first seen with In-111 octreotide imaging with SPECT [8]. This is because of the overexpression of SSTR and neuroendocrine features seen in some sarcomas. Modern applications have demonstrated feasibility of better viewing these malignancies with Ga-68 SSTR analogues with PET [9]. Since the advent of FDG PET, both diagnostic and response prediction are evaluated by this modality. Nevertheless, some tumours do not demonstrate significant FDG activity, so it's important to keep these other modalities and strategies in mind, and thus there may still be an ongoing role for the other older tracers [10].

More modern tracer development shows great promise in the evaluation of sarcomas with target metabolic derangements or receptor over expressions associated with malignancies. Proliferative indices are high in sarcomas and can be assessed by agents that reflect DNA synthesis. ^{18}F-3-fluoro-3-deoxy-thymidine (FLT) is a pyrimidine analogue whose uptake is a measure of cell replication and has been shown as an agent that can image increased proliferation in sarcomas and other malignancies [11]. Furthermore, it can also be used to monitor therapeutic response similar to FDG [12]. There is some evidence suggesting that FLT is less affected by inflammation compared to FDG and thus more specific for tumour activity; however, it is still not specific enough to be able to completely differentiate between the two entities, and thus has not been widely adopted. Another tracer, ^{18}F-fluoromisonidazole (FMISO), is able to assess tumour hypoxia levels that make them more resistant to cytotoxicity during radiotherapy and other treatments. Uptake with FMISO and FDG is frequently discordant, and studies have demonstrated a correlation of FMISO uptake with poor outcomes following therapies [13]. FMISO is a tracer more suited for monitoring therapy than for initial diagnostic and staging workup. This has also not gained traction as a practical clinical imaging tool despite its favourable performance demonstrated in the literature. There is also a class of quinoline-based agents which act as inhibitors of fibroblast-activated proteins (FAP) which are overexpressed by many cancer-associated fibroblasts in many tumours. A new tracer recently developed in this class is a Ga-68 fibroblast-activated protein inhibitor which not only shows great promise as a diagnostic agent in a variety of tumours including sarcomas, but if successful as an imaging agent, could be converted to an effective radiotheragnostic one [14]. This is due to their great target to non-target tissue ratios, although again there is variable uptake depending on tumour

type. Of the patients studied, sarcomas appear to have amongst the most robust uptake, and thus this tracer holds great promise in the near future.

With the increasing success of radiotheragnostics, there is some renewed interest in developing this modality in different malignancies, although there has been little progress in sarcomas in this area. Despite there being few processes specific to sarcoma, there are still some entities that can used as targets for therapy. An area that has undergone clinical trials relies on the uptake of bone-seeking agents in osteosarcomas. Since these radiopharmaceuticals may also be taken up by soft tissue metastases, these agents could offer some therapeutic benefit beyond bone disease. Therapeutic agents in this area include β-emitters using strontium-89 chloride, samarium-153 ethylenediamine tetramethylene phosphonate (EDTMP), Re-186 hydroxyethylidene diphosphonate (HEDP) and others that have been used for pain palliation in prostate cancer. High activity therapy followed by peripheral blood stem cell (PBSC) transplant has been used to treat bone metastases that demonstrate uptake on bone scintigraphy. All patients treated in a clinical trial with Sm-153 EDTMP ranging from 0.04 to 1.11 GBq/kg followed by PBSC transplant noted a reduction or elimination of opioids for pain. Hematopoietic recovery occurred in all but two patients treated at the highest dosage level, which suggested that this could be used as a potential pain palliation regimen [15]. There is suggestion that this approach could be therapeutic when used as part of a multimodality agent along with PBSC support, external beam radiotherapy and multiagent chemotherapy and is generally well tolerated [16]. Ra-223 is also a bone-seeking agent but is an α-emitter and, as demonstrated above, has inherent therapeutic potential beyond pain palliation in men with prostate cancer. There has been great interest in its potential as being a therapeutic agent, rather than one involved in primarily pain palliation. A phase I clinical trial with dose escalation demonstrated good tolerance to 0.1 MBq/kg dosage and showed mixed response in 4/18 patients, and 1 patient showed response in a brain metastasis [17]. Tin in the form of Sn-117m diethylenetriamine pentaacetate (DTPA) is an auger emitter with pain palliation potential in prostate cancer and could theoretically also be used in the setting of osteosarcomas [18].

The ganglioside GD2 is frequently overexpressed in osteosarcomas and Ewing sarcomas but also may be seen in other malignancies such as neuroblastomas, melanomas and others. Monoclonal antibodies have a role to target such tumours as a therapeutic modality, such as with I-131 3f8 [19, 20]. Other mAbs such as I-131 8H9 have also been developed, which target the protein 4Ig-B7H3 expressed on a wide range of paediatric solid tumours, such as neuroblastomas, and various sarcomas, such as rhabdomyosarcomas. Phase I clinical trials have been conducted which appear to show increased survival in patients with CNS metastases treated with I-131 8H9 [21].

There is also potential for treatment of many sarcomas with peptide-based radiolabelled therapies. Since they may overexpress somatostatin receptors and, as mentioned above, many tumours demonstrate very good targeting by SSTR analogues, there is a potential role for peptide receptor radionuclide therapy (PRRT). There are case reports demonstrating success in various settings of sarcomas using Lu-177 DOTATATE, which is already clinically available for treating neuroendocrine tumours [22]. Neurotensin subtype 1 is another amino acid peptide that is overexpressed in several human cancers including Ewing sarcomas [23]. Although developed for pancreatic cancer, In-111 based neurotensin targeting analogues could potentially target overexpressed antigens on Ewing sarcomas as imaging agents, with the potential to develop therapeutic ligands if successful kinetics are observed for that purpose [24].

In a subset of more cutaneous tumours, radioactive patches have been used as brachytherapy to treat malignancies such as Kaposi's sarcoma by directly applying it over the site of tumour, with complete response demonstrated at the sites of treated disease [25]. Obviously, this is more suited for localized disease and has almost no role for more disseminated disease.

Evolving Applications in Melanoma

Imaging melanoma with antibodies was also done several decades ago and demonstrated the feasibility of developing specific probes for imaging metastatic disease [26]. These probes have been around for almost 40 years and have developed as antibody constructs have improved. Other probes for melanoma can be divided into broad categories: melanin targeting (including benzamide derivatives), peptide based [targeting of α-melanocyte-stimulating hormone (α-MSH) receptors, integrins, somatostatin receptors, etc.] and various other probes that are not necessarily specific to melanoma (e.g. PD-1/PD-L1 expression, amino acids, etc.) [27].

Melanin is present in 75–90% of melanomas and is a biopolymer containing indole units. Many of the melanin-targeting constructs are benzamide derivatives, which target melanin-secreting tumours but are not as useful for non-melanomatous tumours. The mechanism of targeting is not completely understood, but specificity is limited since melanin is mostly internal to melanoma cells, so that necrotic cells may be targeted by tracer more than viable tumour cells. Some melanin is also found in the extracellular space and in melanophages. Nevertheless, both SPECT and PET tracers have been developed that have high sensitivity, have better specificity and have lower uptake in inflammatory tissue than FDG PET. A clinical trial with a SPECT tracer ^{123}I-N-(2diethylaminoethyl)-2-iodobenzamide (^{123}I-BZA$_2$) was successful in showing high accuracy for disease detection [28]. PET tracers offer greater resolution and thus potentially greater sensitivity than SPECT tracers but again have to be able to perform better generally than FDG, especially for the brain and smaller lymph node metastases. Benzamide derivative PET agents, such as 18F-5-FPN, appear to show greater sensitivity for detecting small lymph node and lung metastases in the preclinical settings [29]. Another tracer, Ga-68 NODAGA-procainamide, appears favourable not only for its high sensitivity but also because its synthesis is simpler than other tracers labelled with F-18 and C-11 [30]. A tracer N-(2-

(diethylamino)ethyl)-6-[F-18]fluoropyridine-3-carboxamide (F-18 MEL050) has the potential for better accuracy than FDG PET in melanotic melanoma, especially for smaller-volume tumour and liver metastases, and has shown good imaging characteristics in initial human studies. In animal studies, it found 100% of the lymph node metastases after subcutaneous administration of the tracer but only 60% of them if the tracer was systemically administered in the lateral tail vein [31, 32]. Hence, more studies will be needed to see if this will prove to be useful and what would be the best way to image the tracer given that it may be dependent on the method of injection.

For peptide-based probes, there has been much interest in imaging α-MSH, which is a ligand specific for melanocortin receptor subtype 1 (MC1R) that has been reported to be overexpressed in both melanotic and amelanotic disease. Many constructs have been created to improve targeting, and copper-64- and yttrium-86-labelled DOTA-ReCCMSH (Arg11) have shown twice the tumour concentration compared to that for FDG [33]. These ligands are highly accurate for detection of melanomas and also hold great promise clinically. Some of the most recent developments have been the creation of Ga-68 labelled agents that have improved pharmacokinetics and biodistribution compared to many of the earlier generation variants [34]. These developments raise hope of being able to develop effective radiotheragnostic agents against metastatic disease.

There is also increasing interest in imaging the integrins in tumours, specifically the αvβ3 with F-18 galacto-RGD [35]. Imaging integrins has been used in many malignancies to assess the degree and state of angiogenesis in tumours. These imaging agents can not only be used to monitor the disease state in melanomas but also help assess the response to antiangiogenic therapies. Future constructs could look at different integrin families and also try and improve overall accuracy, increase renal and whole-body clearance as well as simplify the radiochemistry. Interestingly, there have been hybrid radiotracers developed that target both the integrins and MC1R but have been used for SPECT imaging. The tracer Tc-99m RGD-(Arg11)-CCMSH, or

variants with slight modifications, has shown to have good renal clearance and tumour targeting [36, 37]. Other targets include Vitaxin, a humanized anti-αvβ3 integrin antibody, which is also active in other malignancies such as prostate cancer and holds some promise for imaging therapeutic responses to monoclonal antibody treatments as a SPECT tracer [38].

Merkel cell carcinomas are neuroendocrine malignancies with overexpression of surface membrane amino acid carriers, such as dopamine receptors and transporters, and F-18 6-fluoro-Ldopa (FDOPA) and other analogues have some activity in melanomas, though with lower sensitivity, but could be useful in picking up disease missed by FDG, such as in the liver [39]. Additionally, the abundance of somatostatin receptor presence demonstrates that Ga-68 SSTR tracers can image these tumours better than FDG with PET [40]. Similar work has also been done in uveal melanomas using In-111 octreotide SPECT imaging, which also suggested that this could be used to determine disease that might be appropriate for therapeutic approaches for SSTR targeting [41]. Various other melanomas likewise have shown to demonstrate sufficient expression of SSTR so that they can be well targeted for imaging [42].

Radiotracers have also been evaluated in imaging melanoma that are not necessarily specific to melanoma physiology and have also been used to study a wide range of other malignancies. Indoleamine 2,3-dioxygenase (IDO) inhibitors are a novel class of immunomodulators with therapeutic applications in many cancers including melanoma and thus a target for imaging. The probe 5-[18F]F-AMT has good tumour-to-background ratios with great potential to image both primary and metastatic disease [43]. Checkpoint inhibitors are another relatively newer and effective class of therapeutic agents used in melanomas but are relatively difficult to follow clinically for response with FDG PET scans. Novel PET agents in mice have shown to provide good correlation with therapeutic biologic activity related to PD-1/PD-L1 inhibition [44]. SPECT versions of In-111 labeled antibodies to PD-1/PD-L1 receptors have also been imaged in mice, allowing a more prolonged evaluation of overall kinetics compared to the PET counterparts [45]. Other immune checkpoints such as CTLA-4 are also potential targets for imaging in melanoma by constructs like MDX-010. Next, C-X-C chemokine receptor type 4 (CXCR4, fusin or CD184) is a 7-transmembrane G-coupled receptor belonging to the chemokine receptor family which is overexpressed in melanomas and other malignancies and thus evaluated by the probe ^{68}Ga-pentixafor; however, in a study that included two melanoma patients, the degree of uptake was only at low-moderate levels and exceeded by that for FDG [46]. Hence, it's utility in melanoma imaging is currently uncertain.

Other non-specific agents are metabolites or minerals. Melanoma cells can also be highly proliferative, expressing high Ki-67 levels. Hence, tracers such as FLT have demonstrated increased uptake in melanomas, although, as pointed out earlier, it still has some issues with differentiating inflammation from malignant tissue, but appears to do so somewhat better than FDG [47]. Early amino acid tracers like C-11 methionine have demonstrated uptake in melanomas, but there is concern that they could underestimate disease in the liver due to high underlying physiologic uptake in the organ [48]. Tracers such as F-18 fluoroethyl-tyrosine (F-18 FET) can be used to evaluate metastatic disease, including brain metastases, but lack specificity [49]. Human copper transporter 1 (CTR1) is also overexpressed in both melanotic and amelanotic melanomas and can be imaged by ^{64}CuCl$_2$ since copper is known to be instrumental for cell angiogenesis and proliferation [50]. This needs to be studied further to see if the agent is useful, since in theory ^{64}CuCl$_2$ can be given in higher doses as a therapeutic modality.

Systemic treatments for melanoma have started gaining interest in around the last 10 years. Targets for treating melanoma have been slowly recognized that could be used in therapeutic trials based on the successful targeting of imaging vectors as has been outlined above. These include melanin itself, epidermal growth factor receptor (EGFR), glycoprotein gp57 or the ganglioside GD surface antigens, etc. Many constructs and methodologies have been studied in animals, but only a few have even made it to clinical trials.

The ganglioside GD2 is highly expressed in melanomas, and modern anti-GD2 mAb constructs like ^{64}Cu-SarAr-GD2 mAb ch14.18 have quite successfully and efficiently targeted it on cells for imaging and as a possible therapeutic target [51]. Later developments led to constructs for therapeutic uses targeting glycoprotein gp57 or the ganglioside GD3 surface antigens [52]. Ganglioside receptors are also found in neuroblastomas, so other antibodies such as I-131 3f8 have also been used [53]. Constructs for EGFR receptors have also been developed and show promise as a radiotheragnostic target [54].

A radiolabelled melanin-binding IgM antibody ^{188}Re PTI-6D2 was used in a phase I human clinical trial, showing it was well tolerated and also had an added response potential with the addition of chemotherapy [55–57]. The novelty of this method was that it was done using a pre-targeting approach as a way to enhance the uptake of the antibody into the tumour and thus improve its potential therapeutic efficacy. This therapy, however, would be more specific to treating melanotic malignancy.

The affinity of benzamides for human melanoma tissue has been an additional approach to targeting melanotic tumours, which also has the advantage of being able to target metastases across the blood-brain barrier, overcoming a limitation of many other non-radioactive therapeutics in that setting [58]. When injected intradermally using a lymphoscintigraphy technique, there is evidence that metastatic deposits in sentinel lymph nodes could achieve cytotoxic levels of radiation [59]. In a clinical trial with the melanin-binding construct ^{131}I-BA52, patients who had a higher-dose administration had a longer median survival than those insufficiently dosed or untreated [60]. This probe was an improvement of the iodinated BZA$_2$ construct. Another target for imaging and therapy is the metabotropic glutamate 1 (mGlu1) receptor, a G protein-coupled receptor normally expressed in the central nervous system, which can also be targeted with benzamide derivative probes in melanomas, specifically brain metastases.

The compound [11]C-6 can be used for PET imaging but can also be radioiodinated with I-124 for PET or I-123 for SPECT imaging and even I-131 for the potential for targeted radionuclide therapy [61]. Hence, benzamide derivatives show some promise as a future radiotheragnostic approach that will need to be optimized in its mode of delivery and patient selection.

Another frequently used target is MC1R using the peptide α-MSH, as in imaging mentioned above. One of the potential problems with this approach is that there is increased renal retention as is seen with many peptide-based therapies, leading to nephrotoxicities. Some constructs were created that had decreased uptake compared to previous generation agents, which could subsequently prove to be better agents for therapy [62]. Another strategy would be to give amino acids that would further decrease renal retention, allowing for greater radiation doses to be delivered to tumours. Constructs such as ^{177}Lu-DOTAGGNle-CycMSH$_{hex}$ have high tumour uptake and brisk renal clearance, which improves upon the biodistribution properties needed for a suitable radiotheragnostic agent.

As shown above, integrins are good targets for imaging and have demonstrated that due to their high uptake, these could be used as sites for therapeutic radionuclide delivery as well. The very late antigen-4 (VLA-4; also called integrin $\alpha 4\beta 1$) is overexpressed in many diseases including melanomas, and for which a high-affinity peptidomimetic ligand has been developed. Small animal PET/CT imaging with ^{64}Cu-NE3TA-PEG4-LLP2A demonstrated high tumour to non-target ratios [63]. Substituting the Cu-64 with Lu-177 shows good targeting of primary and metastatic lesions to the extent that there is potential for developing this as a radiotheragnostic agent [64]. A target of interest being investigated is fibrogen, which is expressed during angiogenesis, with the extra-domain B of fibronectin being overexpressed in tumoural vasculature. L19-small immunoprotein (SIP) is a human recombinant antibody fragment that can target tumour neovasculature in many malignancies, including melanomas. A clinical phase I study performed on several malignancies showed observable clinical

benefit in two of seven patients, with acceptable and tolerable toxicities [65].

Interestingly, increased somatostatin receptors can be seen in melanoma, but a small clinical trial using Lu-177 DOTATATE saw no benefit to the injected patients [66]. Nevertheless, this remains a target of interest and could be utilized if therapeutic delivery of cytotoxic radiolabelled SSTR analogues could be optimized.

A novel approach could be used with the suppression of the RAS to MAPK and P13K/Akt signalling pathways. When this is done, the sodium iodide symporter (NIS) which is found in thyroid cells appears to increase in expression and takes up I-131 NaI [67]. Thus, traditional I-131 therapy could be used to treat these tumours. The downside to this is that a patient's normal thyroid would need to be removed in order to undergo this therapy so as to avoid all the I-131 being soaked up by the thyroid rather than the metastatic disease. Nevertheless, this strategy is used in struma ovarii and could be feasible in some patients in which NIS could be made to sufficiently increase in expression in some melanomas so that therapeutic delivery of I-131 could be delivered.

A different form of internal radiation is offered by boron capture therapy. When thermal neutrons irradiate boron, there is the release of an energetic α-particle, providing internal radiation. Metastatic melanotic cells have shown to take up boron-10 paraboronophenylalanine ([10]B-BPA), but not amelanotic cells. This technique has shown to be curative as a case report when administered to a patient [68].

Brachytherapy forms have been used more successfully clinically in melanomas, especially for primary ocular melanomas. A plaque containing radionuclides can be applied adjacent to the tumour on the superficial portion of the globe. A variety of different isotopes can be used, including strontium-90, I-125 or paladium-103, amongst others. A trial of I-125 vs. tumour enucleation showed similar rates of toxicity and survival as brachytherapy [69, 70]. A study using ruthenium-106 in disease with tumour thickness <5 mm in 425 patients showed metastasis related and overall survival to be 76.5% and 79.6%, respectively, at 5 years [71]. This may be preferred in this scenario due to less toxicity to non-target tissue while delivering similar efficacy of treatment to the choroidal melanoma. Nanoparticles could also be used as brachytherapy. When injected directly into the tumour, mouse models have shown up to a 45% volume reduction of tumours [72]. Finally, selective brachytherapy has also been used by the utilization of hepatic arterial injections of Y-90-labelled microspheres for the selective treatment of liver metastases. The results were encouraging, showing at least stable disease in situations that had previously been refractory to other therapies [73].

Optical Imaging and Radiomics

Optical imaging is a set of techniques that use visible light to noninvasively produce images and do so without the use of ionizing radiation. Whereas it is beyond the scope of this material to discuss the various techniques in details, a few will be highlighted for their potential use in clinical imaging and their relationship to molecular imaging, and in particular their possible roles in managing melanomas and sarcomas. Frequently, optical imaging involves injecting a compound that is sensitive to light excitation, which subsequently localizes to the areas of disease, and can highlight that area either visibly or near infrared regions that can be detected by probes. This can lead to the use of photodynamic therapy, when the localized compound is usually excited with light – usually from a laser – and in the process releases energy into the surrounding tissue leading to cytotoxicity of diseased area with relative sparing of uninvolved regions.

One of the simplest forms of optical imaging is able to detect and diagnose disease that is relatively superficial to the surfaces being studied that is amenable to light exposure either externally or by endoscopy. This may be on skin surfaces or aerodigestive and genitourinary tracts. The patient may be injected with a compound that targets abnormal areas. By subsequently shining a light, often with lasers, the targeted area will light up, which allows direct visualization of the primary tumour, or other sites of metastases

such as lymph nodes or soft tissues, above the surrounding normal tissue. As a result, this allows guided biopsy or selective surgical resections, with the added benefit of finding unsuspected sites of disease while potentially sparing other ones not involved with disease.

A simple example of the application of optical imaging is with methylene blue, a compound that is already used in assisting in visual localization of sentinel lymph nodes in conjunction with sentinel node scintigraphy. The technique improves overall accuracy as well as the surgeon's confidence in correctly identifying sentinel nodes for biopsy over just using gamma probes, although no optical imaging is commonly used for this procedure. The problem with the latter is that background radioactivity can sometimes interfere with getting accurate counts from a node, making it difficult to identify which may be the correct node that should be biopsied. Correlation with visual verification with methylene blue assists in the procedure. It so happens that methylene blue also targets melanotic tumours quite well and has been further modified for detection with infrared optical imaging [74]. The modification improves sensitivity of detection of melanomatous deposits and is used with optical imaging but also raises the possibility of targeting areas with photodynamic therapy. As a result, not only visible areas but also micrometastatic areas not clearly visible can also be targeted by therapeutic light therapy, if they are sufficiently near the light source to be able to cause light-stimulated excitation and subsequent cytotoxicity. There is, however, additional historic interest in methylene blue in molecular imaging as well. Due to its targeting of melanomas, there has been some literature of developing it as a molecular imaging compound with PET and SPECT [75]. Furthermore, this can be modified so that therapeutic halogen radioisotopes can be added to target sites of disease [76]. Since the compound can be radiolabelled with α-particles, it could be used to treat micrometastatic disease quite effectively as this would be very effective in synergistically targeting sites amenable to photodynamic therapy as well while also targeting sites which may not be accessible to laser light. Additionally, α-particles provide greater cell kill than β-particles, although the latter have the advantage of being able to handle larger and heterogeneous tumour distributions better. Hence, methylene blue can be modified in ways to be able to combine the uses of optical imaging and photodynamic therapies, along with molecular imaging and radiotheragnostics to significantly improve staging, targeting and treating metastatic melanomas.

Other techniques include optical coherence tomography (OCT) which has great potential for doing real-time imaging and helping guide surgery. This technique allows in vivo imaging at the microscopic level and thus could be used in the operating room to delineate margins of disease resection in order to obtain better surgical outcomes. There have been several studies showing that OCT could be a clinically feasible technique, such as the resection of liposarcomas, but by extension could really be used in a wide variety of malignancies, with several applications also noted in uveal melanomas and others [77, 78]. Likewise, photoacoustic imaging and diffuse optical tomography are other techniques that also offer promise in the management of these diseases.

Radiomics is a field that uses conventional images to examine the distribution of information in the image of tumours and other lesions and uses that information to determine clinical parameters such as histology, tumour responsiveness to therapy, prognosis, etc. Each voxel in the image contains information specific to the scan modality, such as density in CT scans, physiologic activity in PET and SPECT scans, etc. The image texture can be studied by analysing the distribution of the voxel-based information over an area of interest and involves several parameters including heterogeneity, uniformity, kurtosis, coarseness, busyness as well as many others. Although the bulk of the work has been done with CT and MR imaging, some developing data uses image analysis from FDG PET-CT. Again, a detailed discussion of all the parameters is beyond this chapter, but this is a developing field that holds some promise in providing useful information for patient clinical management and has been studied in melanomas and sarcomas.

Like optical imaging, radiomics can be used to better differentiate benign from malignant histology on tissue seen on images but also potentially use the image texture to predict disease response to treatment. In a study attempting to discriminate between uterine sarcomas from leiomyomas, textural analysis of the FDG PET images found that combining traditional quantitation such as standardized uptake value (SUVmax) with specific radiomics features significantly improved the diagnostic performance of the scan [79]. Another study evaluated the predictive capability of FDG PET textural analysis in correlating with traditional parameters in evaluating treatment response to immunotherapy in melanomas and found good association between them, thus suggesting that radiomics could be used on the pre-therapy scan to help guide clinical management [80]. Consequently, it is possible that other molecular imaging tracers might also yield additional information; however, a study that evaluated the value of radiomics analysis in conjunction with FDG PET, FMISO PET and MRI in the management of soft tissue sarcomas found value in using FDG PET but found little incremental benefit in combining any information provided by FMISO PET [81]. Hence even though at times molecular imaging may add clinical information by using different imaging modalities, radiomics may be able to take existing data and provide information that could supplement some of the imaging and thus improve the cost-effectiveness of any study. Nevertheless, work continues to see what tracers in combination with other modalities and radiomics might have an impact in disease management in sarcomas and melanomas, as well as other diseases.

Summary

The field of molecular imaging and radiotheragnostics is steadily evolving and has great potential in studying and assisting in managing diseases such as melanoma and sarcomas. These pathologies have some limitations of FDG imaging due to its variable uptake and can thus be studied by other probes. Several tracers show promise as imaging agents, both in PET and SPECT, which should be considered complimentary modalities rather than competitive ones. When options such as optical imaging and radiomics are added, there is potential to significantly enhance accuracy and cost-effectiveness of the procedures. Some of these tracers have excellent targeting, making them candidates for radiotheragnostic imaging and therapy. These constructs could offer another option as therapy for treating advanced disease and in limited clinical trials appear to be feasible to use. In addition to other possibilities photodynamic therapy also holds promise to improve the therapeutic impact to disease while also significantly limiting toxicity in select cases. There is great potential yet to be realized in all these approaches and could potentially have an important role to play in the future of targeted imaging and therapies.

References

1. Parker C, Nilsson S, Heinrich D, et al. Alpha Emitter radium-223 and survival in metastatic prostate cancer. N Engl J Med. 2013;369:213–23.
2. Strosberg J, El-Haddad G, Wolin E, et al. Phase 3 trial of 177Lu-Dotatate for Midgut neuroendocrine tumors. N Engl J Med. 2017;376:125–35.
3. Pressman D, Korngold L. The in vivo localization of anti-Wagner-osteogenic-sarcoma antibodies. Cancer. 1953;6:619–23.
4. Rosen G, Loren GJ, Brien EW, et al. Serial thallium-201 scintigraphy in osteosarcoma. Correlation with tumor necrosis after preoperative chemotherapy. Clin Orthop Rel Res. 1993;293:302.
5. Wu C, Wang Q, Li Y. Prediction and evaluation of neoadjuvant chemotherapy using the dual mechanisms of 99mTc-MIBI scintigraphy in patients with osteosarcoma. J Bone Oncol. 2019;17:100250.
6. Kairemo K, Rohren EM, Anderson PM, et al. Development of sodium fluoride PET response criteria for solid tumours (NAFCIST) in a clinical trial of radium-223 in osteosarcoma: from RECIST to PERCIST to NAFCIST. ESMO Open. 2019;4(1):e00043.
7. Turgut TH, Akisik MF, Naddaf SY, et al. Tumor and infection localization in AIDS patients: Ga-67 and Tl-201 findings. Clin Nucl Med. 1998;23:446–59.
8. Friedberg JW, Van den Abbeele AD, Kehoe K, et al. Uptake of radiolabeled somatostatin analog is detectable in patients with metastatic foci of sarcoma. Cancer. 1999;86(8):1621–7.
9. Loaiza-Bonilla A, Bonilla-Reyes PA. Somatostatin receptor avidity in gastrointestinal stromal tumors: theranostic implications of Gallium-68 scan and eligibility for peptide receptor radionuclide therapy. Cureus. 2017;9(9):e1710.
10. Chen J, Chang J, Lew P, et al. Nuclear scintigraphy findings for Askin tumor with In111-pentetreotide, Tc99m-MIBI and F18-FDG. Radiology Case. 2012;6(10):32–9.
11. Cobben DC, Elsinga PH, Suurmeijer AJ, et al. Detection and grading of soft tissue sarcomas of the extremities with 18F–3fluoro-3-deoxy-l-thymidine. Clin Cancer Res. 2004;10:1685–90.
12. Leyton J, Latigo JR, Perumal M, et al. Early detection of tumor response to chemotherapy by 3′-deoxy-3′-[18F]fluorothymidine positron emission tomography: the effect of cisplatin on a fibrosarcoma tumor model in vivo. Cancer Res. 2005;65(10):4202–10.
13. Rajendran JG, Wilson DC, Conrad EU, et al. [(18)F]FMISO and [(18)F]FDG PET imaging in soft tissue sarcomas: correlation of hypoxia, metabolism and VEGF expression. Eur J Nucl Med Mol Imaging. 2003;30:695–704.
14. Kratochwil C, Flechsig P, Lindner T, et al. 68Ga-FAPI PET/CT: tracer uptake in 28 different kinds of cancer. J Nucl Med. 2019;60(6):801–5.
15. Anderson PM, et al. High-dose samarium-153 ethylene diamine tetramethylene phosphonate: low toxicity of skeletal irradiation in patients with osteosarcoma and bone metastases. J Clin Oncol. 2002;20(1):189–96.
16. Franzius C, Schuck A, Bielack SS. High-dose samarium-153 ethylene diamine tetramethylene phosphonate: low toxicity of skeletal irradiation in patients with osteosarcoma and bone metastases. J Clin Oncol. 2002;20(7):1953–4.
17. Subbiah V, Anderson PM, Kairemo K, et al. Alpha particle radium 223 dichloride in high-risk osteosarcoma: a phase I dose escalation trial. Clin Cancer Res. 2019;25(13):3802–10.
18. Srivastava SC, Atkins HL, Krishnamurthy GT, et al. Treatment of metastatic bone pain with tin-117m Stannic diethylenetriaminepentaacetic acid: a phase I/II clinical study. Clin Cancer Res. 1998;4(1):61–8.
19. Heiner J, Miraldi FD, Kallick S, et al. Localization of GD2 specific monoclonal antibody 3F8 in human osteosarcoma. Cancer Res. 1987;47:5377–538.
20. Kailayangiri S, Altvater B, Meltzer J, et al. The ganglioside antigen G(D2) is surface-expressed in Ewing sarcoma and allows for MHC-independent immune targeting. Br J Cancer. 2012;106:1123–33.
21. Kramer K, Modak S, Kushner BH, et al. Radioimmunotherapy of metastatic cancer to the central nervous system: phase I study of intrathecal 131I-8H9. Am Assoc Cancer Res. 2007; LB-4. https://www.cancernetwork.com/view/intrathecal-131i-8h9-cns-mets.
22. Crespo-Jara A, González Manzano R, Lopera Sierra M, et al. A patient with metastatic sarcoma was

successfully treated with radiolabeled somatostatin analogs. Clin Nucl Med. 2016;41(9):705–7.

23. Brans B, Linden O, Giammarile F, Tennvall J, Punt C. Clinical applications of newer radionuclide therapies. Eur J Cancer. 2006;42:994–1003.

24. De Visser M, Janssen PJ, Srinivasan A, et al. Stabilized 111In-labelled DTPA- and DOTA-conjugated neurotensin analogues for imaging and therapy of exocrine pancreatic cancer. Eur J Nucl Med Mol Imaging. 2003;30(8):1134–9.

25. Chung YL, Lee JD, Bang D, et al. Treatment of Bowen's disease with a specially designed radioactive skin patch. Eur J Nucl Med. 2000;27(7):842–6.

26. Larson SM, Brown JP, Wright PW, et al. Imaging of melanoma with I-131-labeled monoclonal antibodies. J Nucl Med. 1983;24:123–9.

27. Weijun W, Ehlerding EB, Lan X, et al. PET and SPECT imaging of melanoma: state of the art. Eur J Nucl Med Mol Imaging. 2018;45(1):132–15.

28. Moins N, D'Incan M, Bonafous J, et al. 123I-N-(2diethylaminoethyl)-2-iodobenzamide: a potential imaging agent for cutaneous melanoma staging. Eur J Nucl Med Mol Imaging. 2002;29:1478–84.

29. Wang Y, Li M, Zhang Y, Zhang F, Liu C, Song Y, et al. Detection of melanoma metastases with PET-comparison of 18F-5-FPN with 18F-FDG. Nucl Med Biol. 2017;50:33–8.

30. Kertesz I, Vida A, Nagy G, Emri M, Farkas A, Kis A, et al. In vivo imaging of experimental melanoma tumors using the novel radiotracer 68Ga-NODAGA-procainamide (PCA). J Cancer. 2017;8:774–85.

31. Ware R, Kee D, McArthur G, et al. First human study of N-(2-(diethylamino) ethyl)-6-[F-18]fluoropyridine-3-carboxamide (MEL050). J Nucl Med. 2011;52(Suppl 1):415.

32. Denoyer D, Potdevin T, Roselt P, et al. Improved detection of regional melanoma metastasis using 18F-6-fluoro-N-[2-(diethylamino)ethyl] pyridine-3carboxamide, a melanin-specific PET probe, by perilesional administration. J Nucl Med. 2011;52:115–22.

33. McQuade P, Miao Y, Yoo J, et al. Imaging of melanoma using ^{64}Cu- and ^{86}Y-DOTA-ReCCMSH(Arg11), a cyclized peptide analogue of alpha-MSH. J Med Chem. 2005;48:2985–92.

34. Zhang C, Zhang Z, Lin KS, et al. Preclinical melanoma imaging with 68Ga-labeled alpha-melanocyte-stimulating hormone derivatives using PET. Theranostics. 2017;7:805–13.

35. Beer AJ, Haubner R, Goebel M, et al. Biodistribution and pharmacokinetics of the alphavbeta3-selective tracer 18F-galacto-RGD in cancer patients. J Nucl Med. 2005;46:1333–41.

36. Flook AM, Yang J, Miao Y. Effects of amino acids on melanoma targeting and clearance properties of Tc-99m-labeled Arg-X-Asp-conjugated alpha-melanocyte stimulating hormone peptides. J Med Chem. 2013;56:8793–802.

37. Flook AM, Yang J, Miao Y. Substitution of the Lys linker with the beta-Ala linker dramatically decreased the renal uptake of 99mTc-labeled Arg-X-Asp-conjugated and X-Ala-Asp-conjugated alpha-melanocyte stimulating hormone peptides. J Med Chem. 2014;57:9010–8.

38. Posey JA, Khazaeli MB, DelGrosso A, et al. A pilot trial of Vitaxin, a humanized anti-Vitronectin receptor (anti alpha v Beta 3) antibody in patients with metastatic cancer. Cancer Biother Radiopharm. 2001;16(2):125–32.

39. Dimitrakopoulou-Strauss A, Strauss LG, Burger C. Quantitative PET studies in pretreated melanoma patients: a comparison of 6-[18F] fluoro-L-dopa with 18F-FDG and (15)O-water using compartment and noncompartment analysis. J Nucl Med. 2001;42(2):248–56.

40. Epstude M, Tornquist K, Riklin C, et al. Comparison of (18)F-FDG PET/CT and (68)Ga-DOTATATE PET/CT imaging in metastasized Merkel cell carcinoma. Clin Nucl Med. 2013;38(4):283–4.

41. Valsecchi ME, Coronel M, Intenzo CM, et al. Somatostatin receptor scintigraphy in patients with metastatic uveal melanoma. Melanoma Res. 2013;23(1):33–9.

42. Long Y, Shao F, Lan X. Mediastinal epithelioid Hemangioendothelioma revealed on 68Ga-DOTATATE PET/CT. Clin Nucl Med. 2020;45(5):414–6.

43. Xin Y, Cai H. Improved radiosynthesis and biological evaluations of L- and D-1-[18F]Fluoroethyl-tryptophan for PET imaging of IDO-mediated kynurenine pathway of tryptophan metabolism. Mol Imaging Biol. 2017;19(4):589–98.

44. Hettich M, Braun F, Bartholoma MD, et al. High-resolution PET imaging with therapeutic antibody-based PD-1/PD-L1 checkpoint tracers. Theranostics. 2016;6(10):1629.

45. Nedrow JR, Josefsson A, Park S, et al. Imaging of programmed death ligand-1 (PD-L1): impact of protein concentration on distribution of anti-PD-L1 SPECT agent in an immunocompetent melanoma murine model. J Nucl Med. 2017;58(10):1560–6.

46. Vag T, Gerngross C, Herhaus P, et al. First experience with chemokine receptor CXCR4-targeted PET imaging of patients with solid cancers. J Nucl Med. 2016;57:741–6.

47. Cobben DC, Jager PL, Elsinga PH, et al. 18F–3-fluoro-3deoxy-L-thymidine: a new tracer or staging of metastatic melanoma? J Nucl Med. 2003;44:1927–32.

48. Lindholm P, et al. Carbon-11-methionine PET imaging of malignant melanoma. J Nucl Med. 1995;36(10):1806–10.

49. Unterrainer M, Galldiks N, Suchorska B, et al. 18F-FET PET uptake characteristics in patients with newly diagnosed and untreated brain metastasis. J Nucl Med. 2017;58:584–9.

50. Qin C, Liu H, Chen K, et al. Theranostics of malignant melanoma with 64CuCl2. J Nucl Med. 2014;55:812–7.

51. Voss SD, Smith SV, DiBartolo N, et al. Positron emission tomography (PET) imaging of neuroblastoma

and melanoma with 64Cu-SarAr immunoconjugates. Proc Natl Acad Sci U S A. 2007;104:17489–93.

52. Garin-Chesa P, Beresford HR, Carrato-Mena A, et al. Cell surface molecules of human melanoma. Immunohistochemical analysis of the gp57, GD3 and mel-CSPG antigenic systems. Am J Pathol. 1989;134:295–303.

53. Cheung NK, Lazarus H, Miraldi FD, et al. Ganglioside GD2 specific monoclonal antibody 3F8: a phase I study in patients with neuroblastoma and malignant melanoma. J Clin Oncol. 1987;5:1430–40.

54. Milenic DE, Wong KJ, Baidoo KE, et al. Cetuximab: preclinical evaluation of a monoclonal antibody targeting EGFR for radioimmunodiagnostic and radio-immunotherapeutic applications. Cancer Biother Radiopharm. 2008;23:619–31.

55. Klein M, Lotem M, Peretz T, et al. Safety and efficacy of 188-rhenium-labeled antibody to melanin in patients with metastatic melanoma. J Skin Cancer. 2013;2013:828329.

56. Dadachova E, Revskaya E, Sesay MA, et al. Preclinical evaluation and efficacy studies of a melanin binding IgM antibody labeled with 188 Re against experimental human metastatic melanoma in nude mice. Cancer Biol Ther. 2008;7:1116–27.

57. Revskaya E, Jongco AM, Sellers RS, et al. Radioimmunotherapy of experimental human metastatic melanoma with melanin-binding antibodies and in combination with dacarbazine. Clin Cancer Res. 2009;15(7):2373–9.

58. Joyal JL, Barrett JA, Marquis JC, et al. Preclinical evaluation of an 131I-labeled benzamide for targeted radiotherapy of metastatic melanoma. Cancer Res. 2010;70:4045–53.

59. Denoyer D, Potdevin T, Roselt P, et al. Improved detection of regional melanoma metastasis using 18 F-6- fluoro-N-[2-(diethylamino)ethyl] pyridine-3-carboxamide, a melanin-speci fi c PET probe, by perilesional administration. J Nucl Med. 2011;52:115–22.

60. Mier W, Kratochwil C, Hassel JC, et al. Radiopharmaceutical therapy of patients with metastasized melanoma with the melanin-binding benzamide 131I-BA52. J Nucl Med. 2014;55:9–14.

61. Fujinaga M, Xie L, Yamasaki T, Yui J, et al. Synthesis and evaluation of 4-halogeno-N-[4-[6-(isopropylamino)pyrimidin-4-yl]-1,3-thiazol-2-yl]-N-[11C]methylbenzamide for imaging of metabotropic glutamate 1 receptor in melanoma. J Med Chem. 2015;58:1513–23.

62. Froidevaux S, Calame-Christe M, Tanner H, Eberle AN. Melanoma targeting with DOTA-alphamelanocyte-stimulating hormone analogs: structural parameters affecting tumor uptake and kidney uptake. J Nucl Med. 2005;46:887–95.

63. Gai Y, Sun L, Hui W, Ouyang Q, et al. New bifunctional chelator p-SCN-PhPr-NE3TA for copper-64: synthesis, peptidomimetic conjugation, radiolabeling, and evaluation for PET imaging. Inorg Chem. 2016;55:6892–901.

64. Beaino W, Nedrow JR, Anderson CJ. Evaluation of (68)Ga- and (177)Lu-DOTA-PEG4-LLP2A for VLA-4-targeted PET imaging and treatment of metastatic melanoma. Mol Pharm. 2015;12:1929–38.

65. Del Conte G, Tosi D, Fasolo A, et al. A phase I trial of antifibronecitin 131I-L19-small immunoprotein (L19-SIP) in solid tumors and lymphoproliferative disease. J Clin Oncol. 2008;26(15_suppl):2575.

66. Van Essen M, Krenning EP, Kooij PP, et al. Effects of therapy with [177 Lu-DOTA0, Tyr3] octreotate in patients with paraganglioma, meningioma, small cell lung carcinoma and melanoma. J Nucl Med. 2006;47:1599–606.

67. Hou P, Liu D, Ji M, et al. Induction of thyroid gene expression and radioiodine uptake in melanoma cells: novel therapeutic implications. PLoS One. 2009;4:e6200.

68. Mishima Y, Ichihashi M, Tsuji M, et al. Treatment of malignant melanoma by selective thermal neutron capture therapy using melanoma-seeking compound. J Invest Dermatol. 1989;92:321S–5.

69. Collaborative Ocular Melanoma Study Group. The COMS randomized trial of iodine 125 brachytherapy for choroidal melanoma: V. twelve-year mortality rates and prognostic factors: COMS report no. 28. Arch Ophthalmol. 2006;124:1684–93.

70. Hawkins BS. Collaborative ocular melanoma study randomized trial of I-125 brachytherapy. Clin Trials. 2011;8:661–73.

71. Verschueren KM, Creutzberg CL, Schalij-Delfos NE, et al. Long-term outcomes of eye-conserving treatment with ruthenium(106) brachytherapy for choroidal melanoma. Radiother Oncol. 2010;95:332–8.

72. Khan MK, Minc LD, Nigavekar SS, et al. Fabrication of (198 Au0) radioactive composite nanodevices and their use for nanobrachytherapy. Nanomedicine. 2008;4:57–69.

73. Cianni R, Urigo C, Notarianni E, et al. Radioembolisation using yttrium 90 (Y-90) in patients affected by unresectable hepatic metastases. Radiol Med. 2010;115(4):619–33.

74. Li Z, Wang YF, Zeng C, Hu L, Liang XJ. Ultrasensitive tyrosinase-activated turn-on near-infrared fluorescent probe with a rationally designed urea bond for selective imaging and photodamage to melanoma cells. Anal Chem. 2018;90(6):3666–9.

75. Schweiger LF, Smith TA. Fully-automated radiosynthesis and in vitro uptake investigation of [N-methyl-¹¹C]methylene blue. Anticancer Res. 2013;33(10):4267–70.

76. Link EM. Targeting melanoma with 211At/131I-methylene blue: preclinical and clinical experience. Hybridoma. 1999;18(1):77–82.

77. Carbajal EF, Baranov SA, Manne VG, et al. Revealing retroperitoneal liposarcoma morphology using optical coherence tomography. J Biomed Opt. 2011;16(2):020502.

78. Davila JR, Mruthyunjaya P. Updates in imaging in ocular oncology. F1000Res. 2019;8:F1000 Faculty Rev-1706.

79. Tsujikawa T, Yamamoto M, Shono K, et al. Assessment of intratumor heterogeneity in mesenchymal uterine tumor by an 18F-FDG PET/CT texture analysis. Ann Nucl Med. 2017;31(10):752–7.

80. Dittrich D, Pyka T, Scheidhauer K, et al. Textural features in FGD-PET/CT can predict outcome in melanoma patients to treatment with Vemurafenib and Ipilimumab Nuklearmedizin. 2020.

81. Vallièresa M, Serbana M, Benzyanea I, et al. Investigating the role of functional imaging in the management of soft-tissue sarcomas of the extremities. Phys Imaging Radiat Oncol. 2018;6:53–60.

Index

© Springer Nature Switzerland AG 2021
A. H. Khandani (ed.), *PET/CT and PET/MR in Melanoma and Sarcoma*,
https://doi.org/10.1007/978-3-030-60429-5

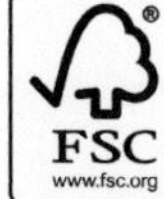

If you have any concerns about our products,
you can contact us on
ProductSafety@springernature.com

In case Publisher is established outside the EU,
the EU authorized representative is:
Springer Nature Customer Service Center GmbH
Europaplatz 3, 69115 Heidelberg, Germany

Printed by Libri Plureos GmbH
in Hamburg, Germany